Medical Management of Diabetes and Heart Disease

Clinical Guides to Medical Management

Consulting Editor

BURTON E. SOBEL, M.D.
Medical Center Hospital of Vermont
University of Vermont
Burlington, Vermont

Medical Management of Heart Disease, edited by Burton E. Sobel

Medical Management of Rheumatic Musculoskeletal and Connective Tissue Diseases, edited by Jan Dequeker, Gabriel Panayi, Theodore Pincus, and Rodney Grahame

Medical Management of Atherosclerosis, edited by John LaRosa

Medical Management of Liver Disease, edited by Edward L. Krawitt

Medical Management of Pulmonary Diseases, edited by Gerald S. Davis; Associate Editors: Theodore W. Marcy and Elizabeth A. Seward

Medical Management of Diabetes Mellitus, edited by Jack L. Leahy, Nathaniel G. Clark, and William T. Cefalu

Medical Management of Kidney and Electrolyte Disorders, edited by F. John Gennari

Medical Management of Thyroid Disease, edited by David S. Cooper

Medical Management of Diabetes and Heart Disease, edited by Burton E. Sobel and David J. Schneider

ADDITIONAL TITLES IN PREPARATION

Medical Management of Diabetes and Heart Disease

edited by

Burton E. Sobel
David J. Schneider
University of Vermont
Burlington, Vermont

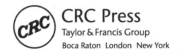

CRC Press
Taylor & Francis Group
Boca Raton London New York

CRC Press is an imprint of the
Taylor & Francis Group, an **informa** business

ISBN: 0-8247-0745-1

Headquarters
Marcel Dekker, Inc.
270 Madison Avenue, New York, NY 10016
tel: 212-696-9000; fax: 212-685-4540

Eastern Hemisphere Distribution
Marcel Dekker AG
Hutgasse 4, Postfach 812, CH-4001 Basel, Switzerland
tel: 41-61-261-8482; fax· 41-61-261-8896

World Wide Web
http://www.dekker.com

The publisher offers discounts on this book when ordered in bulk quantities. For more information, write to Special Sales/Professional Marketing at the headquarters address above.

Preface

Development of this book was stimulated by three sobering facts. First, more than 16 million people in the United States alone are afflicted with diabetes, the large majority with type 2 diabetes. Second, mortality attributable to cancer, heart disease unassociated with diabetes, and stroke has declined markedly since 1980, whereas that associated with diabetes has climbed considerably. Third, coronary disease is the major cause of death in people with diabetes and, in contrast to microangiopathy, progression of macrovascular disease is retarded only modestly by stringent glycemic control. Unfortunately, many still believe that diabetes is simply hyperglycemia, and advances in understanding the pivotal role of insulin resistance in type 2 diabetes are often overlooked. If we are to diminish cardiovascular morbidity and mortality associated with diabetes, we must recognize that, whether covert or overt, diabetes is tantamount to coronary disease. Without early and vigilant interventions by physicians, diabetes will continue to spawn acute coronary syndromes and their enormous toll.

This book was developed to underscore the intimate relationship between diabetes and heart disease, to emphasize targets for prevention and treatment of cardiac manifestations, and to elucidate pathophysiological links that constitute such targets. It is included in the Medical Management program, which is dedicated to providing medical practitioners, whether generalists or specialists, with current and comprehensive information pertinent to the care of patients in a fashion akin to a clinical consultation.

Causal connections between diabetes and heart disease are the editors' point of departure. Chapter 2 discusses different types of diabetes and their implications regarding heart disease. Chapter 3 addresses recognition, assessment, and management of insulin resistance. Relationships between hypertension, diabetes, and the heart are the subject of Chapter 4, and the relationships between hyperlipidemia, diabetes, and the heart are described in Chapter 5. Chapter 6 focuses on derangements in coagulation and fibrinolysis associated with diabetes and their pathogenetic implications regarding coronary disease. Chapter 7 elegantly elucidates the metabolic syndrome of insulin resistance, and Chapter 8 covers its detection and diagnosis. Because the polycystic ovarian syndrome is a syndrome of insulin resistance, its nature and predisposition to coronary disease are considered in Chapter 9. Heart disease associated with diabetes is not confined to coronary disease. Chapter 10 explores cardiomyopathic consequences and their recognition.

Finally, Chapters 11 to 16 deal with prevention and treatment of heart disease in patients with diabetes. Chapter 11 focuses on amelioration of insulin resistance. Chapter 12 discusses treatment of coronary disease in patients with diabetes. Congestive heart failure is covered in Chapter 13, and coronary interventions and surgery are the topics of Chapter 14. Chapter 15 is concerned with nutritional and nonpharmacological reduction of cardiovascular risk.

The armamentarium for retarding progression of heart disease and treating it more effectively is expanding rapidly. Additional opportunities will undoubtedly arise from novel research, some of which we review in Chapter 16.

We are grateful for the authoritative, cogent, and comprehensive contributions from genuine leaders in their fields. We know our readers will benefit from their efforts and expertise.

Burton E. Sobel
David J. Schneider

Contents

Contributors

William E. Boden, M.D.   Director, Division of Cardiology, Hartford Hospital, Hartford, and Professor of Medicine, University of Connecticut School of Medicine, Farmington, Connecticut

Thomas A. Buchanan, M.D.   Professor, Departments of Medicine and Obstetrics–Gynecology, University of Southern California Keck School of Medicine, Los Angeles, California

William T. Cefalu, M.D.   Associate Professor, Department of Medicine, University of Vermont College of Medicine, Burlington, Vermont

Matthew C. Corcoran, M.D.   Fellow, Section of Endocrinology, Department of Medicine, University of Chicago Pritzker School of Medicine, Chicago, Illinois

John S. Douglas, Jr., M.D.   Professor of Medicine; Director, Interventional Cardiology, Department of Medicine, Emory University School of Medicine, Atlanta, Georgia

Tevfik Ecder, M.D.   Research Fellow, Division of Renal Diseases and Hypertension, Department of Medicine, University of Colorado School of Medicine, Denver, Colorado

David A. Ehrmann, M.D.   Department of Medicine, University of Chicago Pritzker School of Medicine, Chicago, Illinois

Henry N. Ginsberg, M.D.   Irving Professor of Medicine, Department of Medicine, Columbia University College of Physicians and Surgeons, New York, New York

Melinda L. Hockensmith, M.D.   Clinical Fellow, Division of Renal Diseases and Hypertension, Department of Medicine, University of Colorado School of Medicine, Denver, Colorado

Howard N. Hodis, M.D.   Associate Professor of Medicine and Preventive Medicine and Director, USC Atherosclerosis Unit, University of Southern California Keck School of Medicine, Los Angeles, California

Edward S. Horton, M.D.   Professor of Medicine, Joslin Diabetes Center, Harvard Medical School, Boston, Massachusetts

Didem Korular, M.D.   Research Fellow, Division of Renal Diseases and Hypertension, Department of Medicine, University of Colorado School of Medicine, Denver, Colorado

Harold E. Lebovitz, M.D.   Professor, Department of Medicine, State University of New York Health Science Center at Brooklyn, Brooklyn, New York

Martin M. LeWinter, M.D.   Professor, Department of Medicine, Unversity of Vermont College of Medicine, Burlington, Vermont

Wendy J. Mack, Ph.D.   Associate Professor, Department of Preventive Medicine, University of Southern California Keck School of Medicine, Los Angeles, California

Virginia Peragallo-Dittko, R.N.   Director, Diabetes Education Center, Winthrop-University Hospital, Mineola, New York

Julio E. Pérez, M.D.   Professor of Medicine, Cardiovascular Division, Department of Internal Medicine, Washington University School of Medicine, and Barnes–Jewish Hospital, St. Louis, Missouri

Gerald M. Reaven, M.D.   Falk Cardiovascular Research Center, Division of Cardiovascular Medicine, Department of Medicine, Stanford University School of Medicine, Stanford, California

David J. Schneider, M.D.   Associate Professor, Department of Medicine, University of Vermont, Burlington, Vermont

Robert W. Schrier, M.D.   Professor and Chairman, Department of Medicine, University of Colorado School of Medicine, Denver, Colorado

Burton E. Sobel, M.D.   E. L. Amidon Professor and Chair, Department of Medicine, University of Vermont, Burlington, Vermont

Srihari Thanigaraj, M.D.   Assistant Professor of Medicine, Cardiovascular Division, Department of Internal Medicine, Washington University School of Medicine, and Barnes–Jewish Hospital, St. Louis, Missouri

Medical Management of Diabetes and Heart Disease

1

Causal Connections

Burton E. Sobel and David J. Schneider
University of Vermont, Burlington, Vermont

This book was inspired by cogent clinical observations and a rapidly expanding body of knowledge implicating diverse, specific, and sometimes paradoxical or unexpected factors in the pathogenesis of accelerated coronary artery disease associated with type 2 diabetes. A clinical example is the initially astounding observation in the BARI I trial of a fourfold increase in 5-year mortality in patients with type 2 diabetes compared with that in nondiabetic subjects after percutaneous transluminal coronary angioplasty (PTCA), and the threefold increase after surgical revascularization. Examples of the unexpected factors include the emerging information strongly implicating insulin resistance in liver, adipose tissue, and skeletal muscle with consequent hyperinsulinemia as a culprit in acceleration of coronary disease and its sequelae independent of the hallmark metabolic abnormalities of diabetes mellitus, including hyperglycemia, hypertriglyceridemia, and elevated concentrations of circulating free fatty acids (FFA).

It is impossible to provide more than a highly selective commentary on some aspects of this area in a brief overview such as this one. Accordingly, we have elected to discuss a few points that often are not considered by cardiovascular or general physicians.

I. SELECTED METABOLIC ASPECTS OF DIABETES

A lay person would describe diabetes as too much sugar in the blood. So would most medical students and physicians. However, hyperglycemia is simply the tip of the iceberg, albeit one of profound pathogenetic impact. Type 2 diabetes is, in fact, a syndrome in which resistance to insulin in peripheral tissues is present for years, if not decades, before hyperglycemia becomes evident. As compensatory pancreatic secretory mechanisms in response to the insulin resistance begin to fail, relative and

1

subsequently absolute insulin deficiency occurs resulting in clinical hyperglycemia. Consequently, the signs and symptoms of polyuria and polydipsia become apparent associated with elevated HbA1c and exacerbation of hyperlipidemia.

Many of the metabolic derangements typical of diabetes can be understood in terms of a few seminal actions of insulin. The dependence of acetyl CoA carboxylase activity on insulin in the liver results, in the case of insulin resistance, in failure of production of malonyl CoA, the first intermediate in fatty acid synthesis. Accordingly, fatty acid synthesis declines in the liver, in turn causing an increase in hepatic gluconeogenesis and hepatic glucose output. The reduction in malonyl CoA concentrations in hepatocytes reduces the inhibition of an enzyme pivotal in fatty acid synthesis, carnitine palmitoyl CoA transferase (CPT-1). Insulin itself inhibits this enzyme and, accordingly, in states of insulin resistance, CPT-1 activity increases markedly. The result is increased FFA oxidation. In the extreme case, when FFA oxidation is excessive and disproportional to FFA synthesis, 2-carbon fragments (acetyl CoA) are formed in abundance and give rise to ketone bodies and potentially ketoacidosis. The latter does not occur generally in type 2 diabetic subjects unless markedly diminished insulin secretory capacity has occurred.

Acetyl CoA is an allosteric inhibitor of pyruvate dehydrogenase. Thus, glucose oxidation diminishes when FFA oxidation is excessive. The decreased glucose oxidation leads to accumulation of citrate, an inhibitor of a rate-limiting enzyme in the glycolytic pathway, fructose 1, 6, phosphatase. Glucose-6-phosphate concentrations consequently increase. This, in turn, diminishes the uptake of glucose contributing to hyperglycemia as does the decreased glycogen synthetase activity in skeletal muscle and decreased glucose transport in the same tissue.

A second key fundamental action of insulin is augmentation of lipoprotein lipase activity. Accordingly, in states of insulin resistance the diminished activity of this enzyme potentiates accumulation of triglycerides, elevation of VLDL in blood, and the hypertriglyceridemia typical of type 2 diabetes.

Beta-cell exhaustion is known to be potentiated by hyperglycemia. Thus, a vicious circle occurs when insulin resistance is followed by a failure of compensatory mechanisms and consequently hyperglycemia. The high blood glucose concentrations exacerbate beta-cell dysfunction and accelerate the evolution of metabolic consequences of type 2 diabetes. The inhibition of insulin secretion induced by hyperglycemia is referred to as "glucose toxicity" and can be reversed by effective treatment that leads to glycemic control.

In the postabsorptive state, patients with insulin resistance are less able to accumulate precursors of triglycerides in adipose tissue such as 3-carbon fragments to which fatty acids can be esterified. The result is elaboration of FFA from adipose tissue contributing to the dyslipidemia.

Insulin mediates the uptake in skeletal muscle of glucose through glucose transporter–mediated functions and activation of enzymes such as hexokinase. In states of insulin resistance, uptake is diminished with consequent exacerbation of hyperglycemia. The major physiological abnormality in whole-body insulin-mediated glucose disposal is a reduction in nonoxidative disposal reflective of an impairment in the muscle glycogen synthesis pathway associated with insulin resistance.

II. THE NATURE OF COMPLICATIONS

The discovery that metabolic consequences of type 1 diabetes (insulin deficiency attributable to failure of pancreatic beta cells, generally induced by autoimmune phenomena) could be corrected by administration of pancreatic extracts and ultimately purified insulin gave rise to a powerful belief system in which insulin deficiency is embraced as the cause of diabetes under all circumstances. We now know that more than 90% of individuals with diabetes have type 2 diabetes, a condition in which insulin resistance is among the primary defects. However, the evolution of diabetes is such that at any given level of insulin resistance the pancreatic compensatory mechanism is inadequate to meet demands and insulin deficiency is a relatively late manifestation of the disorder. Surprisingly, this dichotomy was anticipated in the 1930s. Himsworth was interested in the causes of hyperglycemia in patients with diabetes and performed what Gerald Reaven described as "a series of simple, but elegant experiments aimed at understanding." The results led to the proposal that "the diminished ability of the tissues to utilize glucose is referable either to a deficiency of insulin or to insensitivity to insulin, although it is possible that both factors may operate simultaneously." These remarkably prescient observations led to the development of the concept of the syndrome of insulin resistance (sometimes referred to as metabolic syndrome X).

Only recently have these ideas, developed so effectively by Dr. Reaven, become conventional wisdom. In fact, syndromes of insulin resistance are manifest by impaired responses to insulin in skeletal muscle, adipose tissue, and the liver, clusters of abnormality including dyslipidemia with high triglycerides, low HDL cholesterol, decreased LDL particle size, postprandial lipemia, increased susceptibility to oxidation of LDL, obesity, hypertension, impaired fibrinolysis, and perhaps of most importance to the patient at risk, accelerated coronary artery disease manifested by acute coronary syndromes. Some or all of these derangements are seen in patients with syndromes of insulin resistance even in the absence of the derangements in intermediary metabolism typical of diabetes, including hyperglycemia. Thus, women with the polycystic ovarian syndrome who are insulin resistant have accelerated coronary disease as do normal subjects who are not diabetic but have elevated fasting concentrations of insulin in blood.

Although hyperglycemia per se is a powerful determinant of microvascular disease and may contribute to macrovascular disease, the increasing recognition that macroangiopathy and particularly coronary artery disease is strongly associated with insulin resistance in patients with type 2 diabetes has led to a reformulation of its presumed pathogenesis. Insulin resistance and its consequences, including hyperinsulinemia, have been directly and indirectly linked to the acceleration of coronary artery disease. Thus, even though glycemic control remains the primary objective in therapy of patients with type 2 diabetes, amelioration of insulin resistance is imperative if the rate of evolution of at least some complications, including coronary disease, is to be diminished.

One aspect of insulin resistance that has been implicated directly in accelerating coronary disease includes the effects of insulin on synthesis of plasminogen activator inhibitor type-1 (PAI-1) with consequent augmentation of concentrations of PAI-1 in blood in subjects with insulin resistance, including obese nondiabetic subjects. Impaired fibrinolysis is the result. Another aspect of insulin resistance is endothelial dysfunction that may contribute to hypertension in patients with type 2 diabetes, a strongly associated phenomenon. It occurs in subjects with insulin resistance and hyperinsulinemia without hyperglycemia as well. Thus, it is critical to seek to ameliorate insulin resistance as well as to control hyperglycemia and hyperlipidemia in patients with type 2 diabetes.

Such considerations have led to the initiation of national multicenter randomized patient assignment clinical trials such as the BARI 2D investigation. In this recently initiated investigation, patients with type 2 diabetes and overt coronary artery disease are being randomized in a 2×2 factorial design. One randomization is to treatment of the coronary artery disease itself with coronary intervention (either percutaneous or surgical) as opposed to medical management of the coronary artery disease. The second randomization is to treatment with insulin-providing as opposed to insulin-sensitizing regimens in patients whose coronary disease is being managed in both fashions. The study seeks to determine whether relatively early coronary intervention is or is not beneficial in patients with type 2 diabetes and overt coronary artery disease. In addition, it is designed to determine whether insulin-sensitizing regimens offer an advantage in comparison with insulin-providing regimens with respect to the rate of evolution of coronary artery disease and, if so, whether the advantage is evident in patients whose coronary disease is managed initially medically, initially with intervention, or both. Results in several smaller studies indicate that reduction of insulin resistance with the use of thiazolidinediones diminishes the rate of progression of atherosclerotic disease as judged from ultrasonic interrogation of carotid arteries and assessment of intimal/medial thickness.

III. THE NATURE OF INSULIN RESISTANCE

It is undoubtedly the case that insulin resistance can result from many, many primary defects. Elucidation of insulin receptor action, signal transduction, intracellular mediators, and the molecular genetics determining each is the focus of a prodigious and vigorous area of research. In this overview, only a few aspects can be mentioned.

The specific derangement(s) responsible for insulin resistance in most patients with type 2 diabetes has not been identified. Key factors implicated, however, are docking proteins that interact with the insulin receptor [insulin receptor substrate-1 and -2 (IRS-1 and IRS-2)] that facilitate assembly of complexes of intracellular proteins that initiate signaling through multiple pathways, one of which is mitogenic and one of which gives rise to many of the metabolic actions of insulin. Roles of IRS-1 and IRS-2 appear to be tissue-specific as judged from experiments in knockout mice. These proteins are involved in actions of insulin in adipose tissue, liver, and skeletal muscle among other tissues. IRS-2 has been implicated in growth, development, and function of pancreatic beta cells.

Defects in insulin receptors and glucose transport effector systems have been implicated in syndromes of insulin resistance that are either genetic or secondary to obesity, pregnancy, endocrinopathies, cirrhosis, pancreatic carcinoma, and hepatitis C among other conditions. Cytokines such as tumor necrosis factor-alpha (TNF-α) mediate insulin resistance in general and in adipose tissue particularly. The role of transcription factors in mediating actions of insulin, particularly the peroxisome proliferator-activated receptors (PPAR), is suggested by the beneficial effects on insulin resistance induced by PPAR ligands such as the glitazones. A particularly intriguing potential cause of insulin resistance in women with the polycystic ovarian syndrome is abnormal serine kinase activity resulting in serine phosphorylation as opposed as tyrosine phosphorylation of the insulin receptor with consequent lack of autophosphorylation and functional impairment.

Syndromes of insulin resistance are usually readily detectable based on clinical observation and knowledge of their manifestations. Definitive demonstration of insulin resistance requires sophisticated laboratory testing. The euglycemic insulin clamp procedure is the "gold standard" in a research environment. More universally available procedures such as determination of fasting insulin concentrations in blood in patients not receiving exogenous insulin may be useful, as may the homeostasis model assessment (HOMA) that requires only simultaneous determination of fasting glucose and fasting insulin concentrations. With one iteration of this approach, the concentration of insulin in blood in μU/mL multiplied by the concentration of glucose in blood in mg/dL is divided by 22.5 to provide an index. Results have been correlated with those obtained with sophisticated procedures such as the frequently sampled intravenous glucose tolerance test/minimal model and the insulin tolerance test and found to be robust. In all of these procedures, measurements of insulin concentrations must be performed by laboratories with rigorously standardized reagents and procedures to acquire valid results.

IV. SOME THERAPEUTIC CONSIDERATIONS

The prevention or retardation of coronary artery disease and its sequelae in subjects with type 2 diabetes provides opportunities and challenges. Stringent glycemic control is an imperative. Amelioration of insulin resistance is paramount as well. The armamentarium for treatment of diabetes has expanded recently with the addition to the classical armamentarium of sulfonylureas and insulin of insulin sensitizing agents (glitazones). These agents augment glucose utilization and consequently diminish hyperglycemia, thereby reducing prevailing concentrations of insulin directly and in response to the lowered concentrations of glucose. Other additions include the biguanides, particularly metformin, rapidly acting insulins such as lispro, agonists of first-phase insulin secretion such as Repaglinide, and agents that decrease absorption of glucose from the gastrointestinal track such as α-glucosidase inhibitors. The foundation of effective management of type 2 diabetes includes diet, caloric restriction sufficient to diminish body weight to ideal weight, and exercise. Combinations of oral agents and the use of oral agents plus insulin are often required and frequently constitute the standard of care. With this foundation in place, and optimal pharmacological therapy, glycemic control is generally achievable.

The astute clinician will, however, also address those factors that can contribute to the acceleration of coronary artery disease in type 2 diabetes that are either independent of or linked only indirectly to glycemic control. Thus, assessment and optimal treatment of hyperlipidemia should be undertaken. Control of blood pressure should be vigorous in order to protect the kidney and attenuate progression of coronary disease. In the recently completed UKPDS multicenter investigation, blood pressure was found to be a powerful determinant of complications in type 2 diabetes independent of the adequacy of glycemic control. The use of angiotensin converting enzyme (ACE) inhibitors and angiotensin receptor blockers is supported by their beneficial effects on hypertension, protective effects on the kidney, and reduction of inhibition of fibrinolysis through modulation of elevated PAI-1 concentrations, all of which have been implicated in accelerating coronary artery disease in patients with type 2 diabetes.

Patients with type 2 diabetes who develop manifestations of coronary artery disease must, of course, be assessed and treated vigorously with anti-ischemic agents, myocardial protective agents, and procedures indicated clinically to augment myocardial perfusion. For those who sustain acute myocardial infarction, the use of insulin-glucose infusions and promptly implemented stringent glycemic control can reduce mortality as demonstrated in the DIGAMI studies.

In the following chapters, these and other pathogenetic, diagnostic, and therapeutic aspects of accelerated coronary artery disease in association with type 2 diabetes will be discussed authoritatively by experts with extensive experience.

SUGGESTED READING

1. Alexander GJM. An association between hepatitis C virus infection and type 2 diabetes mellitus: What is the connection? Ann Intern Med 2000; 133:650–651.
2. Alper J. New insights into type 2 diabetes. Science 2000; 289:37–39.
3. Coniff R, Krol A. Acarbose: A review of US clinical experience. Clin Ther 1997; 19:16–26.
4. DeFronzo RA. Pharmacologic therapy for type 2 diabetes mellitus. Ann Intern Med 1999; 131:281–303.
5. Ehrmann DA, Schneider DJ, Sobel BE, Cavaghan MK, Imperial J, Rosenfield RL, Polonsky KS. Troglitazone improves defects in insulin action, insulin secretion, ovarian steroidogenesis, and fibrinolysis in women with polycystic ovary syndrome. J Clin Endocrinol Metab 1997; 82:2108–2116.
6. Feit F, Brooks MM, Sopko G, Keller NM, Rosen A, Krone R, Berger PB, Shemin R, Attubato MJ, Williams DO, Frye R, Detre KM, for the BARI Investigators. Long-term clinical outcome in the Bypass Angioplasty Revascularization Investigation Registry. Circulation 2000; 101:2795–2802.
7. Haffner SM, D'Agostino R, Jr, Saad MF, O'Leary DH, Savage PJ, Rewers M, Selby J, Bergman RN, Nykkanen L. Carotid artery atherosclerosis in type-2 diabetic and nondiabetic subjects with and without symptomatic coronary artery disease (The Insulin Resistance Atherosclerosis Study). Am J Cardiol 2000; 85:1395–1400.
8. Hermans MP, Levy JC, Morris RJ, Turner RC. Comparison of insulin sensitivity tests across a range of glucose tolerance from normal to diabetes. Diabetologia 1999; 42:678–687.
9. Hunter SJ, Garvey WT. Insulin action and insulin resistance: Diseases involving defects in insulin receptors, signal transduction, and the glucose transport effector system. Am J Med 1998; 105:331–345.
10. Inzucchi SE, Maggs DG, Spollett GR, Page SL, Rife FS, Walton V, Shulman GI. Efficacy and metabolic effects of metformin and troglitazone in type II diabetes mellitus. N Engl J Med 1998; 338:867–872.
11. Kido Y, Burks DJ, Withers D, Bruning JC, Kahn CR, White MF, Accili D. Tissue-specific insulin resistance in mice with mutations in the insulin receptor, IRS-1, and IRS-2. J Clin Invest 2000; 105:199–205.
12. Kruszynska Y, Yu JG, Sobel BE, Olefsky JM. Effects of troglitazone on blood concentrations of plasminogen activator inhibitor 1 in patients with type 2 diabetes mellitus and in lean and obese normal subjects. Diabetes 2000; 49:633–639.
13. Lemieux I, Pascot A, Couillard C, Lamarche B, Tchernof A, Almeras N, Bergeron J, Gaudet D, Tremblay G, Prud'homme D, Nadeau A, Despres J-P. Hypertriglyceridemic waist. A marker of the atherogenic metabolic triad (hyperinsulinemia; hyperapolipoproteinB; small, dense LDL) in men? Circulation 2000; 102:179–184.

14. Liu J, Knezetic JA, Strommer L, Permert J, Larsson J, Adrian TE. The intracellular mechanism of insulin resistance in pancreatic cancer patients. J Clin Endocrinol Metab 2000; 85:1232–1239.
15. Malmberg K, Ryden L, Efendic S, Herlitz J, Nicol P, Waldenstrom A, Wedel H, Welin L, on behalf of the DIGAMI Study Group. Randomized trial of insulin-glucose infusion followed by subcutaneous insulin treatmen in diabetic patients with acute myocardial infarction (DIGAMI Study): Effects on mortality and 1 year. J Am Coll Cardiol 1995; 26:57–65.
16. McGill JB, Schneider DJ, Arfken CL, Lucore CL, Sobel BE. Factors responsible for impaired fibrinolysis in obese subjects and NIDDM patients. Diabetes 1994; 43: 104–109.
17. Nordt TK, Bode C, Sobel BE. Stimulation in vivo of expression of intra-abdominal adipose tissue plasminogen activator inhibitor type-1 by proinsulin. Diabetologia 2001; 44:1121–1124.
18. Pessin JE, Saltiel AR. Signaling pathways in insulin action: Molecular targets of insulin resistance. J Clin Invest 2000; 106:165–169.
19. Qiao L-Y, Goldberg JL, Russell JC, Sun XJ. Identification of enhanced serine kinase activity in insulin resistance. J Biol Chem 1999; 274:10625–10632.
20. Reaven GM. Insulin resistance and human disease: A short history. J Basic Clin Physiol Pharmacol 1998; 9:387–406.
21. Saltiel AR. The molecular and physiological basis of insulin resistance: Emerging implications for metabolic and cardiovascular diseases. J Clin Invest 2000; 106:163–164.
22. Saltiel AR, Olefsky JM. Thiazolidinediones in the treatment of insulin resistance and type II diabetes. Diabetes 1996; 45:1661–1669.
23. Schneider DJ, Sobel BE. Augmentation of synthesis of plasminogen activator inhibitor type-1 by insulin and insulin-like growth factor type-1 and its pathogenetic implications for diabetic vascular disease. Proc Natl Acad Sci USA 1991; 88:9959–9963.
24. Schneider DJ, Sobel BE. Plaque vulnerability and acute coronary syndromes: What are the prophylactic and therapeutic implications? In: de Bono D, Sobel BE. Challenges in Acute Coronary Syndromes. London: Blackwell Science, 2001:18–45.
25. Shulman GI. Cellular mechanisms of insulin resistance. J Clin Invest 2000; 106: 171–176.
26. Sobel BE. Potentiation of vasculopathy by insulin: Implications from an NHLBI Clinical Alert. Circulation 1996; 93:1613–1615.
27. Sobel BE. The potential influence of insulin and plasminogen activator inhibitor type-1 on formulation of vulnerable atherosclerotic plaques associated with type 2 diabetes. Proc Assoc Am Physicians 1999; 111:313–318.
28. Sobel BE, Woodcock-Mitchell J, Schneider DJ, Holt RE, Marutsuka K, Gold H. Increased plasminogen activator inhibitor type-1 in coronary artery atherectomy specimens from type 2 diabetic compared with nondiabetic patients: A potential factor predisposing to thrombosis and its persistence. Circulation 1998; 97:2213–2221.
29. Velazquez EM, Mendoza SG, Wang P, Glueck CJ. Metformin therapy is associated with a decrease in plasma plasminogen activator inhibitor-1, lipoprotein(a), and immunoreactive insulin levels in patients with the polycystic ovary syndrome. Metabolism 1997; 46:454–457.

2

Types of Diabetes and Their Implications Regarding Heart and Vascular Disease

Harold E. Lebovitz
*State University of New York Health Science Center at Brooklyn,
Brooklyn, New York*

Diabetes mellitus is a syndrome in which blood glucose levels are inappropriately high for the individual's physiological state. In most populations both fasting and postprandial plasma glucose levels are continuous variables that are skewed toward the higher range. The differentiation between normal and abnormal is therefore arbitrary and must be defined by additional criteria. Diabetic retinopathy is the most common and easily quantified unique complication of diabetes mellitus. Its prevalence increases linearly with duration of diabetes. For these reasons, the diagnosis of diabetes mellitus has been defined operationally as those blood or plasma glucose levels that predict the future development of diabetic retinopathy (1). Three recent epidemiological studies have provided data on such relationships. Accordingly, diabetes mellitus is defined as described in Table 1 by a fasting plasma glucose $\geq$126 mg/dL (7.0 mmol/L) or a 2-h plasma glucose after a 75-g glucose load $\geq$200 mg/dL (11.1 mmol/L) (1). However, a dilemma is presented by the observations that macrovascular complications of diabetes mellitus account for its major morbidity and mortality (2,3); we do not know how to define diabetes mellitus as a function of plasma glucose as it relates to the development of macrovascular disease (4,5).

Diabetes mellitus has many etiologies, all of which cause high plasma glucose as defined above (hyperglycemia) and carry a risk for the development of both microvascular and macrovascular complications. Disorders of glucose metabolism are defined as impaired fasting plasma glucose (IFG), impaired glucose

Table 1 New Diagnostic Criteria for the Diagnosis of Classes
of Glucose Intolerance

	Fasting plasma glucose (mg/dL)	2-h plasma glucose after 75 g of oral glucose (mg/dL)
Normal glucose tolerance	<110	<140
Impaired glucose tolerance	<126	140–199
Impaired fasting glucose	110 to <126	
Diabetes mellitus	≥126	≥200

Source: Ref. 1.

tolerance (IGT), or diabetes mellitus, depending on the level of the fasting and/or
2-h post-glucose-challenge plasma glucose as described in Table 1 (1). Diabetes
mellitus is classified depending on the etiology of the hyperglycemia (Table 2).
Four major categories of diabetes mellitus have been defined: type 1 diabetes,
type 2 diabetes, other specific types of diabetes and gestational diabetes (1). Type
1 diabetes is characterized by severe insulin deficiency that is life threatening
and requires insulin treatment for survival. Both insulin deficiency and insulin
resistance, each of which may vary from minimal through very severe, characterize type 2 diabetes. Other specific types of diabetes are those conditions in which
the underlying etiology is known. Gestational diabetes is hyperglycemia that occurs in the third trimester of pregnancy and usually disappears after delivery only
to reappear as permanent type 2 or type 1 diabetes years later.

Table 2 Classification of Diabetes Mellitus

Type 1 diabetes	Beta-cell destruction usually leading to absolute insulin deficiency. Need exogenous insulin for survival.
Type 2 diabetes	Heterogeneous disorder of unknown etiology characterized by varying degrees of insulin secretory deficiency and insulin resistance.
Other specific types	Genetic abnormalities causing deficient beta-cell function; genetic abnormalities interfering with insulin action; pancreatic diseases causing loss of beta-cell function; endocrinopathies, drug or chemical-induced; infections; uncommon forms of immune-mediated diabetes; other genetic syndromes sometimes associated with diabetes.
Gestational diabetes mellitus	

Source: Ref. 1.

Table 3 Baseline Characteristics of Patients with Type 1 Diabetes at Enrollment into the Diabetes Control and Complications Trial (DCCT)

	Primary prevention	Secondary intervention
Number	726	715
Age (yrs.)	27 ± 8	27 ± 7
Diabetes duration (yrs.)	2.6 ± 1.4	8.8 ± 3.8
Systolic BP (mmHg)	113 ± 12	115 ± 12
Diastolic BP (mmHg)	72 ± 9	73 ± 9
Body weight (% ideal wt.)	103 ± 14	104 ± 12
Serum cholesterol (mg/dL)	174 ± 34	179 ± 33
Plasma triglycerides (mg/dL)	76 ± 50	87 ± 45
Plasma HDL cholesterol (mg/dL)	52 ± 13	49 ± 12
Plasma LDL cholesterol (mg/dL)	107 ± 30	112 ± 29

Source: Ref. 11.
Data are mean ± standard deviation.

From the perspective of cardiovascular disease, a more sensible way to classify diabetes mellitus is to define two variants. One in which there is no significant insulin resistance and the other in which insulin resistance is a dominant pathophysiological abnormality (6–8). The rationale for this classification is that insulin resistance is associated with a cluster of metabolic abnormalities (Table 3), all of which are significant risk factors for cardiovascular disease (9,10), while diabetes mellitus without insulin resistance is only associated with increased risk factors for cardiovascular disease after the diabetes has progressed for many years, and the increased risk factors are usually secondary to the complications of poor control (11,12) or treatment.

I. CARDIOVASCULAR DISEASE IN TYPE 1 DIABETES

Type 1 diabetes is characterized by an absolute loss of beta cells such that there is almost a total absence of insulin secretion (1). The majority of patients who develop type 1 diabetes have an autoimmune process that destroys the beta cells. There is another group of individuals who have type 1 diabetes in which beta-cell function is severely reduced in the absence of autoimmune destruction and in which the etiology of the beta-cell dysfunction is unknown. In type 1 diabetes, there is no significant obesity, the plasma lipid profile is normal, blood pressure is usually not elevated, and there is no evidence of a specific procoagulant state during the first few years of the disease (Table 4) (11). These metabolic abnormalities do not appear to be part of the primary disease process, but they are acquired

Table 4 Differences in Metabolic Profiles Between Insulin-Sensitive
and Insulin-Resistant Type 2 Diabetic Patients

Metabolic parameter	Insulin-sensitive	Insulin-resistant
Hyperglycemia	yes	yes
Hyperinsulinemia	no	yes
Central obesity	no	yes
Diabetic dyslipidemia		
↑ plasma triglycerides	no	yes
↓ plasma HDL cholesterol	no	yes
small, dense LDL pattern	no	yes
Procoagulant state		
↑ plasma fibrinogen	no	yes
↑ plasma PAI-1	no	yes
Hypertension	not ↑ (?)	↑in normal weight but not in obese

Source: The table reflects the results of studies cited in Refs. 6, 7, 26, 29, 30, 41, and 45.

as a consequence of the development of obesity, which appears to be a result of intensive insulin treatment (12) or poorly controlled glycemia that leads to hypertriglyceridemia, excessive activation of vascular cell protein kinase C, increased production of advanced glycosylation end products (AGEs), endothelial dysfunction, and oxidative stress (13). Type 1 diabetic patients have increased cardiovascular risk factors as a consequence of their hyperglycemia and its treatment and not as an intrinsic part of the disease itself. The development of cardiovascular disease is thus a very late complication of type 1 diabetes and manifests itself after age 35 in those with onset of type 1 diabetes prior to age 20 (as shown in Figs. 1 and 2) (14). In cross-sectional studies, the prevalence of cardiovascular disease in type 1 diabetic patients has been between 8 and 10% and did not differ significantly between men and women. The prevalence increases with age (from 6% in patients 15 to 29 years old to 25% in patients 45 to 59 years old) and with duration of diabetes (15,16). In a comparison of 16 European countries, the prevalence of cardiovascular disease in cross-sectional studies in type 1 diabetic populations varied from 3 to 19% (16).

The factors responsible for the increase in cardiovascular disease in type 1 diabetic patients have been investigated recently in several large cohorts. The results vary somewhat depending on the specific cohort, gender, and the age of onset of the diabetes. Patients with type 1 diabetes may develop nephropathy as a consequence of poor glycemic control and extensive data document that

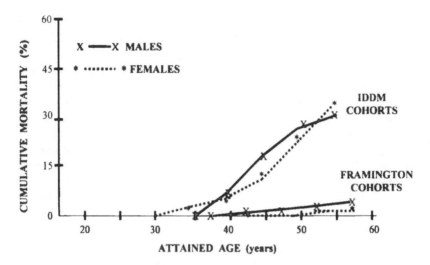

Figure 1 Cumulative mortality from coronary heart disease in patients with type 1 diabetes (IDDM) followed for 20 to 40 years at the Joslin Clinic compared to age- and sex-matched cohorts from the population of the Framingham study. (Reproduced with permission from Ref. 16a.)

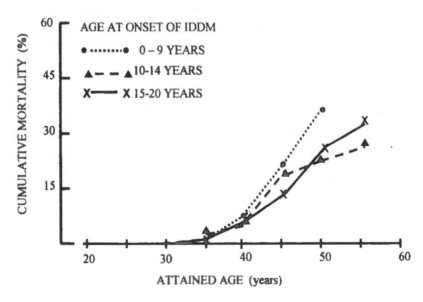

Figure 2 Cumulative mortality from coronary heart disease in type 1 diabetic patients (IDDM) followed at the Joslin Clinic for 20 to 40 years. The data are plotted by age of onset of the diabetes. (Reproduced with permission from Ref. 16a.)

nephropathy is a major risk factor for the development of cardiovascular disease in type 1 diabetic patients (2,3,14). The increase in blood pressure and hyperlipidemia that result from diabetic nephropathy is responsible for a significant proportion of the increased risk. Hypertension in type 1 diabetic patients is itself a major risk factor for cardiovascular disease. It is frequently difficult to determine whether hypertension in type 1 diabetic patients is essential or secondary to early nephropathy.

The impact of nephropathy and hyperglycemia on cardiovascular risk factors in type 1 diabetic patients can be partially dissected by comparing the metabolic consequences of kidney transplantation to those of kidney–pancreas transplantation. A recent Italian study examined atherosclerosis risk factors, endothelial-dependent vasodilation, and changes in carotid artery intimal-media thickness in type 1 diabetic patients with uremia who underwent kidney (30 patients) or kidney–pancreas (60 patients) transplantation (17). Kidney–pancreas transplantation restored glycemia to normal (mean HbA1c 6.2% and fasting plasma glucose 90 mg/dL) and resulted in statistically significant lower fasting plasma homocysteine, von Willebrand factor levels, D-dimer fragments, plasma triglyceride levels, and urinary albumin excretion rate compared to kidney transplant alone. Patients with kidney transplants alone had no endothelium-dependent vasodilation, while those with kidney–pancreas transplants had normal endothelium-dependent vasodilation. Intimal-media thickness of the carotid artery was significantly lower in the patients with the kidney–pancreas transplants than in those with kidney transplants alone. These data support the hypothesis that hyperglycemia in type 1 diabetic patients is a major risk factor for macrovascular disease.

The EURODIAB IDDM Complications Study, a cross-sectional study of 3250 type 1 diabetic patients from 16 European countries, reported that cardiovascular disease in both sexes was associated with high fasting plasma triglyceride and low plasma HDL cholesterol (16). In men, duration of diabetes, waist–hip ratio, and hypertension were also significantly correlated with cardiovascular disease, while in women, a greater body mass index (BMI) was associated with an increased prevalence of cardiovascular disease. No association was found in either gender between insulin dose, HbA1c level, or age-adjusted albumin excretion and cardiovascular disease.

A cross-sectional study of risk factors for cardiovascular disease in 286 men and 281 women from the Pittsburgh Epidemiology of Diabetes Complications Study (EDC) gave somewhat different results (15). The mean age of the population was 28 years and the mean duration of type 1 diabetes was 20 years. The overall prevalence of cardiovascular disease was 8.0 to 8.5% (men vs. women). Fasting plasma triglycerides and hypertension were the major overall predictors of CVD. Waist–hip ratio correlated with CVD in both men and women. HbA1c correlated with CVD in women, but not in men.

Since nephropathy has such a strong relationship to the development of CVD, it is important to evaluate type 1 patients without nephropathy for predictive factors for coronary heart disease (CHD). Lehto et al. performed a prospective study of risk factors for CHD in 177 type 1 diabetic patients with no evidence of clinical nephropathy (18). The study population was restricted to individuals who had developed their diabetes ≥30 years of age and who were between 45 and 64 years of age at baseline (Figs. 3 and 4). They were followed up to 7 years for CHD events. After adjusting for other CV risk factors, a history of a previous myocardial infarction, glycated hemoglobin A1 levels, and duration of diabetes was highly predictive of CHD (hazard ratios for highest tertile 3.4, 2.8, and 3.9, respectively).

Another late-onset population of type 1 diabetic patients that have been evaluated for CVD risk factor relationships are those with latent autoimmune diabetes in adults (LADA) (19). These individuals have the onset of their disease as adults and have a slow progressive loss of beta cells. They have lower BMI, waist-to-hip ratio, and fasting serum C-peptide concentrations, higher plasma HDL_2 cholesterol concentrations, and less hypertension than type 2 diabetic patients. Isomaa et al. reported a comparable prevalence of CHD in their LADA patients as in a matched type 2 diabetic population (19). In multiple regression analysis, glycemic control was associated with CHD in the LADA population but not in the type 2 diabetic population.

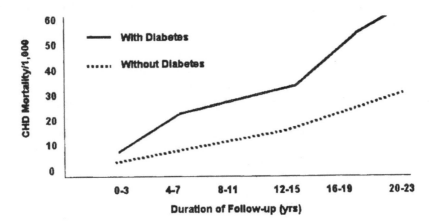

Figure 3 Mortality from coronary heart disease during 24 years of follow-up of a cohort of diabetic men whose diabetes was diagnosed between ages 35 and 64 and who came to the Joslin Clinic soon after the diabetes diagnosis, and in a group of similarly aged nondiabetic male participants of the Framingham study. The increased coronary heart disease mortality in the Joslin cohort, already evident during the first 4 years of follow-up, increased significantly during the subsequent intervals of observation. (Reproduced with permission from Ref. 14.)

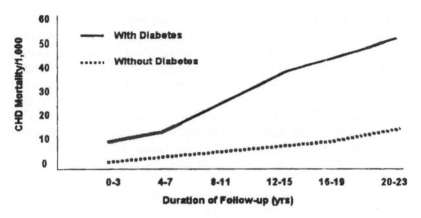

Figure 4 The comparable coronary heart disease mortality in women from the study described in Figure 3. (Reproduced with permission from Ref. 14.)

The inconsistency of the results of the studies that have examined the relationship between glycemic control and CVD in type 1 diabetic patients is difficult to reconcile with other data. Type 1 diabetic patients do not have an increase in the traditional CV risk factors, either proceeding or in the first few years after the onset of their diabetes. CVD occurs only in type 1 diabetics with a long duration of diabetes. These observations indicate that either CV risk factors increase during the course of type 1 diabetes or type 1 diabetes is associated with previously unknown CV risk factors. Considerable circumstantial data support the hypothesis that type 1 diabetic patients develop an increase in cardiovascular risk factors during the course of their disease. The most likely causes of the increase in CV risk are poor glycemic control or treatment-induced obesity (11,12,20,21). Patients with poor glycemic control have a rise in plasma free fatty acids and an increase in VLDL particle synthesis, and a decrease in clearance of chylomicrons and VLDL particles as a result of diminished lipoprotein lipase activity. These alterations lead to elevated plasma triglycerides. Poor glycemic control also results in increases in protein glycosylation and formation of AGEs (advanced glycosylation end products), activation of PKC (protein kinase C), endothelial dysfunction, and increased oxidative stress, all of which increase cardiovascular risk (13,22). On the other hand, patients who are intensively treated with insulin are at significant risk to develop central obesity and the insulin resistance syndrome (12,23,24).

The type 1 diabetic patients in the DCCT (Diabetes Control and Complications Trial) after 6.5 years of treatment had a prevalence of obesity of 33.1% in the intensively treated cohort and 19.1% in the conventionally treated cohort.

Obesity was defined as a BMI $\geq$ 27.8 kg/m^2 for men and $\geq$27.3 kg/m^2 for women (11). The patients were identified at the conclusion of the study by the magnitude of their weight gain and metabolic effects were analyzed by quartiles of weight gain (Table 5) (12). The conventionally treated patients had a mean change in BMI from baseline that ranged from a 4% loss in the lowest quartile to a 13% increase in the highest quartile. The highest quartile had a 3 mmHg rise in mean systolic and diastolic blood pressure and about a 10% increase in plasma triglycerides and total and LDL cholesterol levels. These changes in metabolic parameters occurred with no significant change in HbA1c. The intensively treated patients had an increase in BMI that ranged from no increase in the lowest quartile to a mean 29% increase in the highest quartile. The highest quartile had an absolute 1.9% mean decrease in HbA1c, a 6 mmHg rise in systolic and a 4 mmHg rise in diastolic BP, a 7 to 8% rise in plasma triglycerides and LDL cholesterol levels, and a 4% decrease in plasma HDL cholesterol levels. These data indicate that insulin treatment of type 1 diabetic patients creates the insulin resistance syndrome in a significant number of patients.

The data from the DCCT are not unexpected, as a number of previous studies had reported the development of insulin resistance in treated type 1 diabetic patients. Several reports from the Pittsburgh Epidemiology of Diabetic Complications Study provide additional new information. A family history of type 2 diabetes gave an odds ratio of 1.45 for the presence of CAD in their type 1 cohort (23). The presence of insulin resistance in type 1 diabetic patients was

Table 5 The Effect of Insulin Treatment on Body Weight and Lipid Profiles in Patients with Type 1 Diabetes

Variable	Baseline	Conventionally treated		Intensively treated	
		First quartile	Fourth quartile	First quartile	Fourth quartile
HbA1c (%)	8.6–9.2	9.5	8.9	7.3	7.3
Body mass index (kg/m^2)	23–25	24	27	24	31
Systolic BP (mmHg)	114–116	113	119	113	120
Diastolic BP (mmHg)	72–74	74	76	73	77
Waist–hip ratio		0.82	0.84	0.81	0.83
Plasma triglyceride (mmol/L)	0.86–0.96	0.89	1.05	0.79	0.99
HDL cholesterol (mmol/L)	1.27–1.37	1.32	1.29	1.40	1.27
LDL cholesterol (mmol/L)	2.74–3.00	2.82	3.18	2.74	3.15
LDL R$_f$		0.30	0.30	0.31	0.30

Source: Ref. 12.

shown to be highly correlated with waist–hip ratio, hypertension, and HbA1c level (24). These three parameters can be used to clinically estimate insulin resistance in type 1 diabetic patients.

In summary, the available data suggest that the major factors responsible for CHD and CVD in type 1 diabetic patients are nephropathy, the development of the insulin resistance syndrome or poor glycemic control (Fig. 5). Based on current data, one can speculate that maintaining near-normoglycemia without the development of central obesity from the onset of type 1 diabetes should eliminate the excessive CVD risk as well as microvascular risk. In the event that near-normoglycemia cannot be achieved, aggressive management of blood pressure (systolic <120 mmHg and diastolic <80 mmHg), plasma lipids (LDL cholesterol <100 mg/dL; HDL cholesterol >45 mg/dL; and triglycerides <150 mg/dL), as

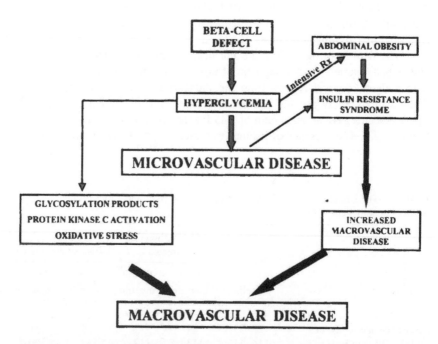

Figure 5   A hypothesis for the pathogenesis of macrovascular disease in type 1 diabetic patients. Absent beta-cell function leads to fasting and postprandial hyperglycemia. If inadequately controlled, hyperglycemia leads to microvascular disease (nephropathy) and biochemical abnormalities such as formation of AGEs, excessive activation of protein kinase C, oxidative stress, etc., which accelerate atherosclerosis. If the hyperglycemia is intensively but not physiologically controlled, visceral obesity develops and, with it, the insulin resistance syndrome that can itself accelerate atherosclerosis.

well as the best glycemic control that can be achieved without significant side effects should be major targets for reducing cardiovascular morbidity and mortality in type 1 diabetic patients (25).

II. CARDIOVASCULAR DISEASE IN TYPE 2 DIABETES

Type 2 diabetes is very different from type 1 diabetes in its underlying etiology and its natural history. Insulin resistance, which is defined as a less than normal effect of insulin on in vivo glucose uptake and metabolism, occurs in a high proportion of the population of societies embracing western culture (10,26). Factors responsible for the development of insulin resistance are only partially understood. Fetal malnutrition predisposes to insulin resistance in postnatal life (27). Excess calorie intake and reduced physical activity lead to exaggerated lipid deposits and obesity. The proportion of excess calories deposited as lipids in subcutaneous adipose tissue relative to visceral adipose tissue is both genetically and hormonally determined (28). An increase in visceral adiposity but not subcutaneous adiposity is highly correlated with insulin resistance and the components of the metabolic syndrome (29,30). There is a significant correlation between visceral adiposity and both liver and muscle triglycerides so that it is difficult to dissect the contribution that each of these makes to the insulin resistance (31,32). The normal compensatory response to insulin resistance is an increase in insulin secretion sufficient to overcome the insulin resistance. As long as the compensatory increase in insulin secretion is sufficient to overcome the insulin resistance, glucose metabolism and plasma glucose levels will remain normal (8,26). However, such individuals will have a cluster of metabolic abnormalities (Table 3) that are associated with the insulin resistance (10,26). These metabolic abnormalities are cardiovascular risk factors and the cluster is referred to as the insulin resistance syndrome, the metabolic syndrome, or, more recently, the dysmetabolic syndrome. This syndrome leads to the development of type 2 diabetes in those individuals with genetically predisposed beta cells (9).

Cardiovascular disease is two to four times more prevalent in patients with type 2 diabetes than in age-matched nondiabetic persons. The time course of the increase in cardiovascular disease is exemplified in Figures 3 and 4 which plot cumulative mortality from coronary heart disease during 24 years of follow-up of a cohort of patients whose diabetes was diagnosed between 35 and 64 years of age (type 2 diabetics) (14). The striking difference between the cumulative mortality curves in the type 2 diabetic patients as contrasted to the type 1 diabetic patients shown in Figures 1 and 2 are the early mortality noted at diagnosis and through the third year. That is, there is no latent period as in the type 1 diabetic patients. Coronary heart disease mortality increased progressively with duration of diabetes. These types of curves suggested that accelerated atherosclerosis was already present at the time of diagnosis of type 2 diabetes and that it progresses with duration of the diabetes.

That concept had been suggested earlier by the prospective data from the Whitehall study of approximately 18,000 civil servant men that showed almost a twofold increase in CHD mortality in nondiabetic men in the upper 5% of the 2-h blood glucose value (>5.3 mmol/L or 95 mg/dL) after a 50-g oral glucose load (33). The Paris Prospective Study followed 7164 working men for a mean of 11.2 years and observed annual CHD mortality rates of 1.4, 2.7, and 3.2 per 1000 persons in normoglycemic persons, impaired glucose tolerance individuals, and new and known type 2 diabetic patients, respectively (34). Many subsequent studies have confirmed that individuals with IGT have approximately a 1.5- to 2.0-fold increased risk of death from CVD when compared to normoglycemic individuals. Coutinho et al. have examined in detail the relationship between nondiabetic plasma glucose values and incident cardiovascular events by doing a metaregression analysis of published data from 20 studies of 95,783 individuals followed for a mean of 12.4 years (5). Their analysis indicated that a fasting plasma glucose of 6.1 mmol/L (110 mg/dL) and a 2-h plasma glucose of 7.8 mmol/L (140 mg/dL) were associated with a relative cardiovascular event risk of 1.33 and 1.58, respectively. Thus, there are overwhelming data to support the concept that accelerated atherosclerosis occurs many years prior to the onset of type 2 diabetes. The data can be interpreted to mean that subdiabetic levels of plasma glucose are responsible for the vascular disease or that type 2 diabetes is preceded by some metabolic state that causes both type 2 diabetes and accelerated atherosclerosis.

Many population-based epidemiological studies published in the 1980s had suggested that high fasting or postprandial plasma insulin levels predicted the development of type 2 diabetes. In 1990, Haffner and associates presented data from the ongoing San Antonio Heart Study that indicated that individuals who were going to develop type 2 diabetes had an increase in many of the components of the insulin resistance syndrome years before the onset of their diabetes (35). The prediabetic individuals were older, more generally and centrally obese, had a dyslipidemia that manifested itself as higher plasma triglyceride and a lower plasma HDL cholesterol, higher (though still normal) systolic and diastolic blood pressure, and a greater prevalence of hypertension. The mean fasting and 2-h post-glucose-challenge plasma glucoses were approximately 5.6 mmol/L (101 mg/dL) and 8.3 mmol/L (149 mg/dL) as compared to 5.0 mmol/L (91 mg/dL) and 5.3 mmol/L (95 mg/dL) in the normal population. The prediabetic individuals had fasting plasma insulin levels that were 66% higher in the men and 102%

higher in the women than in the normal population. Their data indicated that the insulin resistance syndrome preceded the development of type 2 diabetes by many years and that impaired glucose tolerance was associated with the insulin resistance syndrome. Recently, they have further analyzed their prediabetic cohort by defining insulin resistance at baseline by the HOMA model and insulin secretion by the incremental increase in plasma insulin 30 min after an oral glucose load divided by the incremental increase in plasma glucose. Of 195 individuals who developed diabetes, 161 were insulin resistant at baseline and 34 were insulin sensitive. The components of the insulin resistance syndrome were present only in those with insulin resistance as determined by HOMA (36).

Insulin resistance occurs very commonly in societies that have acquired western cultural patterns. In Europe, it is estimated that 16% of the adult population has the insulin resistance syndrome. In a recent analysis of the Botnia population in Finland, the prevalence of the metabolic syndrome as defined by WHO was assessed in individuals with normal glucose tolerance, impaired glucose tolerance, or impaired fasting plasma glucose (IFG), and type 2 diabetes (37). The WHO definition of the metabolic syndrome is (1) hypertension (BP >160/90 mmHg or treatment for hypertension); (2) dyslipidemia, defined as plasma triglyceride ≥1.7 mmol/L (150 mg/dL) and/or HDL cholesterol <0.9 mmol/L (35 mg/dL) in men or <1.0 mmol/L (38.5 mg/dL) in women; (3) obesity, defined as BMI ≥30 kg/m² and/or WHR >0.90 in men or >0.85 in women; and (4) microalbuminuria (urinary albumin excretion ≥20 µg/min). Fifteen (10%) of normal glucose-tolerant men and women aged 35 to 70 years had the metabolic syndrome as compared to 64 (42%) of those with IFG/IGT and 84 (78%) of those with type 2 diabetes.

A routine health examination of 2113 middle-aged men and women in Tokyo in the early 1990s revealed the following prevalence of components of the insulin resistance syndrome: obesity 20.9%; hypertension 23.1%; hyperinsulinemia 11.0%; hypertriglyceridemia 24.4%; low HDL cholesterol 23.0% (38). The individuals with hyperinsulinemia had higher plasma triglycerides, lower plasma HDL cholesterol, higher systolic and diastolic blood pressure, and higher area-under-the-plasma glucose curve during the oral glucose tolerance than those with normoinsulinemia matched for age, sex, and BMI. Individuals with glucose intolerance (defined as 2-h plasma glucose ≥133 mg/dL after a 100-g oral glucose load) had higher plasma triglycerides, higher systolic and diastolic blood pressures, and higher area-under-the-2-h plasma glucose curve during the OGTT as compared to the normal glucose-tolerant individuals matched for age, sex, and BMI.

As noted previously, fasting plasma glucose as well as post-glucose-challenge plasma glucose predicts the future development of type 2 diabetes. This was the reason for the definition of the new category of glucose intolerance called impaired fasting glucose. IFG is defined as a fasting plasma glucose ≥110 mg/ dL (6.2 mmol/dL) and <126 mg/dL (7.0 mmol/dL). The introduction of this category has created much controversy. Many analyses of data bases, including those in the DECODE study, have shown that IFG consists of some who would be diagnosed as type 2 diabetics by the 2-h post-glucose-challenge plasma glucose ≥200 mg/dL (11.1 mmol/L), some who have IGT, and a small subset who have only IFG (39,40). Some series show that IFG predicts CV disease while others show little or no predictive value (41). In studies where IFG predicts future CVD (as in the CARE secondary prevention study employing pravastatin in patients post myocardial infarction), the IFG cohort has the insulin resistance syndrome with increased BMI and waist circumference, increased systolic blood pressure, and the characteristic dyslipidemia (42).

Insulin resistance can occur very early in life. Data from an ongoing prospective study of low-birth-weight infants in India indicate that these children can develop the insulin resistance syndrome as early as 8 years of age. Many studies have found insulin resistance in young adults who are first degree relatives of individuals who have type 2 diabetes. Insulin resistance is a characteristic of individuals who have visceral obesity. Individuals who are obese as assessed by BMI are not necessarily insulin resistant nor do they have the insulin resistance syndrome. Brochu et al. examined the metabolic characteristics of 43 obese, sedentary, postmenopausal women (44). Despite comparable BMI (31.5 vs. 34.7 kg/ m²) and fat mass (37.3 vs. 39.0 kg), 17 individuals had normal insulin sensitivity and 26 were insulin resistant as assessed by the euglycemic hyperinsulinemic clamp. The obese individuals with normal insulin sensitivity had 49% less visceral adipose tissue than the resistant individuals, and had normal fasting and post-glucose-challenge plasma glucose and insulin and mean plasma triglycerides of 1.50 mmol/L (133 mg/dL) and plasma HDL cholesterol of 1.16 mmol/L (45 mg/dL). The insulin-resistant individuals had hyperinsulinemia and the classic dyslipidemia of insulin resistance as well as borderline increases in fasting and post-glucose-challenge plasma glucose levels.

The evidence suggesting that the insulin resistance syndrome plays a central role in the development of macrovascular disease in type 2 diabetic patients comes from many sources. In 1989, Banerji and Lebovitz described two variants of type 2 diabetes: one with impaired insulin action (insulin-resistance variant) and one with normal insulin action (insulin-sensitive variant) (6). Their insulin-sensitive patients had none of the components of the insulin resistance syndrome, while the insulin-resistant patients had the classic insulin resistance syndrome (17). These observations were extended by Haffner et al., who showed that insulin-sensitive type 2 diabetic patients had lower BMI and waist circumference, lower plasma triglyceride and higher plasma HDL cholesterol levels and larger, more buoyant, LDL particles, and lower plasma fibrinogen and plasminogen activator inhibitor 1 (PAI-1) levels than insulin-resistant type 2 patients (45). In essence, the insulin-sensitive type 2 diabetic patients had none of the characteristics of the insulin resistance syndrome. In the United Kingdom Prospective Diabetes Study (UKPDS), newly diagnosed type 2 diabetic Caucasian, Asian, Indian, and Afro-Caribbean patients were randomized to either intensive or conventional glucose control treatment programs and the effects on clinical diabetic complications were assessed over a mean of 11 years. At baseline, the Afro-Caribbean population had less insulin resistance and insulin resistance components and more beta-cell deficiency than the Caucasian population (46). The relative risk of the Afro-Caribbean patients developing a fatal or nonfatal myocardial infarction over the 11-year follow-up was 0.4 that of the Caucasian population (47).

Two large, long-term prospective studies from Finland have examined the relationship between the insulin resistance syndrome and the development of coronary heart events in nondiabetic men. An analysis of 22-year follow-up data from the Helsinki Policemen Study (48) showed that a factor analysis including six risk factor variables that are considered to be components of the insulin resistance syndrome (BMI, subscapular skinfold, areas under the plasma glucose and insulin curves during the oral glucose tolerance test, mean blood pressure, and plasma triglyceride) independently predict the risk of CHD (hazard ratio 1.48) and stroke (hazard ratio 2.02). A 7-year follow-up study of 1069 subjects aged 65 to 74 years from eastern Finland assessed the relationship of various clusters of risk factors to predict CHD events in men and women (49). An insulin resistance factor (BMI, WHR, fasting plasma glucose, insulin, and triglycerides) predicted CHD events in elderly men (hazard ratio 1.33), but not in elderly women.

In the Botnia population, cardiovascular outcomes were assessed in 2401 subjects. The adjusted relative risk of developing CHD was 2.96 and of stroke 2.27 in those whom at baseline had the metabolic syndrome as defined by WHO. Cardiac mortality in 3606 subjects with a mean follow-up of 6.9 years was 12.0% in those who had the metabolic syndrome and 2.2% in those who did not (37).

Outcome studies indicate a statistical relationship between CVD events and each of the various components of the insulin resistance syndrome (37,50–56). The extensive interrelationships among the various components of the insulin resistance syndrome (9,10,37,48) have prevented identifying with certainty whether certain independent individual components underlie the syndrome or, more importantly, whether specific major components are responsible for the accelerated atherosclerosis and increased macrovascular disease.

The mechanism by which insulin resistance is created and the consequences of insulin resistance that contribute to macrovascular and perhaps microvascular disease have been the subjects of intensive investigations and numerous speculations. Considerable new data have suggested that insulin resistance and its dyslipidemia are related to the metabolic consequences of visceral adiposity (8,26,28,30,44,57). It is likely that adipose tissue releases circulating factors that both facilitate and inhibit insulin action (58–61). Free fatty acids (62) and tumor necrosis factor-α (63) inhibit insulin action by blocking activation of the insulin receptor substrate (IRS) phosphoinositide-3 kinase (PI-3 kinase) pathway. This limb of the intracellular insulin action cascade is responsible for regulating insulin's action on glucose transport and lipid metabolism (64). The other limb of the intracellular insulin action cascade is the MAP kinase pathway, which regulates insulin's mitogenic and growth activities (64). This pathway is not inhibited in the insulin resistance syndrome (37,65). Insulin acts on endothelial cells to regulate vascular tone and other aspects of endothelial function (66). Insulin action on endothelial cells is mediated by the intracellular IRS PI-3 kinase pathway and this action is inhibited in the insulin resistance syndrome just as are the intermediary metabolism effects (67–69). The ability of insulin to generate nitric oxide by activating endothelial cell nitric oxide synthase is markedly decreased (67). The result is that endothelial dysfunction is a characteristic finding in the insulin resistance syndrome (66,68–70). The disturbance of endothelial function results in increased synthesis of growth factors and adhesion molecules, proliferation of matrix and smooth muscle cell, and increased expression of PAI-1 gene (66). Increased peripheral resistance and increases in mean arterial blood pressure are probably due in part to an imbalance of the angiotensin-2 and endothelin actions on the endothelial cells predominating over those of insulin and other vasodilators (68–69). The procoagulant and antifibrinolytic state results from abnormalities of the coagulation cascade and the increase in PAI-1 activity (54,71–73). Associated with, and probably part of, the insulin resistance syndrome is an increase in arterial inflammatory processes that are marked by elevated levels of fibrinogen and plasma CRP levels as measured by a highly sensitive assay (74–76).

Many studies have documented the association between insulin resistance and endothelial dysfunction (66,69), the dyslipidemia of high plasma triglycerides, low plasma HDL cholesterol, and a pattern of small dense LDL particles (77–79), the procoagulant state, the low-grade inflammatory state, and, in some populations, increased blood pressure and microalbuminuria (80). These same metabolic abnormalities have all been shown to increase CVD morbidity and mortality risk (37,42,48,49,80). Thus insulin resistance is a metabolic abnormality that increases cardiovascular disease risk. In the type 2 diabetic, cardiovascular risks are due to two factors, the insulin resistance syndrome and poorly controlled hyperglycemia (Fig. 6). In contrast to type 1 diabetic patients, type 2 diabetic patients require treatment of both abnormalities from the onset of the illness.

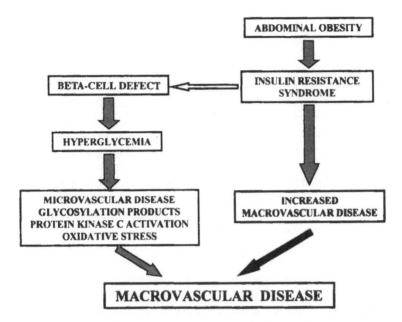

Figure 6 A hypothesis for the pathogenesis of macrovascular disease in type 2 diabetic patients. Visceral obesity leads to the development of insulin resistance and the other components of the insulin resistance syndrome. The insulin resistance syndrome itself causes accelerated atherosclerosis, which increases clinical macrovascular disease events. In those individuals with the genetic predisposition for type 2 diabetes, the insulin resistance, which increases the requirement for insulin secretion, accelerates beta-cell functional failure and this eventually results in first postprandial and later fasting hyperglycemia. The hyperglycemia further contributes to atherogenesis and macrovascular disease by the mechanisms shown in the figure. (Adapted from Ref. 8.)

III. CONCLUSIONS AND THERAPEUTIC IMPLICATIONS

From the point of view of understanding and preventing or treating the macrovascular complications of diabetes mellitus, it is important to differentiate whether the diabetes is or is not associated with insulin resistance. If it is not initially associated with insulin resistance, as in type 1 or insulin-sensitive type 2 diabetes, then the primary goal should be to treat to and maintain the fasting and postprandial plasma glucose as close to normal as possible, while minimizing the development of visceral obesity. Such a strategy, if it can be implemented, should maintain atherosclerosis progression at the prediabetic level.

If, however, insulin resistance is the early event, it should be treated as aggressively as possible in order to prevent accelerated atherosclerosis and the possible progression to type 2 diabetes. The rate of development of atherosclerosis varies in different populations depending on their genetic background and lifestyle (3,81). The acquisition of insulin resistance or diabetes mellitus increases the intrinsic rate of atherosclerosis (82). Populations such as the Pima Indians, who have a low rate of CHD, increase the prevalence two- to threefold with the development of IGT or type 2 diabetes. The absolute prevalence, however, is still significantly lower than that in most nondiabetic populations who have relatively high intrinsic rates of CHD (83).

Insulin resistance usually starts and has been accelerating atherosclerosis years before glucose intolerance and type 2 diabetes become evident. By the time IGT or type 2 diabetes is diagnosed, individuals already have advanced atherosclerosis and are on their way to developing clinical macrovascular disease. This likely explains the observations that a diabetic without any preceding clinical CVD has the same likelihood of having a myocardial infarction in a 7-year follow-up as a nondiabetic individuals who already has had a myocardial infarction (84). The suggestion has been made that all type 2 diabetic patients should be treated to prevent progression of their atherosclerosis and that this would be comparable to secondary intervention rather than primary prevention.

There are data to suggest that such a strategy, while probably good, may not be good enough. The results of the 6.4-year mean follow-up of the Cardiovascular Health Study indicated "that most of the traditional cardiovascular risk factors were not significant predictors of the risk of CVD among diabetics after adjusting for the extent of subclinical disease" (Table 6) (85). Subclinical disease was defined as an ankle-arm index ≤0.9; internal carotid artery wall thickness >80th percentile; carotid stenosis >25%; major ECG abnormalities (based on Minne-

Table 6 Multivariate Analysis of Clinical Endpoints as a Function of Subclinical Disease and CVD Risk Factors in Diabetic Participants Without a History of Baseline Clinical Disease

Variables	Outcome[a]	
	CVD mortality	Incident CHD
Subclinical disease	2.51	1.99
Serum creatinine (per 1 mg/dL)	2.15	
Fasting plasma glucose (per 20 mg/dL)		1.06
Diastolic BP (per 10 mmHg)	1.18	1.18
Plasma triglycerides (per 20 mg/dL)		1.07

Source: Ref. 85.
[a] Adjusted relative risk.

sota code); and a Rose Questionnaire positive for claudication or angina pectoris in the absence of clinical diagnosis of angina pectoris or claudication. Subclinical disease was present in 60% of participants with IGT. One can interpret these types of data to provide the following chronology. The insulin resistance syndrome starts at a relatively young age (young adulthood) and causes accelerated atherosclerosis. By middle age, subclinical macrovascular disease is present. In those individuals with the genetic propensity, beta-cell insulin secretory function decreases and impaired glucose tolerance and finally type 2 diabetes develop. By the time type 2 diabetes does develop, subclinical and, in some cases, clinical macrovascular disease is well established and will continue to progress. Poorly controlled hyperglycemia even further accelerates the rate of atherosclerosis.

The implications of this hypothesis have far-reaching clinical implications. It means that accelerated atherosclerosis starts at a relatively young age, long before there is any clinical disease and before we would traditionally intervene. This is the stage at which treatment of insulin resistance and cardiovascular risk factors are likely to be most effective in reducing macrovascular disease. At the time of diagnosis of type 2 diabetes, many or perhaps most patients will already have moderately advanced subclinical or even clinical cardiovascular disease. Intervention strategies to reduce cardiovascular risk factors in type 2 diabetic patients will be of value but may have somewhat limited effectiveness since the subclinical cardiovascular abnormalities may be more important in determining the future course of the CVD than the risk factors themselves.

REFERENCES

1. Report of the expert committee on the diagnosis and classification of diabetes mellitus. Diabetes Care 2001; 24(suppl 1):S5–S20.
2. Wingard DL, Barrett-Cannor E. Heart disease and diabetes. In: Diabetes in America, 2nd ed. NIH Publication No. 95–1468, 1995:429–448.
3. Tuomilehto J, Rastenyté D. Epidemiology of macrovascular disease and hypertension in diabetes mellitus. In: Alberti KGMM, Zimmet P, DeFronzo RA, Keen H, eds. International Textbook of Diabetes Mellitus, 2nd ed. Chichester: John Wiley & Sons Ltd, 1997:1559–1583.
4. Gerstein HC. Is glucose a continuous risk factor for cardiovascular mortality? Diabetes Care 1999; 22:659–660.
5. Coutinho M, Gerstein HC, Wang Y, Yusuf S. The relationship between glucose and incident cardiovascular events: A metaregression analysis of published data from 20 studies of 95,783 individuals followed for 12.4 years. Diabetes Care 1999; 22: 233–240.
6. Banerji MA, Lebovitz HE. Insulin sensitive and insulin resistant variants in NIDDM. Diabetes 1989; 38:784–792.

7. Banerji MA, Lebovitz HE. Coronary heart disease risk factor profiles in black patients with non-insulin-dependent diabetes mellitus: paradoxic patterns. Am J Med 1991; 91:51–58.

8. Lebovitz HE, Banerji MA, Chaiken RL. The relationship between type II diabetes and syndrome X. Curr Opin Endocrinol Diabetes 1995; 2:307–312.

9. Stern M. The insulin resistance syndrome. In: Alberti KGMM, Zimmet P, DeFronzo RA, Keen H, eds. International Textbook of Diabetes Mellitus, 2nd ed. Chichester: John Wiley & Sons Ltd, 1997:255–283.

10. Lebovitz HE. Insulin resistance: Definition and consequences. Exp Clin Endocrinol Diabetes 2001; 109(suppl 2):S135–S148.

11. Diabetes Control and Complications Trial Research Group. The effect of intensive treatment of diabetes on the development and progression of long-term complications in insulin-dependent diabetes mellitus. N Engl J Med 1993; 329:977–986.

12. Purnell JQ, Hokanson JE, Marcovina SM, Steffes MW, Cleary PA, Brunzell JD. Effect of excessive weight gain with intensive therapy of type 1 diabetes on lipid levels and blood pressure results from the DCCT. JAMA 1998; 280:140–146.

13. King GL, Wakasaki H. Theoretical mechanisms by which hyperglycemia and insulin resistance could cause cardiovascular diseases in diabetes Diabetes Care 1999; 22(suppl 3):C31–C37.

14. Krolewski AS, Warram JH, Valsania P, Martin BC, Laffel LMB, Christlieb AR. Evolving natural history of coronary artery disease in diabetes mellitus. Am J Med 1991; 90(suppl 2A):56S–61S.

15. Orchard TJ, Stevens LK, Forrest KY-Z, Fuller JH. Cardiovascular disease in insulin dependent diabetes mellitus: Similar rates but different risk factors in the US compared with Europe. Int J Epidemiol 1998; 27:976–983.

16. Kolvisto VA, Stevens LK, Mattock M, Ebeling P, Muggeo M, Stephenson J, Idzior-Walus B, The EURODIAB IDDM Complications Study Group. Cardiovascular disease and its risk factors in IDDM in Europe. Diabetes Care 1996; 19:689–697.

16a. Krolewski AS, Kosinski EJ, Warram JH, Leland OS, Busick EJ, Asmal AC, et al. Magnitude and determinants of coronary heart disease in juvenile-onset insulin-dependent diabetes mellitus. Am J Cardiol 1987; 59:750–755

17. Fiorina P, LaRocca E, Venturini M, Minicucci F, Fermo I, Paroni R, D'Angelo A, Sblendido M, Di Carlo V, Cristallo M, Del Maschio A, Pozza G, Secchi A. Effects of kidney-pancreas transplantation on atherosclerotic risk factors and endothelial function in patients with uremia and type 1 diabetes. Diabetes 2001; 50:496–501.

18. Lehto S, Rönnemaa T, Pyörälä K, Laakso M. Poor glycemic control predicts coronary heart disease events in patients with type 1 diabetes without nephropathy. Arterioscler Thromb Vasc Biol 1999; 19:1014–1019.

19. Isomma B, Almgren P, Henricsson M, Taskinen M, Tuomi T, Groop L, Sarelin L. Chronic complications in patients with slowly progressing autoimmune type 1 diabetes (LADA). Diabetes Care 1999; 22:1347–1353.

20. Williams KV, Erbey JR, Becker D, Orchard TJ. Improved glycemic control reduces the impact of weight gain on cardiovascular risk factors in type 1 diabetes. Diabetes Care 1999; 22:1084–1091.

21. Lawson ML, Gerstein HC, Tsui E, Zinman B. Effect of intensive therapy on early macrovascular disease in young individuals with type 1 diabetes: A systematic review and meta-analysis. Diabetes Care 1999; 22(suppl 2):B35–B39.

22. Lebovitz HE. The effect of the postprandial state on nontraditional risk factors. Am J Cardiol 2001; 88(Suppl):20H–25H.

23. Erbey JR, Kuller LH, Becker DJ, Orchard TJ. The association between a family history of type 2 diabetes and coronary artery disease in a type 1 diabetes population. Diabetes Care 1998; 21:610–614.

24. Williams KV, Erbey JR, Becker D, Arslanian S, Orchard TJ. Can clinical factors estimate insulin resistance in type 1 diabetes? Diabetes 2000; 49:626–632.

25. Orchard TJ, Forrest KY-Z, Kuller LH, Becker DJ. Lipid and blood pressure treatment goals for type 1 diabetes: 10 year incidence data from the Pittsburgh Epidemiology of Diabetes Complications Study. Diabetes Care 2001; 24:1053–1059.

26. Lebovitz HE, Banerji MA. Insulin resistance and its treatment by thiazolidinediones. Recent Prog Horm Res 2001; 56:265–294.

27. Bavdekar A, Chittaranjan S, Yajnik S, Fall CHD, Bapat S, Pandit AN, Deshpande V, Bhave S, Kellingray SD, Joglekar C. Insulin resistance syndrome in 8-year-old Indian children. Diabetes 1999; 48:2422–2429.

28. Montague CT, O'Rahilly S. The perils of portliness. Causes and consequences of visceral adiposity. Diabetes 2000; 49:883–888.

29. Banerji MA, Chaiken RL, Gordon D, Kral JG, Lebovitz HE. Does intra-abdominal adipose tissue in black men determine whether NIDDM is insulin resistant or insulin sensitive. Diabetes 1995; 44:141–146.

30. Banerji MA, Lebowitz J, Chaiken RL, Gordon D, Kral JG, Lebovitz HE. Relationship of visceral adipose tissue and glucose disposal is independent of sex in black NIDDM subjects. Am J Physiol 1997; 273E:425–432.

31. Banerji MA, Buckley C, Chaiken RL, Gordon D, Lebovitz HE, Kral JG. Liver fat, serum triglycerides and visceral adipose tissue in insulin-sensitive and insulin-resistant black men with NIDDM. Int J Obesity 1995; 19:846–850.

32. Pan DA, Lillioja S, Kritketos AD, Milner MR, Bauer LA, Bogardus C, Jenkins AB, Storlien LH. Skeletal muscle triglyceride levels are inversely related to insulin action. Diabetes 1997; 46:983–988.

33. Fuller JH, Shipley MJ, Rose G, Jarrett RJ, Keen H. Coronary heart disease and impaired glucose tolerance: The Whitehall Study. Lancet 1980; I:1373–1376.

34. Eschwege E, Richard JL, Thibult N, Ducimetiere P, Warnet JM, Claude JR, Rosselin GE. Coronary heart disease mortality in relation with diabetes, blood glucose and plasma insulin levels: The Paris Prospective Study, ten years later. Horm Metab Res 1985; 15(suppl):41–46.

35. Haffner SM, Stern MP, Hazuda HP, Mitchell BD, Patterson JK. Cardiovascular risk factors in confirmed prediabetic individuals. Does the clock for coronary heart disease start ticking before the onset of clinical diabetes? JAMA 1990; 263:2893–2898.

36. Haffner SM, Mykkänen L, Festa A, Burke JP, Stern MP. Insulin-resistant prediabetic subjects have more atherogenic risk factors than insulin-sensitive prediabetic subjects. Implications for preventing coronary heart disease during the prediabetic state. Circulation 2000; 101:975–980.

37. Isomaa B, Almgren P, Tuomi T, Forsén B, Lahti K, Nissén M, Taskinen M-R, Groop L. Cardiovascular morbidity and mortality associated with the metabolic syndrome. Diabetes Care 2001; 24:683–689.

38. Yamada N, Yoshinaga H, Sakurai N, Shimano H, Gotoda T, Ohashi Y, Yazaki Y, Kosaka K. Increased risk factors for coronary artery disease in Japanese subjects with hyperinsulinemia or glucose intolerance. Diabetes Care 1994; 17:107–114.

39. DECODE study group. Will new diagnostic criteria for diabetes mellitus change phenotype of patients with diabetes? Reanalysis of European epidemiological data. Br Med J 1998; 317:371–375.

40. DECODE study group. Consequences of the new diagnostic criteria for diabetes in older men and women. The DECODE Study (Diabetes Epidemiology: Collaborative Analysis of Diagnostic Criteria in Europe). Diabetes Care 1999; 22:1667–1671.

41. Tominaga M, Eguchi H, Manaka H, Igarashi K, Kato T, Sekikawa A. Impaired glucose tolerance is a risk factor for cardiovascular disease but not impaired fasting glucose. The Funagata Diabetes Study. Diabetes Care 1999; 22:920–924.

42. Goldberg RB, Mellies MJ, Sacks FM, Moyé LA, Howard BV, Howard WJ, Davis BR, Cole TG, Pfeffer MA, Braunwald E, for the CARE Investigators. Cardiovascular events and their reduction with pravastatin in diabetic and glucose-intolerant myocardial infarction survivors with average cholesterol levels. Subgroup analyses in the Cholesterol and Recurrent Events (CARE) Trial. Circulation 1998; 98:2513–2519.

43. Vauhkonen I, Niskanen L, Vanninen E, Kainulainen S, Uusitupa M, Laakso M. Defects in insulin secretion and insulin action in non-insulin-dependent diabetes mellitus are inherited: Metabolic studies on offspring of diabetic probands. J Clin Invest 1998; 101:86–96.

44. Brochu M, Tchernof A, Dionne IJ, Sites CK, Eltabbakh GH, Sims EA, Poehlman ET. What are the physical characteristics associated with a normal metabolic profile despite a high level of obesity in postmenopausal women? J Clin Endocrinol Metab 2001; 86:1020–1025.

45. Haffner SM, D'Agostino RD Jr, Mykkänen L, Tracy R, Howard B, Rewers M, Selby J, Savage PJ, Saad MF. Insulin sensitivity in subjects with type 2 diabetes: Relationship to cardiovascular risk factors: the Insulin Resistance Atherosclerosis Study. Diabetes Care 1999; 22:562–568.

46. U.K. Prospective Diabetes Study Group. UK Prospective Diabetes Study XII: Differences between Asian, Afro-Caribbean and white Caucasian type 2 diabetic patients at diagnosis of diabetes. Diabetes Med 1994; 11:670–677.

47. U.K. Prospective Diabetes Study Group. Ethnicity and cardiovascular disease. The incidence of myocardial infarction in white South Asian, and Afro-Caribbean patients with type 2 diabetes (U.K. Prospective Diabetes Study 32). Diabetes Care 1998; 21:1271–1277.

48. Pyörälä M, Miettinen H, Halonen P, Laakso M, Pyörälä K. Insulin resistance syndrome predicts the risk of coronary heart disease and stroke in healthy middle-aged men. The 22-year follow-up results of the Helsinki policemen study. Arterioscler Thromb Vasc Biol 2000; 20:538–544.

49. Lempiäinen P, Mykkänen L, Pyörälä K, Laakso M, Kuusisto J. Insulin resistance syndrome predicts coronary heart disease events in elderly nondiabetic men. Circulation 1999; 100:123–128.
50. Després J-P. The insulin resistance-dyslipidemia syndrome: The most prevalent cause of coronary artery disease? Can Med Assoc J 1993; 148:1339–1340.
51. Lamarche B, Tchernof A, Mauriége P, Cantin B, Degenais GR, Lupien PJ, Després J-P. Fasting insulin and apolipoprotein B levels and low-density lipoprotein particle size as risk factors for ischemic heart disease. JAMA 1998; 279:1955–1961.
52. Kannel WB. Lipids, diabetes, and coronary heart disease: Insights from the Framingham Study. Am Heart J 1985; 110:1100–1107.
53. Kannel WB, D'Agostino RB, Wilson PWF, Belanger AJ, Gagnon DR. Diabetes, fibrinogen, and the risk of cardiovascular disease: The Framingham experience. Am Heart J 1999; 120:672–676.
54. Kohler HP, Grant PJ. Plasminogen-activator inhibitor type 1 and coronary artery disease. N Engl J Med 2000; 342:1792–1801.
55. Danesh J. Smoldering arteries? Low-grade inflammation and coronary heart disease. JAMA 1999; 282:2169–2170.
56. Danesh J, Collins R, Appleby P, Peto R. Association of fibrinogen, C-reactive protein, albumin, or leukocyte count with coronary heart disease. Meta-analyses of prospective studies. JAMA 1998; 279:1477–1482.
57. Brunzell JD, Hokanson JE. Dyslipidemia of central obesity and insulin resistance. Diabetes Care 1999; 22(suppl 3):C10–C13.
58. Nadler ST, Stoehr JP, Schueler KL, Tanimoto G, Yandell BS, Attie AD. The expression of adipogenic genes is decreased in obesity and diabetes mellitus. PNAS(USA) 2000; 92:11371–11376.
59. Moitra J, Mason MM, Olive M, Krylov D, Gavrilova O, Marcus-Samuels B, Feigenbaum L, Lee E, Aoyama T, Eckhaus M, Reitman ML, Vinson C. Life without white fat: a transgenic mouse. Genes Devel 1998; 12:3168–3181.
60. Willson TM, Brown PJ, Sternbach DD, Henke BR. The PPARs: from orphan receptors to drug discovery. J Med Chem 2000; 43:527–550.
61. Willson TM, Lambert MH, Kliewer SA. Peroxisome proliferator-activated receptor γ and metabolic disease. Annu Rev Biochem 2001; 70:341–367.
62. Dresner A, Laurent D, Marcucci M, Griffin ME, Dufour S, Cline GW, Slezak LA, Andersen DK, Hundal RS, Rothman DL, Petersen KF, Shulman GI. Effects of free fatty acids on glucose transport and IRS-1-associated phosphatidylinositol 3-kinase activity. J Clin Invest 1999; 103:253–259.
63. Hotamisligil GS, Spiegelman BM. Tumor necrosis factor α: A key component of the obesity-diabetes link. Diabetes 1994; 43:1271–1278.
64. Virkamaki A, Ueki K, Kahn CR. Protein-protein interaction in insulin signaling and the molecular mechanisms of insulin resistance. J Clin Invest 1999; 103:931–943.
65. Dib K, Whitehead JP, Humphreys PJ, Soos MA, Baynes KCR, Kumar S, Harvey T, O'Rahilly S. Impaired activation of phosphoinositide 3-kinase by insulin in fibroblasts from patients with severe insulin resistance and pseudoacromegaly: A disorder characterized by selective postreceptor insulin resistance. J Clin Invest 1998; 101:1111–1120.

66. Calles-Escandon J, Cipolla M. Diabetes and endothelial dysfunction: A clinical perspective. Endocrine Rev 2001; 22:36–52.

67. Zeng G, Nystrom FH, Ravichandran LV, Cong L-N, Kirby M, Mostowski H, Quon MJ. Roles for insulin receptor, PI 3-kinase, and Akt in insulin-signaling pathways related to production of nitris oxide in human vascular endothelial cells. Circulation 2000; 101:1539–1545.

68. Thomas GD, Ahang W, Victor RG. Nitric oxide deficiency as a cause of clinical hypertension: Promising new drug targets for refractory hypertension. JAMA 2001; 285:2055–2057.

69. Tooke JE. Endotheliopathy precedes type 2 diabetes. Diabetes Care 1998; 21:2047–2049.

70. Yudkin JS, Panahloo A, Stehouwer C, Emeis JJ, Bulmer K, Mohamed-Ali V, Denver AE. The influence of improved glycaemic control with insuln and sulphonylureas on acute phase and endothelial markers in Type II Diabetic subjects. Diabetologia 2000; 43:1099–1106.

71. Yudkin JS. Abnormalities of coagulation and fibrinolysis in insulin resistance. Evidence for a common antecedent? Diabetes Care 1999; 22(suppl 3):C25–C30.

72. Carr ME. Diabetes mellitus: A hypercoagulable state. J Diabetes Complications 2001; 15:44–54.

73. Meigs JBJ, Mittleman MA, Nthan DM, Tofler GH, Singer DE Murphy-Sheehy PM, Lipinska I, D'Agostino RB, Wilson PWF. Hyperinsulinemia, hyperglycemia, and impaired hemostasis: The Framingham Offspring Study. JAMA 2000; 283:221–228.

74. Visser M, Bouter LM, McQuillan GM, Wener MH, Harris TB. Elevated C-reactive protein levels in overweight and obese adults. JAMA 1999; 282:2131–2135.

75. Festa A, D'Agostino R Jr, Howard G, Mykkänen L, Tracy RP Haffner SM. Chronic subclinical inflammation as part of the insulin resistance syndrome: The Insulin Resistance Atherosclerosis Study (IRAS). Circulation 2000; 102:42–47.

76. Festa A, D'Agostino R Jr, Howard G, Mykkänen L, Tracy RP, Haffner SM. Inflammation and microalbuminuria in nondiabetic and type 2 diabetic subjects: The Insulin Resistance Atherosclerosis Study. Kidney Int 2000; 58:1703–1710.

77. Feingold KR, Grunfeld C, Pang M, Doerrier W, Krauss RM. LDL subclass phenotypes and triglyceride metabolism in non-insulin-dependent diabetes. Arterioscler Thromb 1992; 12:1496–1502.

78. Festa A, D'Agostino R Jr, Mykkänen L, Tracy RP, Hales CN Howard BV, Haffner SM. LDL particle size in relation to insulin, proinsulin, and insulin sensitivity. Diabetes Care 1999; 22:1688–1693.

79. Ginsberg HN, Tuck C. Diabetes and dyslipidemia. In: Lebovitz HE, ed. Educational Review Manual in Endocrinology and Metabolism. New York: Castle Connolly Graduate Medical Publishing, 2000:1–47.

80. Mykkänen L, Zaccaro DJ, Wagenknecht LE, Robbins DC, Gabriel M, Haffner SM. Microalbuminuria is associated with insulin resistance in nondiabetic subjects: The Insulin Resistance Atherosclerosis Study. Diabetes 1998; 47 793–800.

81. Wagenknecht LE, D'Agostino RB Jr, Haffner SM Savage PJ. Rewers M. Impaired glucose tolerance, type 2 diabetes, and carotid wall thickness: The Insulin Resistance Atherosclerosis Study. Diabetes Care 1998; 21:1812–1818.

82. Laakso M, Rönnemaa T, Lehto S, Puukka P, Kallio V, Pyörälä K. Does NIDDM

increase the risk for coronary heart disease similarly in both low- and high-risk populations? Diabetologia 1995; 38:487–493.

83. Liu QZ, Knowler WC, Nelson RG, Saad MS, Charles MA, Liebow IM, Bennett PH, Pettitt DJ. Insulin treatment, endogenous insulin concentration, and ECG abnormalities in diabetic Pima Indians. Cross-sectional and prospective analyses. Diabetes 1992; 41:1141–1150.

84. Haffner SM, Lehto S, Rönnemaa T, Pyörälä K, Laakso M. Mortality from coronary heart disease in subjects with type 2 diabetes and in nondiabetic subjects with and without prior myocardial infarction. N Engl J Med 1998; 339:229–234.

85. Kuller LH, Velentgas P, Barzilay J, Beauchamp NJ, O'Leary DH, Savage PJ. Diabetes mellitus: Subclinical cardiovascular disease and risk of incident cardiovascular disease and all-cause mortality. Arterioscler Thromb Vasc Biol 2000; 20:823–829.

3

Recognition and Assessment of Insulin Resistance

William T. Cefalu
University of Vermont College of Medicine, Burlington, Vermont

I. INTRODUCTION

Insulin resistance, defined as an attenuation of normal insulin action, is a key pathogenic phenomenon observed in the natural history of type 2 diabetes (1,2). Development of this condition in insulin-sensitive peripheral tissues (e.g., muscle and fat) results in hyperinsulinemia, a compensatory mechanism required to maintain normal or near-normal glucose levels. This "compensated" state may be maintained for many years. Once pancreatic β-cell dysfunction occurs, however, inability to compensate for the increased insulin resistance results in clinical hyperglycemia and the diagnosis of type 2 diabetes is then apparent and can be made on clinical grounds. As such, insulin resistance can be considered an initial pathophysiological event leading to, and premonitory of, type 2 diabetes (3–5). Intensive research has been aimed at identifying the cellular mechanisms responsible for insulin resistance and providing a framework for designing pharmacological therapies to alleviate the condition. This chapter will review basic research studies evaluating the cellular defects contributing to insulin resistance, describe methods to clinically assess this variable, discuss associated clinical risk factors, and provide an overview of management options.

The concept of "insulin resistance" originated well over 50 years ago and the understanding of this condition has continued to evolve, as outlined from a historical perspective by Hunter and Garvey (6). Specifically, early observations noted with the clinical use of insulin therapy for treatment of diabetes suggested that there were two groups of diabetic patients, roughly divided by their glycemic response to exogenously administered insulin (6). Using present-day terms, these two groups may correspond to the classes conforming to current definitions of type 1 and type 2 diabetes. The term insulin resistance continued to evolve to describe diabetic patients with markedly elevated insulin requirements (≥ 200 units of insulin a day). This elevated exogenous insulin demand was often associated with antibodies induced by the insulin preparations available at the time (i.e., bovine and porcine insulin) (6). With the advent in the 1960s of the radioimmunoassay for insulin (which distinguished type 1 diabetic patients with absolute insulin deficiency from type 2 diabetic patients who were found to have relatively normal or elevated insulin levels), it became readily apparent that a cohort of individuals existed with euglycemia, but at the expense of elevated insulin levels. Clinical research studies in the 1970s and 1980s took advantage of more sophisticated techniques to assess glucose disposal in vivo, and added greatly to the understanding. Specifically, results from these investigations demonstrated conclusively that insulin resistance was due to impaired insulin action in insulin-sensitive peripheral tissues such as fat, muscle, and liver (1). These studies referred to abnormalities in the insulin signaling cascade after stimulation of the insulin receptor and defined insulin resistance as a "postreceptor" defect. Therefore, the most accepted and current-day definition of insulin resistance stems from these studies and defines insulin resistance as "a clinical state in which a normal or elevated insulin level produces an impaired biological response" (6).

Insulin, by definition, is a growth factor and would be expected to elicit myriad biological responses; the biological response could result in changes in carbohydrate, lipid, or protein metabolism (i.e., altering metabolic processes) or result in alterations in growth, differentiation, DNA synthesis, or regulation of gene transcription (i.e., altering mitogenic processes) (6). Therefore, insulin resistance could apply to any of these pleiotrophic effects of insulin. The term insulin resistance, however, is classically applied to insulin's primary role to stimulate glucose uptake in adipose tissue and skeletal muscle. It is this biological response that is most directly relevant to the clinical manifestations (e.g., hyperinsulinemia and impaired glucose tolerance). Further, insulin resistance although generally referring to the glucose–insulin relationship, should not be confused with the clinical concept of the "insulin resistance syndrome" (i.e., syndrome X, deadly quartet), which refers to additional biological actions of insulin (including its effects on lipid and protein metabolism, endothelial function, and gene expression) and consists of a cluster of clinical disorders and biochemical abnormalities (6–10). The associated clinical and laboratory abnormalities that represent this syndrome consist of type 2 diabetes mellitus, central obesity, dyslipidemia (increased triglycerides, decreased HDL, and increased small dense LDL), hypertension, increased prothrombotic and antifibrinolytic factors (i e., hypercoagulability), and a predilection for heart disease (see Fig. 1) (7–10). There are a number of other conditions that refer to specific clinical presentations (such as polycystic ovarian syndrome, pregnancy, or glucocorticoid therapy) and are associated with

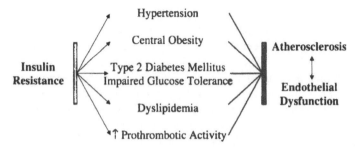

Figure 1 Clinical and laboratory abnormalities associated with the insulin resistance syndrome.

insulin resistance. However, these conditions include some or none of the features of the insulin resistance syndrome or syndrome X. (From Ref. 6.)

II. INSULIN RESISTANCE IN THE NATURAL HISTORY OF TYPE 2 DIABETES

Reduced insulin-dependent glucose transport is frequently found in nondiabetic relatives and offspring of patients with type 2 diabetes (5). This observation, as demonstrated in families and populations with a high incidence of type 2 diabetes, suggests that insulin resistance may be a primary factor in the development of type 2 diabetes and the early development of accelerated atherosclerosis. As such, the natural history of type 2 diabetes suggests that patients may be euglycemic and have normal insulin levels for many years before the development of the disease. In the presence of obesity and a family history of diabetes, insulin resistance typically is present and the individual will need to increase insulin secretion, particularly after meals, to compensate for the insulin resistance (1–4). Euglycemia is maintained, therefore, as long as the individual continues to sustain the compensatory hyperinsulinemia required to overcome the resistance (1–4). As recently reviewed from the Consensus Development Conference on Insulin Resistance, plasma insulin levels, whether measured fasting or postprandially, appear to be predictive for development of type 2 diabetes, and this risk appears independent of obesity or waist circumference (5). In addition, this risk is particularly strong for individuals with a known family history of type 2 diabetes. However, as pancreatic beta-cell dysfunction becomes apparent, leading to a relative decrease in secretion of insulin, the individual is unable to compensate for the insulin resistance (3). Increased hepatic gluconeogenesis occurs and fasting blood glucose begins to rise such that the clinician can now make the diagnosis of type 2 diabetes. Results from both cross-sectional and longitudinal studies have supported this concept that the natural history of type 2 diabetes begins with insulin resistance and, subsequently, a decreasing insulin secretion resulting in fasting hyperglycemia (11,12). Specifically, a longitudinal study in the Pima Indians demonstrated that the transition from normal to impaired glucose tolerance was associated with insulin resistance and a decline in the acute insulin secretory response (11). The progression of the disease from impaired glucose tolerance to clinically overt type 2 diabetes was associated with further worsening of the insulin resistance and a markedly diminished pancreatic insulin secretion (11).

The period in the patient's life associated with insulin resistance and impaired glucose tolerance is felt to represent the prediabetic phase, as insulin resistance appears highly predictive of development of type 2 diabetes (2–5). It is at this prediabetic stage in the natural history of type 2 diabetes where prevention trials are currently evaluating interventions that improve insulin sensitivity by both pharmacological and nonpharmacological means, in the hope that type 2 diabetes can be prevented or delayed (13). It is also at this stage that the clustering of clinical risk factors (e.g., syndrome X, cardiovascular dysmetabolic syndrome, "deadly quartet") is observed (7–10). Therefore, we now recognize that insulin resistance occurs early in the development of type 2 diabetes and may be present many years before the diagnosis of type 2 diabetes is made. Further, insulin resistance is associated with a clustering of risk factors that predisposes a patient to accelerated atherosclerosis (7–10,14–20). A schematic representing the natural history of type 2 diabetes (i.e., insulin resistance and compensatory hyperinsulinemia, associated risk factors, and when a diagnosis of type 2 diabetes is likely to be made) is outlined in Figure 2 [adapted from the results of the Paris Prospective Study (15)].

A. Cellular Events Defining Insulin Action

Understanding the cellular mechanism(s) of action in the insulin-sensitive tissues responsible for insulin resistance would be important in the goal of identifying its genetic basis. Further, an understanding of the cellular defect would allow both the development of effective therapies and optimal use of current therapies. As stated, the aspect of insulin resistance that has been the most well described is inefficient glucose uptake and utilization in peripheral tissues in response to insulin stimulation (1,5). Specifically, this is represented by a reduction in the insulin-stimulated storage of glucose as glycogen in both muscle and liver in vivo (1,5). The primary mechanism in muscle appears to be a block in the glucose transport and phosphorylation step and both genetic and environmental factors appear to induce this defect (5). A brief overview of the cellular factors regulating insulin action will be presented in order to fully understand the potential cellular abnormalities contributing to insulin resistance.

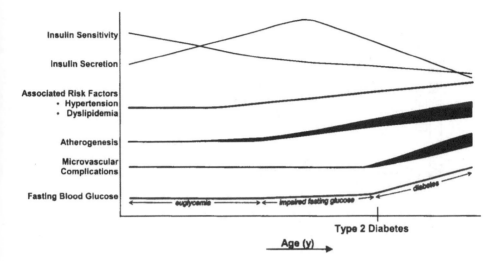

Figure 2 Schematic representing clinical and laboratory findings in the natural history of type 2 diabetes. (Reprinted with permission from Ref. 92.)

The insulin signaling cascade, which results in the biological action of insulin in insulin-sensitive peripheral tissues (e.g., fat or muscle) begins with specific binding to high-affinity receptors on the plasma membrane of the target tissue (Fig. 3) (21,22). The insulin receptor is a large transmembrane protein consisting of α- and β-subunits. Insulin initiates its cellular effects by binding to the α-subunit of its receptor (whose structure establishes the specificity for insulin binding) and thus leads to the autophosphorylation of specific tyrosine residues of the β-subunit (21,22). The β-subunit possesses tyrosine kinase activity and this process enhances the tyrosine kinase activity of the receptor toward other protein substrates. Considerable evidence demonstrates that activation of insulin receptor kinase plays an essential role for many, if not all, of the biological effects of insulin (21–24). Further, insulin receptor tyrosine kinase plays a major role in signal transduction distal to the receptor, as activation results in tyrosine phosphorylation of insulin receptor substrates (IRSs), including IRS-1, IRS-2, IRS-3, IRS-4, Grb-2, and SHC (21,22,25–29). The IRS proteins are cytoplasmic proteins with multiple tyrosine phosphorylation sites that, following insulin stimulation, serve as "docking sites" for cytosolic substrates that contain specific recognition domains, termed SH2 domains (Fig. 3) (30–32). These structural domains on the IRS proteins provide an extensive potential for interaction with downstream signaling molecules via the multiple phosphorylation motifs, including p85α/β, p50, Grb-2, SHP-2, and Nck (21,22,25–32). Thus, since the divergence

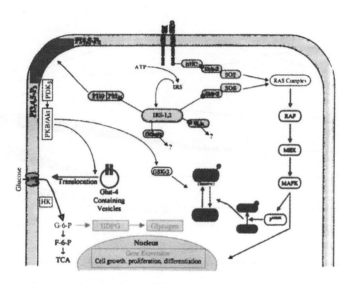

Figure 3   Schematic representing proposed signals in the insulin signaling cascade. (Reprinted with permisson from Ref. 117.)

of insulin signaling pathways within the cell may reside at the level of the IRS docking proteins, the IRS proteins have been appropriately referred to as the "metabolic switches" of the cell.

The specific cellular events promoting glucose uptake after insulin stimulation are less well defined but appear to involve the enzyme phosphatidylinositol-3 kinase (PI-3 kinase). Insulin stimulation increases the amount of PI-3 kinase associated with IRS, and PI-3 kinase activity is directly activated by docking with the IRS proteins (21,22,26,27,31). Specifically, binding of IRSs to the regulatory subunit of phosphatidylinositol-3-OH kinase at SHC homology 2 domains results in activation of PI-3 kinase, which appears necessary for insulin action on glucose transport (33–36), glycogen synthesis (37), protein synthesis (38), antilipolysis (34), and gene expression (39). As activation of PI-3 kinase appears to be of crucial importance for glucose transporter (e.g., Glut-4) translocation from intracellular vesicles to the plasma membrane after insulin stimulation (34,40,41) and glycogen synthase (GS) activation (two major cellular events of insulin action), the study of upstream intracellular signals (e.g., IRS phosphorylation, PI-3 kinase activity) that regulate glucose uptake and glycogen synthesis would provide a cellular basis for understanding insulin resistance. Activation of PI-3 kinase also appears to be critical for transducing the metabolic effects of insulin, as inhibition of PI-3 kinase activation blocks insulin's ability to stimulate glucose transport. However, other growth factor receptors have been shown to activate PI-3 kinase to the same extent as the insulin receptor, but they do not stimulate glucose transport. Therefore, it appears that, although PI-3 kinase is necessary for the action of insulin, it is not sufficient in and of itself to account for the glucose uptake process. Thus, current evidence suggests that IRS proteins increase tyrosine phosphorylation after insulin stimulation and bind to and regulate intracellular enzymes containing SH2 domains. As such, the IRS proteins serve as a "docking site" for several adaptor proteins and this allows the cellular signal to diverge throughout the target cell (21,22,26,27,30–32).

B. Insulin-Stimulated Glucose Transport

The generation of the second messengers following insulin receptor binding and activation promotes cellular glucose transport into the cell. The enhanced insulin-stimulated glucose transport is mediated by translocation of a large number of glucose transporters from an intracellular pool to the plasma membrane (42). The glucose transporters consist of at least five homologous transmembrane proteins (Glut-1, -2, -3, -4, and -5) encoded by distinct genes, and have distinct specificities, kinetic properties, and tissue distribution that define their clinical role (42). Glut-1 and Glut-4 are two major glucose transporters that have been identified in skeletal muscle. Whereas Glut-1 may be primarily involved in basal glucose uptake, Glut-4 is considered the major insulin-responsive glucose transporter. In addition to skeletal muscle, Glut-4 is expressed in insulin target tissues such as cardiac muscle and adipose tissue. In normal muscle cells, Glut-4 is recycled between the plasma membrane and intracellular storage pools; thus it differs from other transporters in that approximately 90% of it is sequestered intracellularly in the absence of insulin (42). With stimulation by insulin, the equilibrium of this recycling process is altered to favor translocation (regulated movement) of Glut-4 from intracellular stores to the plasma membrane and transverse tubules in the muscle, resulting in a rise in the maximal velocity of glucose transport into the cell (42).

As outlined, cellular trafficking of Glut-4 in insulin-sensitive tissues follows insulin receptor binding and activation of tyrosine kinase phosphorylation at the intracellular portion of the receptor. In addition, subsequent activation of PI-3 kinase by insulin-stimulated IRS phosphorylation appears to be a necessary step for glucose transport (33–36), glycogen synthesis (37), and Glut-4 translocation (34,40–43). Specifically, activation of PI-3 kinase has been reported to be necessary for insulin-stimulated glucose uptake in rat adipocytes (34,44), 3T3-L1 adipocytes (33,45–47), L6 muscle cells (48), and rat skeletal muscle (49). Further, specific inhibitors of PI-3 kinase inhibited insulin-stimulated glucose uptake in 3T3-L1 adipocytes (45) and a P85 mutant lacking the binding site for P110 inhibited insulin-stimulated glucose uptake in CHO cells, providing additional support for the role of PI-3 kinase on Glut-4 translocation (36). However, despite excellent studies suggesting potential cellular mechanisms, the specific downstream pathway by which PI-3 kinase activation results in Glut-4 translocation remains unknown. A candidate molecule that has received recent interest is the serine/threonine kinase Akt, also known as protein kinase B, or Rac (50,51). PI-3 kinase appears to be an upstream regulator of Akt, as demonstrated by studies showing that wortmannin, dominant-negative PI-3 kinase mutants, and growth factor point mutations prevent the activation of Akt (50–53), and constitutively active mutants of PI-3 kinase are sufficient to stimulate Akt in cells (54,55).

C. Signaling Pathways Regulating Glycogen Synthesis

In addition to promoting glucose uptake, another major cellular effect of insulin is the production of glycogen. Thus, a reduction in glycogen synthesis is reflected by a decrease in nonoxidative glucose disposal assessed during clamp studies (see Sec. IV) and is a hallmark of insulin resistance. Glycogen synthesis involves the conversion of UDP-glucose to glycogen by GS, which is considered the rate-limiting step (43). GS is regulated by both allosteric and phosphorylation–dephosphorylation mechanisms (43,56,57). This enzyme has been shown to be serine phosphorylated on multiple sites. Insulin stimulation results in dephosphorylation of several of these sites, which activates the enzyme and results in increased glycogen synthesis (57). Insulin stimulation may also regulate GS activity by protein phosphatase-1 (PP1) activation and glycogen synthase kinase-3 (GSK-3) inhibition (57,58). Results of recent studies have questioned that insulin signaling to GS is mediated exclusively through the ras-MAP kinase transduction, but have indicated the presence of yet another parallel pathway likely involving PI-3 kinase.

The specific pathway by which PI-3 kinase activation relays the insulin signal to activation of GS is not known, but it may be secondary to the interaction of the lipid products of PI-3 kinase with the serine/threonine kinase protein kinase B (PKB)/Akt (50,51). Thus, the lipid products of PI-3 kinase appear to play a role in Akt activation. Specifically, the PI-3,4-P$_3$ lipid products of PI-3 kinase activate and recruit PtdIns 3,4,5-triphosphate-dependent protein kinase 1, which phosphorylates Akt (Fig. 3) (50,51). Support of this mechanism is found in studies whereby inhibitors of PI-3 kinase prevent activation of PKB/Akt (59) Akt has been shown to mediate the effects of PI-3 kinase on cellular events such as apoptosis (60) and protein synthesis (61,62). Further, it is thought to mediate the phosphorylation and inactivation of GSK-3 by insulin (63). Specific inhibition of PI-3 kinase by wortmannin in rat L6 cells, which also decreases Glut-4 translocation and activation, prevented the inactivation of insulin on GSK-3 and the activation of p90^{RSK}, p70^{S6K}, and the MAP-kinases (64). The activation of protein kinase B (PKB) is prevented by blocking PI-3 kinase (63). These results demonstrate a link between PI-3 kinase and PKB to the insulin-dependent glycogen synthesis.

In summary, the formation of muscle glycogen following insulin stimulation appears to be mediated through two complementary cellular pathways. The cellular pathway involving PI-3 kinase and PKB with inhibition of GSK-3 and thereby activation of GS has been proposed in addition to the pathway involving dephosphorylation (activation) of GS through activation of PP1. However, the most interesting signal protein is probably PI-3 kinase, which, when associated with the IRS proteins, seems to be deleterious in type 2 diabetes for Glut-4 translocation and activation of glycogen synthesis.

III. IDENTIFYING THE RESPONSIBLE CELLULAR EVENT

The cellular abnormality accounting for clinical insulin resistance could theoretically involve any one of the multiple steps of the insulin signaling cascade as described above. Alterations in insulin production, insulin binding, or intracellular signaling each have the potential to induce an insulin-resistant state. For example, an abnormal beta-cell product resulting from a mutation in the gene coding for the insulin molecule (i.e., mutant insulin syndromes) may be associated with impaired insulin action (6). These conditions may arise secondary to single amino acid substitutions in regions of the molecule that interact with the insulin receptor with reduced affinity and ultimately result in an impaired biological action (6). An example of an acquired defect associated with insulin resistance is the development and presence of "anti-insulin antibodies." In this state, antibodies directed against the insulin molecule can complex with insulin and reduce the amount available to target insulin receptors (6). Fortunately, due to the common use of recombinant human insulin in clinical practice, high titers of insulin antibodies are now rare. The conditions outlined above may be referred to as prereceptor causes of insulin resistance, since these defects occur prior to or at the binding of insulin to the receptor. The insulin resistance most commonly observed clinically is referred to as a postreceptor defect, referring to alterations in the insulin signaling cascade following insulin receptor activation.

Insulin resistance is also frequently observed in clinical conditions associated with overproduction of counter-regulatory hormones such as cortisol, epinephrine, and growth hormone (6). Specifically, acromegaly, Cushing's syndrome, and pheochromocytoma, on clinical grounds, are associated with attenuated insulin action and may present with impaired carbohydrate metabolism. A number of other human diseases and conditions characterized by insulin resistance have been described, as recently reviewed by Hunter and Garvey; these are listed in Table 1 (6).

Table 1 Human Diseases and Conditions Characterized by Insulin Resistance

Insulin resistance may be primary	Insulin resistance may be secondary	Insulin resistance associated with genetic syndromes
Type 2 diabetes mellitus	Obesity	Progeroid syndromes (e.g., Werner's syndrome)
Insulin resistance syndrome (syndrome X)	Type 1 diabetes mellitus	Cytogenetic disorders (Down's, Turner's, and
	Type B severe insulin resistance	Klinefelter's)
Gestational diabetes mellitus	Hyperlipidemias	Ataxia telangiectasia
Type A severe insulin resistance	Pregnancy	Muscular dystrophies
Lipoatrophic diabetes	Acute illness and stress	Friedreich's ataxia
Leprechaunism	Cushing's disease and syndrome	Alstrom syndrome
Rabson–Mendenhall syndrome	Pheochromocytoma	Laurence-Moon-Biedl syndrome
Hypertension	Acromegaly	Pseudo-Refsum's syndrome
Atherosclerotic cardiovascular disease	Hyperthyroidism	Other rare hereditary neuromuscular disorders
	Liver cirrhosis	
	Renal failure	

Source: From Ref. 6.

From a clinical perspective, the aspect of insulin resistance most studied is defective insulin-mediated glucose uptake and utilization (1,43,65,66). In patients, this defect is defined by a reduction in nonoxidative glucose disposal (glycogen synthesis) in muscle and liver. With the observation that the rate-limiting step in cellular glucose metabolism is the plasma membrane transport, Glut-4 defects have the potential to readily result in insulin resistance at the level of the glucose transport effector system. Studies have shown that impaired glucose transport may contribute greatly to the reduced glycogen synthesis observed in insulin resistance (65,66). A decrease in gene expression (i.e., protein content), diminished functional capacity, or impaired translocation of Glut-4 to the plasma membrane are defects that may contribute to the diminished transport. However, this defect in glucose transport cannot be explained by a reduction in the total number of glucose transporter units and studies have not defined whether the intrinsic activity of the glucose transporter is impaired or whether there is a defect in translocation (5).

It is highly likely that defects in intracellular signaling are the cause for the resistance, but a specific defect in any one signaling pathway has not been observed (5). It has been described that a critical threshold level of IRS activity is necessary in order to maximally stimulate PI-3 kinase, and that IRS proteins play a major role in insulin-stimulated glucose uptake (21,27,32). But precise and specific intracellular defects to account for the majority of cases of insulin resistance are not yet described. Therefore, the molecular basis of insulin resistance appears to be polygenic and the relative contribution of any one signaling defect may vary greatly among individuals (5). It is further suggested that the cumulative effects of several mild alterations in signal transduction may be needed to induce insulin resistance, and this remains an area of very active investigation.

IV. ASSESSMENT OF CLINICAL INSULIN RESISTANCE

A number of techniques that differ in sophistication, complexity, and sensitivity are currently available to assess the degree of insulin resistance in patients (67,68).

The most widely accepted research "gold standard" for delineation of insulin resistance is the euglycemic hyperinsulinemic clamp technique (67,68). In this procedure, exogenous insulin is infused to maintain a constant plasma insulin level above fasting while glucose is infused at varying rates to keep the blood glucose within a fixed range. The amount of infused glucose required to maintain the blood glucose at the target level over time is an index of insulin sensitivity. As described, the more glucose that has to be infused per unit time in order to maintain the fixed glucose level, the more sensitive the patient is to insulin. With this procedure, the insulin-resistant patient requires much less infused glucose to maintain the basal level of blood glucose. The clamp procedure, therefore, provides a measure of insulin-stimulated whole-body glucose disposal (M value). More specifically, combined with calorimetry studies, the whole-body glucose disposal obtained from the clamp can be further divided into both oxidative and nonoxidative components. Nonoxidative glucose disposal essentially represents glycogen deposition, and it is a reduction in this measured parameter that has traditionally defined insulin resistance.

The clamp has a number of limitations, however, primarily related to its complexity and expense. Due to the rapid feedback needed from multiple glucose checks during the procedure, a well-staffed clinical research setting is usually required (67,68), making clamps unrealistic for clinical practice or large population-based studies.

A second method used clinically to assess insulin resistance is the "frequently sampled intravenous glucose tolerance test" (FSIVGTT) or the so-called "minimal model." The FSIVGTT is less invasive and more practical than the clamp and can be applied to larger populations (67,68). However, it is less specific and precise. With this procedure, glucose is injected as an intravenous bolus and blood levels of glucose and insulin are assessed frequently from an indwelling catheter over the next several hours. The results reflect glucose disappearance over time and are entered in a mathematical model that generates a value considered an index of insulin sensitivity, termed S_I units. This measure of insulin resistance has been shown to correlate well with the euglycemic hyperinsulinemic clamp in nondiabetic subjects, but its accuracy deteriorates in diabetic subjects because the immediate plasma insulin response to the glucose challenge, a major determinant for this analysis, is diminished. This problem has been addressed in diabetic subjects by analysis after administration of exogenous insulin or a secretagogue (i.e., tolbutamide) during the early parts of testing.

The homeostasis model assessment (HOMA) of insulin sensitivity is another procedure that has received interest (69,70). This approach was proposed approximately 10 years ago as a simple, inexpensive alternative to more sophisticated techniques and derives an estimate of insulin sensitivity from the mathematical modeling of fasting plasma glucose and insulin concentrations. Specifically, an estimate of insulin resistance by HOMA score (70) is calculated with the formula:

[fasting serum insulin (μU/mL) $\times$ fasting plasma glucose (mmol/L)]/22.5

The HOMA method has been shown to correlate strongly to glucose disposal methods as assessed by clamp studies (69).

The total integrated insulin response to a 75-g oral glucose challenge was recently found to be the best surrogate marker of insulin resistance, accounting for over two-thirds in the variability in insulin-mediated glucose disposal in 490 healthy, nondiabetic volunteers (71).

However, from a clinical perspective, the most practical way of assessing insulin resistance is the measurement of plasma insulin levels (5). It is suggested that these levels be assessed in the overnight fasting condition, since glucose levels in the postprandial state are changing rapidly and confound the simultaneous measure of insulin. There is a significant correlation between fasting insulin levels and insulin action as measured by the clamp technique. In addition, it is generally true that very high plasma insulin values in the setting of normal glucose tolerance are very likely to reflect insulin resistance. The utility of assessment of fasting insulin is limited by the fact that, again, there is considerable overlap between results in insulin-resistant and in nondiabetic patients. Another major limitation is the lack of standardization of the insulin assay procedure. However, if the insulin assay were definitive, it would be useful to detect insulin resistance early and before clinical disease appears (5).

Studies that have used any or all of these techniques have demonstrated that there is a wide range of insulin sensitivity in nondiabetic individuals and these values overlap with similar values in type 2 diabetics. Therefore, it is very difficult to distinguish between nondiabetic and diabetic individuals on the basis of insulin resistance (5).

V. SYNDROME OF INSULIN RESISTANCE

A clustering of clinical risk factors (e.g., obesity, dyslipidemia, and hypertension) are associated with insulin resistance and this clinical state is referred to as the cardiovascular dysmetabolic syndrome or syndrome X. Cause and effect is difficult to establish, and significant interaction exists between multiple risk factors (7–10).

A. Obesity/Body Composition

Obesity is clearly associated with chronic diseases such as type 2 diabetes, coronary heart disease, and dyslipidemia, yet the underlying mechanisms are not well defined. However, the evidence is strong that insulin resistance contributes greatly to the pathophysiology of these observed metabolic abnormalities and their associated morbidity (72). Insulin resistance is observed frequently in obese subjects and is considered an independent risk factor for the development of both type 2 diabetes and coronary artery disease (72–75). Although it is established that hyperinsulinemia, insulin resistance, and other obesity-related metabolic abnormalities are significantly associated with overall accumulation of fat in the body, there is considerable evidence that the specific fat distribution is important.

Excessive accumulation of fat in the upper body's abdominal area is referred to as "truncal" or "central" obesity. Central obesity appears to be a better predictor of morbidity than excess fat in the lower body, the so-called lower body segment obesity (72,74,75). Such types of body composition have been clinically separated based on a waist-to-hip circumference ratio (WHR) and individuals are referred to as having apple- or pear-shaped bodies, based on having an elevated or decreased WHR, respectively. The importance of body composition was first reported over 40 years ago by Vague, who noted that the incidence of metabolic complications among equally obese subjects varied depending on their physique (76). Morbidity was clearly shown to be higher in "android-type" obesity than in "gynoid-type" obesity and this heterogeneity was supported by results in several studies suggesting regional differences in adipose tissue metabolism (77–79). The heterogeneity of fat distribution has led investigators to accept the concept of morbid regional adiposity (i.e., that accumulation of fat in certain adipose tissue regions appears to be more deleterious than accumulation of fat in other adipose tissue regions). The hypothesis that has been put forward is that mesenteric adipose tissues constitute the morbid areas of the body and accumulation of fat in these regions has major implications for metabolism and particularly for insulin sensitivity (72,74,75).

Specific abdominal fat depots do appear to have clinical relevance and efforts have been directed to assessing quantity of these fat depots by precise methods. Sonography has been used to measure intra-abdominal tissue (80,81), but has not been as widely used in clinical research settings as magnetic resonance imaging (MRI) and computer tomography (CT) scans. Both CT scans and MRI allow direct visualization of internal adipose tissue compartments and have been tested and validated in human subjects for assessment of intra-abdominal fat stores (82). The quantity of intra-abdominal fat, as assessed with MRI and CT scans, is significantly correlated to insulin resistance (83,84). In particular, it was observed in studies evaluating the insulin resistance of aging that insulin resistance related more to the visceral fat depot than to the subcutaneous fat depot (84). Additional studies have evaluated adipose tissue distribution in other areas, such as thigh skeletal muscle, and have shown significant correlation to insulin sensitivity (85). Thus, it is well established that obesity, in particular central obesity, appears to be the depot most associated with insulin resistance.

B. Dyslipidemia

The increased risk for cardiovascular disease observed with insulin-resistant states is multifactorial, but unfavorable changes in lipoproteins contribute greatly (86–91). An elevation in triglyceride-rich lipoproteins, often accompanied by a decreased HDL cholesterol level (88), is the quantitative change most frequently associated with the insulin resistance syndrome. Thus, this dyslipidemic pattern (by its association with insulin resistance) may be observed in the prediabetic state and may precede the diagnosis of type 2 diabetes. LDL cholesterol levels in insulin-resistant patients and those with type 2 diabetes may be comparable to those seen in the general population. However, LDL compositional differences may make these particles more atherogenic (89,91). Specifically, hyperinsulinemia appears to be significantly associated with both quantitative changes (e.g., increased triglycerides, high Apo B, low Apo A1 levels) in the lipoproteins and also qualitative changes (e.g., low LDL cholesterol/Apo B and low HDL cholesterol/low Apo A1) (88–92). It is further established that insulin levels appear not to be associated with the absolute concentration of the LDL cholesterol, but are associated with the relative decrease in the small dense LDL particles termed LDL subclass pattern B. Insulin resistance has also been associated with this preponderance of small dense LDL particles (86,87). It is the small dense LDL particle that has been suggested to be the more atherogenic LDL. The association of lipoprotein abnormalities to insulin resistance has generated investigation as to whether improvement in insulin sensitivity with pharmacological agents can improve the dyslipidemia. Studies have suggested that insulin sensitizers (e.g., thiazolidinediones) may favorably improve LDL size. Although it has been shown that the ratio of LDL to HDL cholesterol may not change with treatment with insulin sensitizers, the qualitative properties of LDL may change with their use: large (buoyant) LDL is increased and small dense LDL is decreased (93). Whether the compositional change in LDL is indeed secondary to improvement in insulin resistance or secondary to other characteristics of insulin sensitizers (e.g., antioxidant effect) is an area of great debate because there appears to be no relationship between the effect of glitazones on lipoproteins and on insulin sensitivity.

C. Endothelial Dysfunction

The primary role of the vascular endothelium is to modulate the underlying blood vessel tone by producing a number of vasoconstrictors and vasodilators (94–96). Agents that preferentially dilate the vascular wall include nitric oxide (NO), prostacyclin, bradykinin, and endothelium-derived hyperpolarization factor. Agents that have been found to constrict blood vessel tone include endothelin, superoxide anion, endothelium-derived constricting factor, locally produced angiotensin II, and thromboxane. These agents have been described not only to control and regulate arterial tone, but to affect other parameters (i.e., platelet adhesion, aggregation, and thrombogenicity of the blood) that contribute to development of atherosclerosis (94–96). Therefore, if endothelial damage results in more production of vasoconstrictors and less of vasodilators, particularly NO, circulating platelets may aggregate in these particular areas, releasing cytokines and growth factors, and may initiate the inflammatory reaction. After the initial inflammatory reaction, LDL cholesterol is taken up into the vessel wall (via a direct mechanism or possibly in the form of foam cells, i.e., lipid-laden macrophages) and may result in the formation of a fatty streak. Ultimately, vascular smooth muscle cells participate in the process by migrating into the intima, proliferating, and increasing their production of extracellular matrix proteins. The summation of these processes results in the formation of organized atherosclerotic plaque (94–96). Therefore, from the evidence outlined above one can appreciate the potential of the endothelium to participate in cell proliferation contributing to the development and progression of atherosclerosis and, as such, endothelial function has received considerable research interest.

It has been shown that endothelial dysfunction may be secondary to insulin resistance and hyperinsulinemia, in addition to the multiple other components of the cardiovascular dysmetabolic syndrome. Hyperlipidemia, hyperglycemia, hypertension, smoking, and homocysteine have all been reported to damage the endothelium. The resulting endothelial dysfunction leads to an imbalance in the endothelial production of the vasoconstrictors versus the vasodilators. Studies have evaluated clinical intervention, both pharmacological and nonpharmacological, in the treatment of endothelial dysfunction. In particular, the role of an insulin sensitizer was evaluated in individuals felt to have impaired glucose tolerance and insulin resistance and who had attenuated brachial artery vasoactivity (97). After 2 months of therapy, vasoactivity was shown to improve with glitazone treatment and appeared to normalize after 4 months (97). Although this demonstrates that pharmacological treatment of insulin resistance may have favorable effects on endothelial dysfunction, this should not imply that insulin resistance is the sole factor in the development of endothelial dysfunction. As stated above, risk factors associated with the syndrome (i.e., lipids, glucose, and hypertension) have all been shown to damage the endothelium, and studies that have treated these particular components have also shown favorable effects on endothelial dysfunction.

D. Atherosclerosis

It is clear from epidemiological studies that hyperinsulinemia is strongly associated with coronary artery disease, as several large-scale prospective trials have clearly shown that insulin levels correlate with coronary artery disease in multivariate analyses (15–20). However, it is still unclear whether insulin itself is a pathogenic factor in the development of atherosclerosis. A prospective study of men in Quebec found that fasting insulin levels were indeed associated with ischemic heart disease after adjustment for coexisting factors such as hypertension, medications, family history, and lipid levels (17). In the MR-FIT (Multiple Risk Factor Intervention Trial) it was demonstrated that fasting insulin levels were a risk factor for coronary artery disease only in men with a certain lipid phenotype (apolipoprotein E3/2 phenotype) (98). However, in the Caerphilly Prospective Study, the effect of insulin levels on heart disease event rates appeared to be present only in the setting of hypertriglyceridemia (99). Therefore, the possibility exists that hyperinsulinemia is a risk factor only in certain ethnic groups or in patients with certain risk factor abnormalities. Another explanation is that it may simply be a marker for insulin resistance (95).

Despite the conflicting data with insulin levels, insulin resistance appears to be a better correlate with coronary artery disease (95). The number of patients studied to date with direct measurement of insulin resistance is small, but many studies have shown a relationship between insulin resistance and specific measures of atherosclerosis such as arterial lesion size. In particular, the Insulin Resistance and Atherosclerosis Study (IRAS) suggested that insulin resistance had an independent effect on the development of atherosclerosis. In the IRAS, insulin resistance was measured by minimal model analysis in three groups of subjects: Hispanics, non-Hispanic whites, and African-Americans (73). Insulin resistance was found to correlate with intimal medial wall thickness of the carotid artery in non-Hispanic whites, after adjustment for factors such as smoking, lipids, hypertension, medications, and gender (73). In African-Americans, however, there appeared to be no detectable relationship between insulin resistance and the carotid artery intimal wall thickness. Another report from the same group of investigators demonstrated an association between insulin resistance and definite coronary artery disease, even after adjusting for demographics, hypertension, smoking, and dyslipidemia (100).

It is important to note from IRAS that over 50% of the subjects in the study were women (and most of these women were postmenopausal), therefore providing substantial evidence that insulin resistance and coronary artery disease are indeed related in women (73). The clinical observations to date clearly suggest that a more precise measure of insulin action is critical for investigating and defining the relationship between insulin resistance and coronary artery disease (95).

E. Hypertension

Hypertension is a well-described risk factor in insulin-resistant clinical states, but correlation between blood pressure and plasma insulin levels appears to be inconsistent and relatively weak. Specifically, there appears to be little scientific evidence that chronic hyperinsulinemia causes blood pressure elevations in humans (101). Both acute and chronic hyperinsulinemia lasting for several weeks did not cause a hypertensive shift of pressure natriuesis or increased arterial pressure in animal and human studies (102,103). The insulin infusions required to raise concentrations of insulin to those comparable to levels found in obesity tended to reduce arterial pressure by inducing peripheral vasodilation (102,103).

Insulin has also been found not to potentiate the blood pressure or kidney effects of other vasoactive substances, such as norepinephrine or angiotensin-II (102,103). Further, in obese subjects who are resistant to the metabolic and vaso-dilator effects of insulin, elevated insulin did not appear to increase arterial pressure (104). Therefore, the results of several clinical research studies strongly suggest that hyperinsulinemia does not explain the increased renal tubular NaCl reabsorption, shifts of pressure natriuesis, or the hypertension associated with obesity in both animals and humans (101).

In contrast to the above, results from rodent studies suggest that long-term elevated insulin levels may result in significant elevations in arterial pressure. This effect may be mediated through interactions with the RAS and thromboxane (101). Studies have suggested that inhibition of thromboxane synthesis or ACE inhibition did indeed abolish the insulin-induced rise in arterial pressure in rodents (105,106). Further, blockade of endothelial-derived NO synthesis appears to enhance insulin-induced hypertension in rodents (107). It is unclear whether these findings in rodents are relevant to the hypertension noted in obese humans, but summation of the currently available studies does suggest that chronic elevated insulin levels cannot account for obesity-induced increases in blood pressure. Therefore, the very close correlation between hyperinsulinemia and hypertension in obese subjects may be because obesity itself not only elevates arterial pressure but also induces peripheral insulin resistance in hyperinsulinemia through parallel but independent mechanisms (101).

The question that remains, therefore, is the mechanism by which obesity contributes to hypertension. A recent review by Hall et al. (101) outlines a summary of mechanisms by which obesity may cause hypertension and glomerulosclerosis by activation of the renin-angiotensin and sympathetic nervous systems, including metabolic abnormalities and compression of the renal medulla. A summary of these mechanisms is outlined in Figure 4 (101).

F. Prothrombotic Activity

An additional mechanism proposed to explain the accelerated atherosclerosis observed with insulin resistance and type 2 diabetes is a hypercoagulable state. The body's fibrinolytic system normally limits vascular thrombosis and appears responsible for dissolution of thrombi after vascular repair has occurred. However, a disturbance of the fibrinolytic system favors the development of vascular damage and the final occlusion event in the progress of coronary heart disease (108–113).

A balance normally exists between plasminogen activators and inhibitors, and diminished fibrinolysis secondary to elevated concentrations of plasminogen activator inhibitors may help to explain the exacerbation and persistence of thrombosis observed in acute events. A diminished release of tissue plasminogen

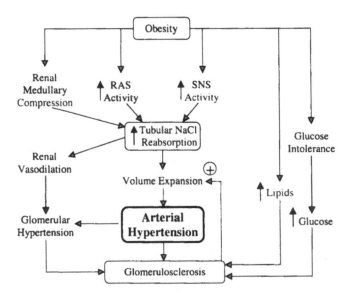

Figure 4 Schematic outlining postulated mechanisms by which obesity contributes to hypertension. (Adapted from Ref. 101; used with permission.)

activator (t-PA) or increased levels of PAI-1 (Fig. 5) may both contribute to impaired fibrinolysis (108–112). PAI-1, a major regulator of the fibrinolytic system, is a serine protease inhibitor and binds to and inhibits t-PA and u-PA (urokinase plasminogen activator). Sources of PAI-1 include hepatocytes, endothelial cells, adipocytes, and smooth muscle cells. PAI-1 is also present in the alpha granules of platelets.

Elevated PAI-1 activity or reduced t-PA resulting in defective fibrinolysis may predispose individuals to sequela from thrombotic events and contribute to the development and progression of atherosclerosis (108–114). PAI-1 appears to modulate vessel wall proteolysis, and increased production of PAI-1 has been observed in components of the atherosclerotic plaque and the vessel wall (111). Diminished vessel wall proteolysis may predispose to accumulation of extracellular matrix. Further, cell migration is dependent on cell surface expression of u-PA. Thus, overexpression of PAI-1 in the vessel wall may limit migration of smooth muscle cells into the neointima. This limitation of migration may predispose to the development of a thin cap overlying the lipid core, a feature associated with increased risk of evolution of vulnerable plaque rupture, when acute events trigger proteolysis (112,113).

The fibrinolytic variables (PAI-1 and t-PA antigen) are strongly associated with components of the insulin resistance syndrome in cross-sectional studies

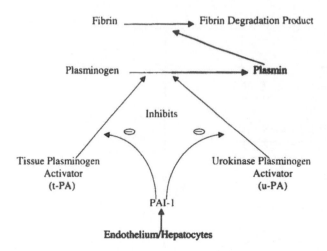

Figure 5 Schematic demonstrating components of the fibrinolytic system. (Reprinted with permission from Ref. 117.)

(115,116). Further, the observed association between insulin resistance and PAI-1 or t-PA antigen levels has also been confirmed in intervention studies aimed at reducing insulin resistance (113). The improvement in insulin resistance is paralleled by improvement of the metabolic abnormalities altering the concentrations of these moieties. Among those subjects who manifested insulin resistance and components of the syndrome (i.e., excess body weight increased WHR, hypertension, and elevated lipids), treatment of insulin resistance was associated with a decrease in PAI-1 and improvement of the fibrinolytic activity in the majority of these studies.

VI.   CLINICAL INTERVENTIONS IN THE MANAGEMENT OF THE INSULIN RESISTANCE SYNDROME

On the basis of convincing clinical studies, it is no longer questioned that the insulin resistance syndrome is associated with an increased morbidity and mortality. A more relevant question is whether improvement of insulin resistance with effective clinical interventions will decrease mortality and morbidity associated with the syndrome. Addressing the question will be problematic, as a clinically practical and reliable test to assess insulin resistance, or a way to serially measure clinical resistance with less invasive techniques for large-scale studies, is not well established (5). We do know, however, that there are a number of clinical interventions that increase insulin sensitivity. These interventions include a calorie-restricted diet, weight reduction, exercise, and pharmacological intervention with agents such as metformin and glitazones (5). Most clinicians will readily agree that, in those subjects who do comply, a calorie-restricted diet will markedly ameliorate insulin resistance. Insulin sensitivity, in these cases, is significantly increased very early after initiating the calorie-restricted diet and this reduction is observed even before significant weight loss has occurred. Clinically, a reduction in insulin resistance is reflected by an improvement in glycemic control or a marked decrease in the need for exogenous insulin or higher doses of oral antidiabetic medications to maintain glycemic control. It has also been firmly established that weight reduction over a longer time frame continues to improve insulin sensitivity. Should a patient not be able to lose weight, the most efficient means of preventing insulin resistance and worsening morbidity may be to avoid additional weight gain (5). A current controversy regarding nutritional recommendations for weight loss is whether caloric distribution among carbohydrates and the various fats is a critical parameter. A general consensus is that total calorie intake is the critical parameter responsible for the weight loss. However, others would argue that the distribution of calories is the key. Unfortunately, comparison trials evaluating such diets have not been done (5).

Exercise is an effective intervention in the management of the insulin-resistant syndrome, as vigorous exercise has been demonstrated to improve insulin sensitivity, even in elderly patients. Unfortunately, the effect on insulin sensitivity is known to diminish quickly (within 3 to 5 days) after stopping the exercise. Exercise should be considered a necessary adjunct to diet, as long-term exercise would result in little weight reduction unless caloric restriction is also part of the regimen.

Pharmacological treatment of insulin resistance is an area of active investigation. Two specific pharmacological approaches in the treatment of insulin resistance have been made available over the past several years. A class of compounds called biguanides, as represented by the agent metformin, has been available for a number of years and has a predominant effect of diminishing hepatic glucose production. The biguanides also have a moderate effect on skeletal muscle insulin resistance. On the other hand, drugs referred to as thiazolidinediones, represented by agents such as troglitazone, rosiglitazone, and pioglitazone, represent a class of drugs considered true insulin sensitizers, as insulin-stimulated glucose disposal is enhanced in insulin-sensitive tissues. Although both classes of drugs are currently available in the United States for treatment of the type 2 diabetic condition, neither class is approved to treat insulin resistance in the absence of the type 2 diabetic state.

Both classes of drugs have been postulated to be beneficial in either delaying or preventing the progression to type 2 diabetes. In particular, the Diabetes Prevention Program, sponsored by the National Institutes of Health, is designed to determine if any treatment (nutrition, exercise, or pharmacological) is effective in the primary prevention of type 2 diabetes in people who have been diagnosed with impaired glucose tolerance (13). As originally designed, there was to be a control group that employed intensive lifestyle changes to effect an approximately 7% reduction in body weight through caloric restriction and exercise. The second and third groups were to consist of pharmacological treatments to reduce insulin resistance, mainly metformin and troglitazone. The troglitazone arm was dropped from study due to an adverse event involving the liver. Because of the hepatic concern, troglitazone was removed from the market in March 2000.

It is not currently recommended that providers prescribe pharmacological treatment to their patients who are felt to be insulin resistant before the diagnosis is established for type 2 diabetes. Depending on the outcome of the current prevention trials, this may be a recommendation in the future. However, until the ongoing prevention trials are completed and the results made available, a nonpharmacological approach is probably the most reasonable option the clinician can offer to the patient in order to achieve a reduction in insulin resistance and prevent the development of type 2 diabetes. Appropriate candidates for such therapy include those who are centrally obese, have a strong family history of diabetes or gestational diabetes, demonstrate impaired fasting glucose on testing, or manifest other clinical symptoms associated with insulin resistance (e.g., hypertension, dyslipidemia).

VII. SUMMARY

This chapter has summarized current concepts regarding insulin resistance and its associated clinical risk factors. Insulin resistance is very much a part of the natural history of type 2 diabetes and may precede the clinical diagnosis by many years. The responsible cellular mechanisms that contribute to insulin resistance are not clearly defined, yet it is well established that cardiovascular risk factors are strongly related to insulin resistance. Whether specific treatment of insulin resistance will delay or prevent development of type 2 diabetes and reduce morbidity and mortality from cardiovascular disease will need to be answered in well-defined clinical studies.

REFERENCES

1. Reaven GM. Banting lecture 1988. Role of insulin resistance in human disease. Diabetes 1988; 37:1595–1607.
2. Haffner SM. The prediabetic problem: development of non-insulin-dependent diabetes mellitus and related abnormalities. J Diabetes Complications 1997; 11:69–76.

3. Lillioja S, Mott DM, Spraul M, Ferraro R, Foley JE, Ravussin E, Knowler WC, Bennett PH, Bogardus C. Insulin resistance and insulin secretory dysfunction as precursors of non-insulin-dependent diabetes mellitus. Prospective studies of Pima Indians. N Engl J Med 1993; 329:1988–1992.

4. Martin BC, Warram JH, Krolewski AS, Bergman RN, Soeldner JS, Kahn CR. Role of glucose and insulin resistance in development of type 2 diabetes mellitus: results of a 25-year follow-up study. Lancet 1992; 340:925–929.

5. Consensus Development Conference on Insulin Resistance. 5–6 November 1997. American Diabetes Association. Diabetes Care 1998; 21:310–314.

6. Hunter SJ, Garvey WT. Insulin action and insulin resistance: diseases involving defects in insulin receptors, signal transduction, and the glucose transport effector system. Am J Med 1998; 105:331–345.

7. Deedwania PC. The deadly quartet revisited. Am J Med 1998; 105(1A):1S–3S.

8. DeFronzo RA. Insulin resistance, hyperinsulinemia, and coronary artery disease: a complex metabolic web. J Cardiovasc Pharmacol 1992; 20(suppl 11):S1–S16.

9. Haffner SM, Valdez RA, Hazuda HP, Mitchell BD, Morales PA, Stern MP. Prospective analysis of the insulin-resistance syndrome (syndrome X). Diabetes 1992; 41:715–722.

10. Opara JU, Levine JH. The deadly quarter—the insulin resistance syndrome. South Med J 1997; 90:1162–1168.

11. Weyer C, Bogardus C, Mott DM, Pratley RE. The natural history of insulin secretory dysfunction and insulin resistance in the pathogenesis of type 2 diabetes mellitus. J Clin Invest 1999; 104:787–794.

12. Bogardus C. Insulin resistance in the pathogenesis of NIDDM in Pima Indians. Diabetes Care 1993; 16:228–231.

13. The Diabetes Prevention Program Design and methods for a clinical trial in the prevention of type 2 diabetes. Diabetes Care 1999; 22:623–634.

14. Haffner SM, Miettinen H. Insulin resistance implications for type II diabetes mellitus and coronary heart disease. Am J Med 1997; 103:152–162.

15. Eschwege E, Richard JL, Thibult N, Ducimetiere P, Warnet JM, Claude JR, Rosselin GE. Coronary heart disease mortality in relation with diabetes, blood glucose and plasma insulin levels. The Paris Prospective Study, ten years later. Horm Metab Res 1985; 15:41–46.

16. Fontbonne AM, Eschwege EM. Insulin and cardiovascular disease. Paris Prospective Study. Diabetes Care 1991; 14:461–469.

17. Després JP, Lamarche B, Mauriège P, Cantin B, Dagenais GR, Moorjani S, Lupien PJ. Hyperinsulinemia as an independent risk factor for ischemic heart disease. N Engl J Med 1996; 334:952–957.

18. Ducimetiere P, Eschwege E, Papoz L, Richard JL, Claude JR, Rosselin G. Relationship of plasma insulin levels to the incidence of myocardial infarction and coronary heart disease mortality in a middle-aged population. Diabetologia 1980; 19:205–210.

19. Welborn TA, Wearne K. Coronary heart disease incidence and cardiovascular mortality in Busselton with reference to glucose and insulin concentrations. Diabetes Care 1979; 2:154–160.

20. Pyörälä K. Relationship of glucose tolerance and plasma insulin to the incidence

of coronary heart disease: results from two population stud es in Finland. Diabetes Care 1979; 2:131–141.

21. White MF, Kahn CR. The insulin signaling system. J Biol Chem 1994; 269:1–4.

22. Cheatham B, Kahn CR. Insulin action and the insulin signaling network. Endocr Rev 1995; 16:117–142.

23. Ebina Y, Araki E, Taira M, Shimada F, Mori M, Craik CS, Siddle K, Pierce SB, Roth RA, Rutter WJ. Replacement of lysine residue 1030 in the putative ATP-binding region of the insulin receptor abolishes insulin- and antibody-stimulated glucose uptake and receptor kinase activity. Proc Natl Acad Sci USA 1987; 84: 704–708.

24. Chou CK, Dull TJ, Russell DS, Gherzi R, Lebwohl D, Ullrich A, Rosen OM. Human insulin receptors mutated at the ATP-binding site lack protein tyrosine kinase activity and fail to mediate postreceptor effects of insulin. J Biol Chem 1987; 262: 1842–1847.

25. Kim YB, Nikoulina SE, Ciaraldi TP, Henry RR, Kahn BB Normal insulin-dependent activation of Akt/protein kinase B, with diminished ac tivation of phosphoinositide 3-kinase, in muscle in type 2 diabetes. J Clin Invest 1999; 104:733–741.

26. Heesom KJ, Harbeck M, Kahn CR, Denton RM. Insulin action on metabolism. Diabetologia 1997; 40(suppl 3):B3–B9.

27. White MF. The insulin signalling system and the IRS proteins. Diabetologia 1997; 40(suppl 2):S2–17.

28. Lavan BE, Fantin VR, Chang ET, Lane WS, Keller SR, Lienhard GE. A novel 160-kDa phosphotyrosine protein in insulin-treated embryonic kidney cells is a new member of the insulin receptor substrate family. J Biol Chem 1997; 272:21403–21407.

29. Lavan BE, Lane WS, Lienhard GE. The 60-kDa phosphotyrosine protein in insulin-treated adipocytes is a new member of the insulin receptor substrate family. J Biol Chem 1997; 272:11439–11443.

30. Sun XJ, Rothenberg P, Kahn CR, Backer JM, Araki E, Wilden PA, Cahill DA, Goldstein BJ, White MF. Structure of the insulin receptor substrate IRS-1 defines a unique signal transduction protein. Nature 1991; 352:73–77.

31. White MF. The IRS-signalling system in insulin and cytokine action. Philos Trans R Soc Lond B Biol Sci 1996; 351:181–189.

32. Kahn CR. Diabetes. Causes of insulin resistance. Nature 1995; 373:384–385.

33. Cheatham B, Vlahos CJ, Cheatham L, Wang L, Blenis J, Kahn CR. Phosphatidylinositol 3-kinase activation is required for insulin stimulation of pp70 S6 kinase, DNA synthesis, and glucose transporter translocation. Mol Cell Biol 1994; 14: 4902–4911.

34. Okada T, Kawano Y, Sakakibara T, Hazeki O, Ui M. Essential role of phosphatidylinositol 3-kinase in insulin-induced glucose transport and antilipolysis in rat adipocytes. Studies with a selective inhibitor wortmannin. J Biol Chem 1994; 269:3568–3573.

35. Le Marchand-Brustel Y, Gautier N, Cormont M, Van Obberghen E. Wortmannin inhibits the action of insulin but not that of okadaic acid in skeletal muscle: comparison with fat cells. Endocrinology 1995; 136:3564–3570.

36. Hara K, Yonezawa K, Sakaue H, Ando A, Kotani K, Kitamura T, Kitamura Y, Ueda

H, Stephens L, Jackson TR. 1-Phosphatidylinositol 3-kinase activity is required for insulin-stimulated glucose transport but not for RAS activation in CHO cells. Proc Natl Acad Sci USA 1994; 91:7415–7419.

37. Shepherd PR, Nave BT, Siddle K. Insulin stimulation of glycogen synthesis and glycogen synthase activity is blocked by wortmannin and rapamycin in 3T3-L1 adipocytes: evidence for the involvement of phosphoinositide 3-kinase and p70 ribosomal protein-S6 kinase. Biochem J 1995; 305:25–28.

38. Mendez R, Myers MGJ, White MF, Rhoads RE. Stimulation of protein synthesis, eukaryotic translation initiation factor 4E phosphorylation, and PHAS-I phosphorylation by insulin requires insulin receptor substrate 1 and phosphatidylinositol 3-kinase. Mol Cell Biol 1996; 16:2857–2864.

39. Sutherland C, Waltner-Law M, Gnudi L, Kahn BB, Granner DK. Activation of the ras mitogen-activated protein kinase-ribosomal protein kinase pathway is not required for the repression of phosphoenolpyruvate carboxykinase gene transcription by insulin. J Biol Chem 1998; 273:3198–3204.

40. Frevert EU, Kahn BB. Differential effects of constitutively active phosphatidylinositol 3-kinase on glucose transport, glycogen synthase activity, and DNA synthesis in 3T3-L1 adipocytes. Mol Cell Biol 1997; 17:190–198.

41. Tanti JF, Gremeaux T, Grillo S, Calleja V, Klippel A, Williams LT, Van Obberghen E, Le Marchand-Brustel Y. Overexpression of a constitutively active form of phosphatidylinositol 3-kinase is sufficient to promote Glut 4 translocation in adipocytes. J Biol Chem 1996; 271:25227–25232.

42. Shepherd PR, Kahn BB. Glucose transporters and insulin action—implications for insulin resistance and diabetes mellitus. N Engl J Med 1999; 341:248–257.

43. Beck-Nielsen H. Mechanisms of insulin resistance in non-oxidative glucose metabolism: the role of glycogen synthase. J Basic Clin Physiol Pharmacol 1998; 9(2–4):255–279.

44. Quon MJ, Chen H, Ing BL, Liu ML, Zarnowski MJ, Yonezawa K, Kasuga M, Cushman SW, Taylor SI. Roles of 1-phosphatidylinositol 3-kinase and ras in regulating translocation of GLUT4 in transfected rat adipose cells. Mol Cell Biol 1995; 15:5403–5411.

45. Clarke JF, Young PW, Yonezawa K, Kasuga M, Holman GD. Inhibition of the translocation of GLUT1 and GLUT4 in 3T3-L1 cells by the phosphatidylinositol 3-kinase inhibitor, wortmannin. Biochem J 1994; 300:631–635.

46. Herbst JJ, Andrews GC, Contillo LG, Singleton DH, Genereux PE, Gibbs EM, Lienhard GE. Effect of the activation of phosphatidylinositol 3-kinase by a thiophosphotyrosine peptide on glucose transport in 3T3-L1 adipocytes. J Biol Chem 1995; 270:26000–26005.

47. Katagiri H, Asano T, Ishihara H, Inukai K, Shibasaki Y, Kikuchi M, Yazaki Y, Oka Y. Overexpression of catalytic subunit p110alpha of phosphatidylinositol 3-kinase increases glucose transport activity with translocation of glucose transporters in 3T3-L1 adipocytes. J Biol Chem 1996; 271:16987–16990.

48. Tsakiridis T, McDowell HE, Walker T, Downes CP, Hundal HS, Vranic M, Klip A. Multiple roles of phosphatidylinositol 3-kinase in regulation of glucose transport, amino acid transport, and glucose transporters in L6 skeletal muscle cells. Endocrinology 1995; 136:4315–4322.

49. Yeh JI, Gulve EA, Rameh L, Birnbaum MJ. The effects of wortmannin on rat
     skeletal muscle. Dissociation of signaling pathways for insulin- and contraction-
     activated hexose transport. J Biol Chem 1995; 270:2107-2111.

50. Coffer PJ, Jin J, Woodgett JR. Protein kinase B (c-Akt): a multifunctional mediator
     of phosphatidylinositol 3-kinase activation. Biochem J 1998; 335:1-13.

51. Burgering BM and Coffer PJ. Protein kinase B (c-Akt) in phosphatidylinositol-3-
     OH kinase signal transduction. Nature 1995; 376:599-602.

52. Franke TF, Yang SI, Chan TO, Datta K, Kazlauskas A, Morrison DK, Kaplan DR,
     Tsichlis PN. The protein kinase encoded by the Akt proto-oncogene is a target of
     the PDGF-activated phosphatidylinositol 3-kinase. Cell 1995; 81:727-736.

53. Kohn AD, Kovacina KS, Roth RA. Insulin stimulates the kinase activity of RAC-
     PK, a pleckstrin homology domain containing ser/thr kinase. EMBO J 1995; 14:
     4288-4295.

54. Didichenko SA, Tilton B, Hemmings BA, Ballmer-Hofer K, Thelen M. Constitu-
     tive activation of protein kinase B and phosphorylation of p47phox by a membrane-
     targeted phosphoinositide 3-kinase. Curr Biol 1996; 6:1271-1278.

55. Klippel A, Reinhard C, Kavanaugh WM, Apell G, Escobedo MA, Williams LT.
     Membrane localization of phosphatidylinositol 3-kinase is sufficient to activate
     multiple signal-transducing kinase pathways. Mol Cell Biol 1996; 16:4117-4127.

56. Markuns JF, Wojtaszewski JF, Goodyear LJ. Insulin and exercise decrease glyco-
     gen synthase kinase-3 activity by different mechanisms in rat skeletal muscle. J
     Biol Chem 1999; 274:24896-24900.

57. Lawrence JCJ and Roach PJ. New insights into the role and mechanism of glycogen
     synthase activation by insulin. Diabetes 1997; 46:541-547.

58. Vestergaard H. Studies of gene expression and activity of hexokinase, phospho-
     fructokinase and glycogen synthase in human skeletal muscle in states of altered
     insulin-stimulated glucose metabolism. Dan Med Bull 1999; 46:13-34.

59. Alessi DR, Andjelkovic M, Caudwell B, Cron P, Morrice N, Cohen P, Hemmings
     BA. Mechanism of activation of protein kinase B by insulin and IGF-1. EMBO J
     1996; 15:6541-6551.

60. Franke TF, Kaplan DR, Cantley LC. PI3K: downstream AKTion blocks apoptosis.
     Cell 1997; 88:435-437.

61. Kitamura T, Ogawa W, Sakaue H, Hino Y, Kuroda S, Takata M, Matsumoto M,
     Maeda T, Konishi H, Kikkawa U, Kasuga M. Requirement for activation of the
     serine-threonine kinase Akt (protein kinase B) in insulin stimulation of protein syn-
     thesis but not of glucose transport. Mol Cell Biol 1998; 18:3708-3717.

62. Hajduch E, Alessi DR, Hemmings BA, Hundal HS. Constitutive activation of pro-
     tein kinase B alpha by membrane targeting promotes glucose and system A amino
     acid transport, protein synthesis and inactivation of glycogen synthase kinase 3 in
     L6 muscle cells. Diabetes 1998; 47:1006-1013.

63. Cross DA, Alessi DR, Cohen P, Andjelkovich M, Hemmings BA. Inhibition of
     glycogen synthase kinase-3 by insulin mediated by protein kinase B. Nature 1995;
     378:785-789.

64. Cross DA, Alessi DR, Vandenheede JR, McDowell HE, Hundal HS, Cohen P. The
     inhibition of glycogen synthase kinase-3 by insulin or insulin-like growth factor 1 in
     the rat skeletal muscle cell line L6 is blocked by wortmannin, but not by rapamycin:

evidence that wortmannin blocks activation of the mitogen-activated protein kinase pathway in L6 cells between Ras and Raf. Biochem J 1994; 303:21–26.

65. Shulman GI. Cellular mechanisms of insulin resistance in humans. Am J Cardiol 1999; 84(1A):3J–10J.

66. Cline GW, Petersen KF, Krssak M, Shen J, Hundal RS, Trajanoski Z, Inzucchi S, Dresner A, Rothman DL, Shulman GI. Impaired glucose transport as a cause of decreased insulin-stimulated muscle glycogen synthesis in type 2 diabetes. N Engl J Med 1999; 341:240–246.

67. Ferrannini E, Mari A. How to measure insulin sensitivity. J Hypertens 1998; 16: 895–906.

68. Del Prato S. Measurement of insulin resistance in vivo. Drugs 1999; 58(suppl 1): 3–6.

69. Bonora E, Targher G, Alberiche M, Bonadonna RC, Saggiani F, Zenere MB, Monauni T, Muggeo M. Homeostasis model assessment closely mirrors the glucose clamp technique in the assessment of insulin sensitivity. Diabetes Care 2000; 23: 57–63.

70. Matthews DR, Hosker JP, Rudenski AS, Naylor BA, Treacher DF, Turner RC. Homeostasis model assessment: insulin resistance and beta-cell function from fasting plasma glucose and insulin concentrations in man. Diabetologia 1985; 28:412–419.

71. Yeni-Komshian H, Carantoni M, Abbasi F, Reaven GM. Relationship between several surrogate estimates of insulin resistance and quantification of insulin-mediated glucose disposal in 490 healthy nondiabetic volunteers. Diabetes Care 2000; 23: 171–175.

72. Abate N. Insulin resistance and obesity. The role of fat distribution pattern. Diabetes Care 1996; 19:292–294.

73. Howard G, O'Leary DH, Zaccaro D, Haffner S, Rewers M, Hamman R, Selby JV, Saad MF, Savage P, Bergman R. Insulin sensitivity and atherosclerosis. The Insulin Resistance Atherosclerosis Study (IRAS) Investigators. Circulation 1996; 93: 1809–1817.

74. Kaplan NM. The deadly quartet. Upper-body obesity, glucose intolerance, hypertriglyceridemia, and hypertension. Arch Intern Med 1989; 149:1514–1520.

75. Yamashita S, Nakamura T, Shimomura I, Nishida M, Yoshida S, Kotani K, Kameda-Takemuara K, Tokunaga K, Matsuzawa Y. Insulin resistance and body fat distribution. Diabetes Care 1996; 19:287–291.

76. Vague J. La différenciation sexuelle facteur déterminant des formes de l'obésité. Presse Med 1947; 55:339–340.

77. Rebuffe-Scrive M, Andersson B, Olbe L, Bjorntorp P. Metabolism of adipose tissue in intraabdominal depots of nonobese men and women. Metabolism 1989; 38:453–458.

78. Rebuffe-Scrive M, Lonnroth P, Marin P, Wesslau C, Bjorntorp P, Smith U. Regional adipose tissue metabolism in men and postmenopausal women. Int J Obes 1987; 11:347–355.

79. Rebuffe-Scrive M, Anderson B, Olbe L, Bjorntorp P. Metabolism of adipose tissue in intraabdominal depots in severely obese men and women. Metabolism 1990; 39: 1021–1025.

80. Armellini F, Zamboni M, Rigo L, Bergamo-Andreis IA, Robbi R, De Marchi M, Bosello O. Sonography detection of small intra-abdominal fat variations. Int J Obes 1991; 15:847–852.

81. Armellini F, Zamboni M, Rigo L, Todesco T, Bergamo-Andreis IA, Procacci C, Bosello O. The contribution of sonography to the measurement of intra-abdominal fat. J Clin Ultrasound 1990; 18:563–567.

82. Ohsuzu F, Kosuda S, Takayama E, Yanagida S, Nomi M Kasamatsu H, Kusano S, Nakamura H. Imaging techniques for measuring adipose-tissue distribution in the abdomen: a comparison between computed tomography and 1.5-tesla magnetic resonance spin-echo imaging. Radiat Med 1998; 16:99–107.

83. Sites CK, Calles-Escandon J, Brochu M, Butterfield M, Ashikaga T, Poehlman ET. Relation of regional fat distribution to insulin sensitivity in postmenopausal women. Fertil Steril 2000; 73(1):61–65.

84. Cefalu WT, Wang ZQ, Werbel S, Bell-Farrow A, Crouse JR, Hinson WH, Terry JG, Anderson R. Contribution of visceral fat mass to the insulin resistance of aging. Metabolism 1995; 44:954–959.

85. Goodpaster BH, Thaete FL, Kelley DE. Thigh adipose tissue distribution is associated with insulin resistance in obesity and in type 2 diabetes mellitus. Am J Clin Nutr 2000; 71:885–892.

86. Grundy SM. Small LDL, atherogenic dyslipidemia, and the metabolic syndrome. Circulation 1997; 95:1–4.

87. Fagan TC, Deedwania PC. The cardiovascular dysmetabolic syndrome. Am J Med 1998; 105:77S–82S.

88. Grundy SM. Hypertriglyceridemia, insulin resistance, and the metabolic syndrome. Am J Cardiol 1999; 83:25F–29F.

89. Lamarche B, Lemieux I, Despres JP. The small, dense LDL phenotype and the risk of coronary heart disease: epidemiology, patho-physiology and therapeutic aspects. Diabetes Metab 1999; 25:199–211.

90. Sheu WH, Jeng CY, Young MS, Le WJ, Chen YT. Coronary artery disease risk predicted by insulin resistance, plasma lipids, and hypertension in people without diabetes. Am J Med Sci 2000; 319:84–88.

91. MacLean PS, Vadlamudi S, MacDonald KG, Pories WJ, Houmard JA, Barakat HA. Impact of insulin resistance on lipoprotein subpopulation distribution in lean and morbidly obese nondiabetic women. Metabolism 2000; 49:285–292.

92. Cefalu WT. Insulin resistance. In: Leahy JL, Clark NG, Cefalu WT, eds. Medical Management of Diabetes Mellitus. New York: Marcel Dekker, Inc., 2000:57–76.

93. Tack CJ, Smits P, Demacker PN, Stalenhoef AF. Troglitazone decreases the proportion of small, dense LDL and increases the resistance of LDL to oxidation in obese subjects. Diabetes Care 1998; 21:796–799.

94. Hsueh WA, Quinones MJ, Creager MA. Endothelium in insulin resistance and diabetes. Diabetes Rev 1997; 5:343–352.

95. Hsueh WA, Law RE. Cardiovascular risk continuum: implications of insulin resistance and diabetes. Am J Med 1998; 105:4S–14S.

96. Quyyumi AA. Endothelial function in health and disease: new insights into the genesis of cardiovascular disease. Am J Med 1998; 105(A):32S–39S.

97. Avena R, Mitchell ME, Nylen ES, Curry KM, Sidawy AN. Insulin action enhancement normalizes brachial artery vasoactivity in patients with peripheral vascular disease and occult diabetes. J Vasc Surg 1998; 28:1024–1031.
98. Orchard TJ, Eichner J, Kuller LH, Becker DJ, McCallum LM, Grandits GA. Insulin as a predictor of coronary heart disease: interaction with apolipoprotein E phenotype. A report from the Multiple Risk Factor Intervention Trial. Ann Epidemiol 1994; 4:40–45.
99. Yarnell JW, Sweetnam PM, Marks V, Teale JD, Bolton CH. Insulin in ischaemic heart disease: are associations explained by triglyceride concentrations? The Caerphilly prospective study. Br Heart J 1994; 71:293–296.
100. Rewers M, D'Agostino RJ, Burke GL, et al. Coronary artery disease is associated with low insulin sensitivity independent of insulin levels and cardiovascular risk factors. Diabetes 1996; 45(suppl 2):52A.
101. Hall JE, Brands MW, Henegar JR. Mechanisms of hypertension and kidney disease in obesity. Ann NY Acad Sci 1999; 892:91–107.
102. Hall JE, Brands MW, Zappe DH, Alonso-Galicia M. Cardiovascular actions of insulin: are they important in long-term blood pressure regulation? Clin Exp Pharmacol Physiol 1995; 22:689–700.
103. Hall JE. Hyperinsulinemia: a link between obesity and hypertension? Kidney Int 1993; 43:1402–1417.
104. Hall JE, Brands MW, Zappe DH, Dixon WN, Mizelle HL, Reinhart GA, Hildebrandt DA. Hemodynamic and renal responses to chronic hyperinsulinemia in obese, insulin-resistant dogs. Hypertension 1995; 25:994–1002.
105. Keen HL, Brands MW, Smith MJJ, Shek EW, Hall JE. Inhibition of thromboxane synthesis attenuates insulin hypertension in rats. Am J Hypertens 1997; 10:1125–1131.
106. Brands MW, Harrison DL, Keen HL, Gardner A, Shek EW, Hall JE. Insulin-induced hypertension in rats depends on an intact renin-angiotensin system. Hypertension 1997; 29:1014–1019.
107. Shek EW, Keen HL, Brands MW, et al. Inhibition of nitric oxide synthesis enhances insulin-hypertension in rats. FASEB J 1996; 10:A556.
108. Juhan-Vague I, Alessi MC, Vague P. Thrombogenic and fibrinolytic factors and cardiovascular risk in non-insulin-dependent diabetes mellitus. Ann Med 1996; 28:371–380.
109. Panahloo A, Yudkin JS. Diminished fibrinolysis in diabetes mellitus and its implication for diabetic vascular disease. Coron Artery Dis 1996; 7:723–731.
110. Schneider DJ, Nordt TK, Sobel BE. Attenuated fibrinolysis and accelerated atherogenesis in type II diabetic patients. Diabetes 1993; 42:1–7.
111. Sobel BE, Woodcock-Mitchell J, Schneider DJ, Holt RE, Marutsuka K, Gold H. Increased plasminogen activator inhibitor type 1 in coronary artery atherectomy specimens from type 2 diabetic compared with nondiabetic patients: a potential factor predisposing to thrombosis and its persistence. Circulation 1998; 97:2213–2221.
112. Sobel BE. The potential influence of insulin and plasminogen activator inhibitor type 1 on the formation of vulnerable atherosclerotic plaques associated with type 2 diabetes. Proc Assoc Am Physicians 1999; 111:313–318.

113. Sobel BE. Insulin resistance and thrombosis: a cardiologist s view. Am J Cardiol 1999; 84:37J–41J.
114. Juhan-Vague I, Alessi MC, Vague P. Increased plasma plasminogen activator inhibitor 1 levels. A possible link between insulin resistance and atherothrombosis. Diabetologia 1991; 34:457–462.
115. Festa A, D'Agostino RJ, Mykkanen L, Tracy RP, Zaccaro DJ, Hales CN, Haffner SM. Relative contribution of insulin and its precursors to fibrinogen and PAI-1 in a large population with different states of glucose tolerance. The Insulin Resistance Atherosclerosis Study (IRAS). Arterioscler Thromb Vasc Biol 1999; 19:562–568.
116. Meigs JB, Mittleman MA, Nathan DM, Tofler GH, Singer DE, Murphy-Sheehy PM, Lipinska I, D'Agostino RB, Wilson PW. Hyperinsulinemia, hyperglycemia, and impaired hemostasis: the Framingham Offspring Study. JAMA 2000; 283:221–228.
117. Cefalu WT. Insulin resistance: Cellular and clinical concepts. Exp Biol Med 2001; 226:13–26.

4

Hypertension, Diabetes, and the Heart

Tevfik Ecder, Melinda L. Hockensmith, Didem Korular, and Robert W. Schrier
University of Colorado School of Medicine, Denver, Colorado

I. INTRODUCTION

Diabetes mellitus is a common health problem throughout the world. According to the World Health Organization statistics, the global prevalence of diabetes mellitus is approximately 155 million, which is expected to increase to 300 million in the year 2025 (1). The prevalence of diabetes is increasing significantly in the United States (2). According to the Third National Health and Nutrition Examination Survey (NHANES III), which was conducted between 1988 and 1994, there are 10.2 million diagnosed and 5.4 million undiagnosed diabetic adult patients in the United States based on American Diabetes Association criteria (3). Diabetes is even more common in certain ethnic groups. African Americans, Native Americans, and Hispanic Americans have a two- to sixfold greater prevalence of diabetes when compared with white non-Hispanic Americans (3,4).

Type 1 diabetes comprises 5 to 10% of diagnosed cases, whereas type 2 diabetes accounts for 90 to 95% of the cases in the United States (5). Both type 1 and type 2 diabetes are associated with vascular complications leading to coronary heart disease, peripheral vascular disease, nephropathy, retinopathy, and neuropathy. These complications adversely affect the morbidity and mortality of diabetic patients, in addition to causing an enormous economic burden. Cardiovascular complications are the most common cause of death, accounting for 60 to 70% of all deaths in patients with diabetes mellitus (6,7). Moreover, diabetes is the most common cause of renal failure, adult blindness, and amputations in the United States (7). Thus, patients with diabetes mellitus should be carefully managed both for the prevention and treatment of these complications.

II. PREVALENCE OF HYPERTENSION AND CARDIOVASCULAR COMPLICATIONS IN DIABETES

Diabetes plays a powerful role in the development of cardiovascular diseases (8–10). The incidence of cardiovascular disease is two times higher in men with diabetes and three times higher in women with diabetes than nondiabetic subjects (10). Haffner et al. (11) reported that the risk of developing a myocardial infarction in type 2 diabetic patients without a previous history of myocardial infarction is similar to that of nondiabetic patients who have had a prior myocardial infarction.

Diabetic patients have a twofold increase in the prevalence of hypertension compared with nondiabetic subjects (5). Hypertension is even more common in certain ethnic groups with type 2 diabetes. Almost twice as many African Americans and three times as many Hispanic Americans as compared with white non-Hispanic subjects have coexistent diabetes and hypertension (5). The coexisting hypertension and diabetes continue to rise dramatically in western countries as the overall population ages and as obesity and sedentary lifestyles become more prevalent.

The coexistence of diabetes and hypertension causes a very high risk for the development of macrovascular and microvascular complications. In patients with diabetes, 30 to 75% of complications can be attributed to hypertension (12). Risk for cardiovascular disease increases significantly when hypertension coexists with diabetes mellitus (13,14). Moreover, hypertension has a greater impact on cardiovascular diseases in diabetic as compared with nondiabetic subjects (15). Diabetic patients have a higher incidence of coronary artery disease, congestive heart failure, and left ventricular hypertrophy when hypertension is present. The incidence of other macrovascular complications, such as stroke and peripheral vascular disease, also increases significantly when hypertension exists in diabetic patients. Moreover, in addition to macrovascular complications, hypertension accelerates the risk of microvascular complications. Diabetic nephropathy (16,17), retinopathy (18–20), and neuropathy (21) are much more common when hypertension is found in association with diabetes.

The prevalence and natural history of hypertension differ markedly between patients with type 1 and type 2 diabetes mellitus. The prevalence of hypertension in patients with type 1 diabetes mellitus is similar to that of the general population until the onset of diabetic nephropathy. Hypertension not only develops with the onset of renal disease in these patients but also worsens with the progression of nephropathy. The hypertension in this setting is characterized by elevation of both systolic and diastolic blood pressures. In contrast, nearly 50% of patients with type 2 diabetes mellitus have hypertension at the time of diagnosis of diabetes. The prevalence of hypertension in these patients increases with age. Type 2 diabetic patients constitute more than 90% of those individuals with a dual diagnosis of diabetes and hypertension (5). Hypertension also commonly occurs in association with other components of the insulin resistance syndrome, termed "syndrome X," which includes obesity, dyslipidemia, hyperuricemia, atherosclerotic cardiovascular disease, and microalbuminuria. Isolated systolic hypertension is common in patients with type 2 diabetes mellitus, suggesting decreased vascular compliance due to macrovascular disease. Hypertensive patients with type 2 diabetes also commonly have an attenuated nocturnal decline in blood pressure (i.e., they do not have the normal nighttime fall in blood pressure) (22).

III. PATHOGENESIS OF HYPERTENSION IN DIABETES

Several factors are involved in the pathogenesis of hypertension in patients with diabetes mellitus. These include genetic factors, sodium retention, and hyperinsulinemia.

A. Genetic Factors

Genetic predisposition plays an important role in the development of hypertension in both type 1 and type 2 diabetes. The higher prevalence of hypertension in certain ethnic groups, such as African Americans, suggests the role of genetic factors (5). Diabetic patients with hypertension are reported to have high frequencies of family history of hypertension (23). Elevated levels of sodium–lithium countertransport activity (24,25) and sodium–hydrogen countertransport activity (26) have also been found to play a role in the genetic predisposition to hypertension.

B. Sodium Retention

Diabetic patients have increased total body sodium, which is approximately 10% higher than nondiabetic subjects (27). Diabetic patients also excrete less sodium in response to sodium load compared to nondiabetic subjects (28). This is due to enhanced tubular reabsorption of sodium. Several factors play a role in this phenomenon. In hyperglycemic patients, glucose in the tubular fluid is reabsorbed together with sodium by the glucose–sodium cotransporter (29). Moreover, increased activity of sodium–lithium countertransporter (24,25) and sodium–

hydrogen countertransporter (26) may lead to enhanced tubular sodium reabsorption in diabetes.

The renin-angiotensin-aldosterone system (RAAS) may contribute to sodium retention in diabetes. Although low to normal levels of plasma renin activity (PRA) are reported in diabetic patients, these levels may be inappropriately high, considering the increased total body sodium content (30). In a study on patients with type 2 diabetes mellitus, Price et al. (31) found inappropriately high renin levels on high salt intake compared to healthy subjects. Moreover, increased plasma angiotensin converting enzyme (ACE) levels have been reported in diabetic patients (32,33).

Type 1 diabetic patients, when challenged with a saline infusion, demonstrate less of an increase in atrial natriuretic peptide levels and natriuresis compared to normal subjects (34,35). This may also contribute to sodium retention in diabetes.

C. Hyperinsulinemia and Insulin Resistance

Hyperinsulinemia may play an important role in the development of hypertension in diabetes mellitus because there is a close association between hyperinsulinemia and hypertension (36). There are several mechanisms by which hyperinsulinemia may cause hypertension. Insulin stimulates the renal tubular sodium–potassium ATPase and sodium–hydrogen countertransporter and increases the action of aldosterone on sodium and potassium transport. These actions of insulin promote sodium and water retention that, in turn, increase intravascular volume and thus blood pressure (37).

Hyperinsulinemia also activates the sympathetic nervous system, raises the plasma norepinephrine level, and increases blood pressure by increasing arteriolar vascular resistance, cardiac output, and renal sodium retention (38,39). The mechanism by which insulin activates the sympathetic nervous system appears to be through beta-adrenergic receptors (40).

Insulin affects different transport systems on vascular smooth muscle cells. Hyperinsulinemia causes the activation of the sodium–hydrogen countertransporter, leading to increased levels of intracellular sodium, which in turn enhance the sensitivity of the vascular smooth muscle cells to the vasopressors, such as norepinephrine and angiotensin-II (41). On the other hand, the increased activity of the sodium–hydrogen countertransporter increases intracellular pH, which stimulates protein synthesis and cell proliferation resulting in arteriolar hypertrophy (42).

Enhanced sodium–lithium countertransport activity has been demonstrated to be associated with the development of hypertension in nondiabetic subjects (43,44). Furthermore, an association between the development of diabetic nephropathy and a predisposition to hypertension has also been shown in type 1 diabetic patients with increased sodium–lithium countertransport activity (45). In type 2 diabetes, insulin resistance is also found to be associated with increased sodium–lithium countertransport activity (46,47).

IV. PATHOGENESIS OF CARDIOVASCULAR COMPLICATIONS IN DIABETES: ROLE OF HYPERTENSION

As previously discussed, the combination of hypertension and diabetes is associated with an increased risk of vascular complications. Hypertension confers a higher risk of coronary heart disease, left ventricular hypertrophy, congestive heart failure, peripheral vascular disease, and stroke in patients with diabetes.

Alterations in hemostasis and vascular endothelial structure and function appear to be involved in the vascular complications observed in diabetes. The RAAS appears to play a deleterious role in the development and progression of these complications.

A. Alterations in Hemostasis

In patients with diabetes mellitus, the balance between coagulation and fibrinolysis is affected in favor of coagulation. Coagulation factors, such as von Willebrand factor and fibrinogen, are increased in diabetes mellitus. The increase in von Willebrand factor is associated with endothelial cell injury. Additionally, factor VII, factor VIII, and thrombin–antithrombin complexes are elevated in diabetic patients (48). Fibrinolysis is induced by plasmin which is mediated by plasminogen activators. Plasminogen activator inhibitor-1 (PAI-1) produced by the liver and endothelial cells neutralizes the activity of the plasminogen activators leading to a decrease in fibrinolytic activity and a propensity for thrombosis (49). In this regard, PAI-1 levels have been found to be elevated in both type 1 and 2 diabetes (50,51) and in hypertension (52).

Platelet adhesion and aggregation are increased in both diabetes and hypertension (48). Increased platelet aggregation may be associated with an altered balance of intracellular platelet cations. Elevated levels of intracellular calcium and decreased levels of intracellular magnesium facilitate platelet aggregation. Both hypertensive and diabetic patients have increased platelet intracellular calcium and decreased platelet intracellular magnesium levels (53).

B. Vascular Endothelium Function and Structure

Both diabetes and hypertension cause functional and structural abnormalities in the vascular endothelium that can precipitate the development of diabetic vascular complications. Hyperglycemia activates protein kinase C in endothelial cells (54). Protein kinase C stimulates the synthesis of vasoconstrictor prostaglandins, endothelin, and ACE. Moreover, hyperglycemia induces endothelial cell collagen IV and fibronectin synthesis. Increased activity of enzymes involved in collagen synthesis may also result in basement membrane thickening (55). Insulin and insulinlike growth factors stimulate the proliferation of endothelial cells.

C. The Role of the RAAS

The RAAS may have many detrimental effects on the macrovascular and microvascular complications in diabetic patients. Elevated plasma and tissue levels of angiotensin-II may play an important role in causing endothelial dysfunction, which is an early manifestation of vascular injury. Angiotensin-II may potentiate the effect of endothelin-1, which is a potent endogenous vasoconstrictor (56). Moreover, endothelin-1 stimulates the conversion of angiotensin-I to angiotensin-II, which further increases the activity of angiotensin-II (57). Angiotensin-II also induces oxygen release in vascular endothelial cells via activation of membrane-bound NADH/NADPH oxidase. This leads to increased generation of superoxide anions that can degrade nitric oxide (58). In addition, angiotensin-II is known to increase PAI-1 levels, which may facilitate thrombus formation (59). ACE inhibitors have been shown to decrease both endothelin and PAI-1 in patients with coronary heart disease (60–63). Furthermore, treatment with ACE inhibitors is shown to improve endothelial dysfunction both in nondiabetic patients with coronary atherosclerosis and in diabetic patients (64,65).

V. CLINICAL TRIALS RELEVANT TO TREATMENT OF HYPERTENSION AND PREVENTION OF CARDIOVASCULAR COMPLICATIONS IN DIABETES

Treatment of hypertension is crucial for the reduction of cardiovascular complications. There have been a considerable number of prospective randomized trials showing the benefits of treating hypertension in diabetes. The SHEP (Systolic Hypertension in the Elderly Program) trial showed that treatment of isolated systolic hypertension in elderly type 2 diabetic patients with a diuretic, chlorthalidone, was associated with a significant decrease in the 5-year rates of cardiovascular events and mortality compared to placebo (66). Similarly, in the Systolic Hypertension in Europe (Sys-Eur) Trial, treatment of isolated systolic hypertension in elderly patients with type 2 diabetes with an intermediate-acting calcium channel blocker, nitrendipine, showed a significant decline in cardiovascular events and mortality compared to placebo (67). In both of these studies, the absolute risk reduction with active treatment compared with placebo was significantly larger for diabetic versus nondiabetic patients, reflecting the higher cardiovascular risk seen in diabetic patients.

In the United Kingdom Prospective Diabetes Study (UKPDS), 1148 hypertensive patients with type 2 diabetes were randomized either to tight blood pressure control (defined as <150/85 mmHg) or to less tight blood pressure control (defined as <180/105 mmHg) (68). The less tight control group received treatment that excluded an ACE inhibitor or a beta-blocker, whereas the tight control group received either captopril or atenolol. Achieved mean blood pressure in the tight control group was 144/82 mmHg versus 154/87 mmHg in the less tight group ($p < 0.0001$) (Fig. 1). After a median follow-up of 8.4 years, even this small difference in blood pressure level (10/5 mmHg) yielded a 24% risk reduction in diabetic endpoints, 32% in diabetes-related deaths, 44% in stroke, and 37% in microvascular endpoints in patients in the tight blood pressure control group. Furthermore, these reductions were much greater than those achieved with intensive blood glucose control (69). In a separate analysis of the tight blood

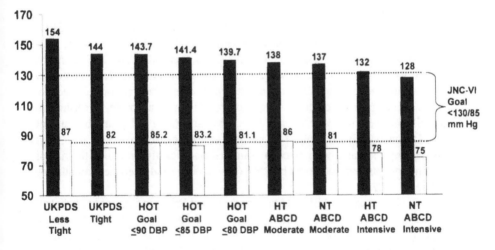

Figure 1 Comparison of the mean systolic and diastolic blood pressures achieved in different target blood control groups of UKPDS, HOT, and ABCD trials. The blood pressures shown for the HOT trial are the means of both diabetic and nondiabetic patients included in this study. The blood pressures shown for the UKPDS and ABCD trials are the means of diabetic patients included in these studies. ■ = systolic blood pressure; □ = diastolic blood pressure; DBP = diastolic blood pressure; HT = hypertensive; NT = normotensive.

pressure control group that used captopril or atenolol as the initial therapy, no significant differences were seen between the two agents (70). Overall, this study indicated that blood pressure reduction is more important than the antihypertensive agent used.

The Hypertension Optimal Treatment (HOT) study included 18,790 hypertensive patients from 26 countries (71). The patients were randomized to diastolic blood pressure goals of ≤90, ≤85, and ≤80 mmHg. Felodipine was used as baseline therapy, but other therapeutic agents were added as needed. The lowest incidence of major cardiovascular events occurred at a mean achieved diastolic blood pressure of 82.6 mmHg and the lowest risk of cardiovascular mortality occurred at 86.5 mmHg, with an average of 3.8 years follow-up. In the subgroup analysis of the 1501 diabetic patients included in the HOT study, there was a 51% reduction in major cardiovascular events in the ≤80 mmHg target group as compared with target group of ≤90 mmHg.

Both the UKPDS and the HOT study showed that reducing diastolic blood pressure by as little as 5 mmHg significantly reduced the risk of cardiovascular complications in diabetic patients. Moreover, no "J-shaped curve" (i.e., increased risk of cardiovascular events with the lower diastolic blood pressure) was observed in these studies. Thus, more intensive treatment of hypertension in diabetic patients is shown to be safe.

The Microalbuminuria, Cardiovascular, and Renal Outcomes (MICRO) substudy from the Heart Outcomes Prevention Evaluation HOPE) study analyzed 3577 patients with diabetes mellitus (72). In this MICRO-HOPE substudy, diabetic patients who had a previous cardiovascular event or at least one other cardiovascular risk factor were randomized to receive either ramipril or placebo. The combined primary outcome was myocardial infarction, stroke, or cardiovascular death. The study was stopped 6 months early (after 4.5 years) because of a significant benefit of ramipril in decreasing cardiovascular events and overt nephropathy compared with placebo. Ramipril significantly decreased the risk of the combined primary outcome by 25% ($p = 0.0004$) and overt nephropathy by 24% ($p = 0.027$).

The hypertensive ABCD (Appropriate Blood Pressure Control in Diabetes) trial was designed to compare the effects of moderate control of blood pressure (target diastolic blood pressure, 80 to 89 mmHg) with those of intensive control of blood pressure (target diastolic blood pressure, 75 mmHg) on the incidence and progression of diabetes complications in 470 hypertensive patients with type 2 diabetes (73). The patients were also randomized to treatment with either an ACE inhibitor, enalapril, or a long-acting dihydropyridine calcium channel blocker, nisoldipine, as first-line antihypertensive agents. After a mean of 5 years of follow-up, the Data and Safety Monitoring Committee of the ABCD trial recommended that the nisoldipine treatment be terminated because of the higher incidence of fatal and nonfatal myocardial infarctions in this group as compared to the enalapril-treated group. This difference was independent of blood pressure control, concentrations of glycosylated hemoglobin and lipids, smoking behavior, and past cardiovascular events. After 5 years of follow-up, the mean blood pressure achieved was 132/78 mmHg in the intensive group and 138/86 mmHg in the moderate group (Fig. 1). No difference was observed between the groups (both intensive versus moderate and nisoldipine versus enalapril) regarding the progression of microvascular complications. However, all-cause mortality was significantly less in the intensive blood pressure control group compared to the moderate blood pressure control group (74).

The normotensive ABCD trial included 480 type 2 diabetic patients, who had baseline blood pressures of less than 140/90 mmHg (75). These patients were randomized to intensive blood pressure control (10 mmHg below the baseline diastolic blood pressure) versus moderate blood pressure control (80–89 mmHg). Patients in the moderate group were given placebo, while the patients randomized to intensive therapy received either nisoldipine or enalapril as the initial antihypertensive medication. Over a 5-year follow-up period, the mean blood pressure achieved was 128/75 mmHg in the intensive group and 137/81 mmHg in the moderate group (Fig. 1). Patients in the intensive blood pressure control group had significantly slower progression to incipient diabetic nephropathy (microalbuminuria 30–300 mg/day) and to overt (albuminuria > 300 mg/day) diabetic nephropathy, slower progression of diabetic retinopathy, and decreased incidence of stroke as compared to moderate blood pressure control group. These findings were independent of whether the initial agent was enalapril or nisoldipine. These results suggest that normotensive type 2 diabetic patients should have a blood pressure goal of less than 130/80 mmHg.

The Fosinopril versus Amlodipine Cardiovascular Events Randomized Trial (FACET) compared the effects of an ACE inhibitor, fosinopril, and a calcium channel blocker, amlodipine, on serum lipids and diabetes control in 380 patients with hypertension and type 2 diabetes (76). If blood pressure was not controlled, the other study drug was added. Prospectively defined cardiovascular events were assessed as secondary outcomes. Although both drugs had similar effects on biochemical measures and blood pressure control, fosinopril alone or in combination with amlodipine was associated with less cardiovascular events than amlodipine alone during a 3.5-year follow-up period. Since blood pressure control, blood glucose and lipid levels, and renal function were similar in both groups, the reduced cardiovascular events in the fosinopril group were independent of these parameters. The authors suggested that one possible mechanism may be due to the suppression of PAI-1 levels by the ACE inhibitor. As discussed previously, increased rates of thrombotic events have been linked to elevated levels of PAI-1 in diabetic patients and angiotensin-II is a potent stimulator of PAI-1 (59).

The Captopril Prevention Project (CAPPP) randomized trial compared the effects of ACE inhibition with captopril versus conventional therapy of diuretics and/or beta-blockers on cardiovascular morbidity and mortality in hypertensive patients (77). Among 10,985 patients included in the study, 572 were diabetic. Although the entire cohort showed little difference between antihypertensive agents regarding cardiovascular morbidity and mortality, the diabetic patients in the captopril group had significantly less total mortality fatal and nonfatal myocardial infarctions, and total cardiovascular events when compared to conventional treatment during a mean follow-up of 6.1 years. This result contrasts with the UKPDS findings, which did not show a difference between captopril and atenolol (68). The lack of difference seen in the UKPDS may be a result of the inadequate dosing of captopril during the study and different levels of achieved blood pressures.

The Swedish Trial in Old Patients with Hypertension-2 (STOP Hypertension-2) was designed to compare conventional antihypertensive drugs (diuretics or beta-blockers), calcium channel blockers, and ACE inhibitors in elderly patients (78). The study included 719 elderly hypertensive patients with diabetes. The analysis of these diabetic patients showed that reduction of blood pressure and prevention of cardiovascular complications were similar in the conventional treatment group compared to the ACE inhibitor or calcium channel blocker group (79). However, patients treated with the ACE inhibitor had a lower risk of myocardial infarction and congestive heart failure than those treated with a calcium channel blocker.

The aforementioned clinical studies show that ACE inhibitors provide a clear benefit in terms of decreasing diabetic complications. In this regard, similar beneficial results can likely be expected from angiotensin-II receptor blockers. Angiotensin-II has been shown to act on two different receptor types, type 1 and 2. All known clinical effects of angiotensin-II are mediated by the type 1 (AT1) receptors. The angiotensin-II receptor blockers mediate their action through inhibition of AT1 receptors. It is known that ACE inhibitors may not completely block the conversion of angiotensin-I to angiotensin-II because of non-ACE pathways. In this regard, angiotensin-II receptor blockers may be more efficacious than ACE inhibitors by more completely blocking the RAAS at the receptor level. On the other hand, the ACE inhibitor effect of increasing nitric oxide levels by decreasing breakdown of bradykinin may be more advantageous. There are ongoing clinical trials to investigate the effects of angiotensin-II receptor blockers on diabetic complications. The Appropriate Blood Pressure Control in Diabetes-Part 2 with Valsartan (ABCD-2V) trial will evaluate the long-term effects of moderate and intensive blood pressure control on the progression of diabetic complications in hypertensive and normotensive patients with type 2 diabetes, comparing valsartan versus placebo as initial antihypertensive therapy (80).

The ongoing Antihypertensive and Lipid Lowering Treatment to Prevent Heart Attack Trial (ALLHAT), which includes approximately 15,000 hypertensive diabetic patients, will compare a thiazide diuretic, a dihydropyridine calcium channel blocker, an ACE inhibitor, and an alpha blocker (81). Because of a greater incidence of congestive heart failure with the alpha blocker versus the thiazide diuretic, the alpha blocker arm has been discontinued.

VI. MANAGEMENT OF HYPERTENSION IN DIABETIC PATIENTS

Blood pressure control decreases both macrovascular and microvascular complications in diabetic patients. Clinical studies have clearly shown that treatment of hypertension reduces cardiovascular morbidity and mortality (66–68,71–77). Moreover, control of blood pressure slows the progression of nephropathy and retinopathy (82–84). Therefore, hypertension should be recognized early and treated aggressively in patients with diabetes mellitus.

The Sixth Report of the Joint National Committee on Prevention, Detection, and Treatment of High Blood Pressure (JNC-VI), World Health Organization, International Society of Hypertension and American Diabetes Association have recommended a goal blood pressure of less than 130/85 mmHg for patients with diabetes (85–87). Optimal blood pressure, with respect to cardiovascular risk, is less than 120/80 mmHg. Furthermore, JNC-VI recommends a target blood pressure of less than 125/75 mmHg for hypertensive diabetic patients with at least 1 g of proteinuria. Intensive treatment of hypertension with a target level of less than 130/85 mmHg is also found to be cost-effective because of the reduced number of vascular complications (88).

Supine, sitting, and standing blood pressures should be measured in all diabetic patients to detect evidence of autonomic dysfunction and orthostatic hypotension. Ambulatory blood pressure monitoring may be useful to detect the 24-h blood pressure profile. The nocturnal decline in blood pressure is typically not observed in diabetic patients with autonomic neuropathy, which must be considered in therapeutic decisions when treating hypertension.

According to the risk stratification of JNC-VI, diabetic patients with high-normal blood pressure (systolic blood pressure 130–139 mmHg or diastolic blood pressure 85–89 mmHg) are considered in the high-risk group. Thus, pharmacological therapy is recommended for the diabetic patient, even with a high-normal blood pressure. Nevertheless, lifestyle modifications and treatment of other risk factors should be considered in every patient together with the pharmacological therapy.

A. Nonpharmacological Therapy

Weight reduction for overweight type 2 diabetic patients is important for improved control of hypertension. It is also useful for the amelioration of insulin resistance and dyslipidemia, which are important cardiovascular risk factors. Reducing dietary intake of sodium is another particularly important factor, considering the increased exchangeable body sodium in these patients. Additionally, cessation of smoking, moderation of alcohol intake, and regular aerobic physical activity are vital measures to be undertaken.

B. Pharmacological Therapy

Patient noncompliance is a major problem in the treatment of hypertension. Thus patients should be reminded of the importance of blood pressure control in the prevention of complications, many of which are life-threatening. Antihypertensive therapy should be tailored so as not to adversely affect blood glucose control and lipid levels in diabetic patients.

A considerable number of clinical trials have demonstrated that ACE inhibitors slow the progression of microvascular complications and decrease the risk of cardiovascular morbidity and mortality in diabetic patients. ACE inhibitors have no adverse effects on serum lipid levels or glycemic control and can decrease insulin resistance. These agents have also been shown to reduce microalbuminuria and proteinuria and delay or prevent diabetic nephropathy. Similarly, they retard the progression of retinopathy (84,89). Therefore, JNC-VI recommends ACE inhibitors as first-line agents for treating hypertension in diabetic patients, especially in the setting of proteinuria.

Renal function should be monitored in patients who initiate therapy with ACE inhibitors. A rapid decline in renal function can occur in patients with bilateral renal artery stenosis or renal artery stenosis to a solitary kidney. With ACE inhibitors, there is the risk of hyperkalemia, especially in patients with renal failure. Cough, and rarely angioedema, can also be seen with ACE inhibitor therapy.

Calcium channel blockers, like ACE inhibitors, have the advantage of not adversely affecting blood glucose and lipid levels. Calcium channel blockers can be combined with ACE inhibitors. This combination may have additive antihypertensive effect and may even improve the side-effect profile (90).

Since diabetic patients are generally volume-expanded and "salt-sensitive," diuretics are particularly useful in this population (91). Thiazide diuretics have been shown to reduce morbidity and mortality in diabetic and nondiabetic hypertensive patients (66). In higher doses, however, diuretics may have detrimental metabolic effects, such as dyslipidemia, hyperinsulinemia, and hyperuricemia. They may cause hypokalemia and hypomagnesemia, as well. These adverse effects are minimized by lowering the dosage. Indapamide, a diuretic that does not have metabolic adverse effects, may be used in diabetic patients. Combination of diuretics with ACE inhibitors can potentiate the antihypertensive effect and reduce adverse metabolic effects. Thiazide diuretics become ineffective in case of renal failure (glomerular filtration rate <25 mL/min). Loop diuretics should be considered in diabetic patients with advanced renal failure. Potassium-sparing diuretics should be used with caution because of the high prevalence of hyporeninemic hypoaldosteronism in diabetic patients and also when the patient is on ACE inhibitor therapy.

Multiple drug combinations are frequently necessary to reach the recommended target blood pressure levels in diabetic patients. Calcium channel blockers or low-dose thiazide diuretics can be added if the target blood pressure level of less than 130/85 mmHg is not achieved with ACE inhibitors alone.

Beta-blockers are helpful in reducing the cardiovascular events in diabetic patients. However, they have adverse effects on blood glucose and lipid levels. They can also interfere with awareness of hypoglycemia and may prolong the recovery from hypoglycemia. Since they decrease peripheral blood flow, they may worsen claudication in patients with peripheral vascular disease. They can also cause vasospasm in asthmatic patients. Therefore, beta-blockers should be considered in diabetic patients only when there is angina or after myocardial infarction.

Alpha-adrenergic blockers have been recommended for the treatment of hypertension in diabetic patients because of the lack of adverse metabolic effects. Moreover, these agents can decrease insulin resistance, improve glucose tolerance, reduce total and LDL cholesterol and triglycerides, and increase HDL cholesterol in nondiabetic and diabetic patients. Orthostatic hypotension may be a side effect in diabetic patients receiving alpha blockers, especially if diabetic neuropathy is present.

Angiotensin-II receptor blockers may be used as an alternative to ACE inhibitors. They are better tolerated than ACE inhibitors and have less side effects and can be used in patients who do not tolerate ACE inhibitors because of the adverse effect of cough. Although they are expected to have beneficial effects similar to those of ACE inhibitors regarding their inhibition of the RAAS, randomized controlled trials are needed to establish their benefit.

VII. SUMMARY

Hypertension occurs frequently in diabetic patients and plays a detrimental role in the development and progression of cardiovascular complications. Control of blood pressure is shown to be effective in decreasing cardiovascular morbidity and mortality, which is the most common cause of death in diabetic patients. Treatment of hypertension decreases the risk of both macrovascular and microvascular complications of diabetes. Therefore, hypertension should be aggressively treated in patients with diabetes. ACE inhibitors should be the first-line antihypertensive agents. Combination of ACE inhibitors with diuretics and/or calcium channel blockers may be necessary to reach the optimal blood pressure goal of less than 130/85 mmHg in diabetic patients.

REFERENCES

1. King H, Aubert RE, Herman WH. Global burden of diabetes, 1995–2025. Prevalence, numerical estimates, and projections. Diabetes Care 1998; 21:1414–1431.
2. Mokdad AH, Ford ES, Bowman BA, Nelson DE, Engelgau MM, Vinicor F, Marks JS. Diabetes trends in the U.S.: 1990–1998. Diabetes Care 2000; 23:1278–1283.
3. Harris MI, Flegal KM, Cowie CC, Eberhardt MS, Goldstein DE, Little RR, Wiedmeyer HM, Byrd-Holt DD. Prevalence of diabetes, impaired fasting glucose, and impaired glucose tolerance in U.S. adults. The Third National Health and Nutrition Examination Survey, 1988–1994. Diabetes Care 1988; 21:518–524.
4. Carter JS, Pugh JA, Monterrosa A. Non-insulin-dependent diabetes mellitus in minorities in the United States. Ann Intern Med 1996; 125:221–232.
5. The National High Blood Pressure Education Program Working Group. National high blood pressure education program working group report on hypertension in diabetes. Hypertension 1994; 23:145–158.
6. Gu K, Cowie CC, Harris MI. Mortality in adults with and without diabetes in a national cohort of the U.S. population, 1971–1993. Diabetes Care 1998; 21:1138–1145.
7. Harris MI. Diabetes in America: Epidemiology and scope of the problem. Diabetes Care 1998; 21:C11–C14.
8. Kannel WB, Hjortland M, Castelli WP. Role of diabetes in congestive heart failure: The Framingham Study. Am J Cardiol 1974; 34:29–34.
9. Kannel WB, McGee DL. Diabetes and cardiovascular disease. The Framingham Study. JAMA 1979; 241:2035–2038.
10. Kannel WB, McGee DL. Diabetes and cardiovascular risk factors: The Framingham Study. Circulation 1979; 59:8–13.
11. Haffner SM, Lehto S, Ronnemaa T, Pyorala K, Laakso M. Mortality from coronary heart disease in subjects with type 2 diabetes and in nondiabetic subjects with and without prior myocardial infarction. N Engl J Med 1998; 339:229–234.
12. Consensus statement. Treatment of hypertension in diabetes. Diabetes Care 1996; 19:S107–S113.
13. The Hypertension in Diabetes Study Group. Hypertension in Diabetes Study (HDS): II. Increased risk of cardiovascular complications in hypertensive type 2 diabetic patients. J Hypertens 1993; 11:319–325.
14. Rossing P, Hougaard P, Borch-Johnsen K, Parving HH. Predictors of mortality in insulin dependent diabetes: 10-year observational follow up study. Br Med J 1996; 313:779–784.
15. Stamler J, Vaccaro O, Neaton JD, Wentworth D. Diabetes, other risk factors, and 12-yr cardiovascular mortality for men screened in the Multiple Risk Intervention Trial. Diabetes Care 1993; 16:434–444.

16. Christensen CK, Mogensen CE. The course of incipient diabetic nephropathy: studies of albumin excretion and blood pressure. Diabetic Med 1985; 2:97–102.
17. Savage S, Schrier RW. Progressive renal insufficiency: the role of angiotensin converting enzyme inhibitors. Adv Intern Med 1992; 37:85–101.
18. Knowler WC, Bennett PH, Ballintine EJ. Increased incidence of retinopathy in diabetes with elevated blood pressure. A six-year follow-up study in Pima Indians. N Engl J Med 1980; 302:645–650.
19. Ishihara M, Yukimura Y, Aizawa T, Yamada T, Ohto K, Yoshizawa K. High blood pressure as risk factor in diabetic retinopathy development in NIDDM patients. Diabetes Care 1987; 10:20–25.
20. Klein R, Klein BE, Moss SE, Davis MD, DeMets DL. Is blood pressure a predictor of the incidence or progression of diabetic retinopathy? Arch Intern Med 1989; 149: 2427–2432.
21. Maser RE, Steenkiste AR, Dorman JS, Nielsen VK, Bass EB, Manjoo Q, Drash AL, Becker DJ, Kuller LH, Greene DA et al. Epidemiological correlates of diabetic neuropathy. Report from Pittsburgh Epidemiology of Diabetes Complications Study. Diabetes 1989; 38:1456–1461.
22. Keller CK, Bergis KH, Fliser D, Ritz E. Renal findings in patients with short-term type 2 diabetes. J Am Soc Nephrol 1996; 7:2627–2635.
23. Barzilay J, Warram JH, Bak M, Laffel LMB, Canessa M, Krolewski AS. Predisposition to hypertension: Risk factor for nephropathy and hypertension in IDDM. Kidney Int 1992; 41:723–730.
24. Krolewski AS, Canessa M, Warram JH, Laffel LM, Christlieb AR, Knowler WC, Rand LI. Predisposition to hypertension and susceptibility to renal disease in insulin-dependent diabetes mellitus. N Engl J Med 1998; 318:140–145.
25. Fujita J, Tsuda K, Seno M, Obayashi H, Fukui I, Seino Y. Erythrocyte sodium-lithium countertransport activity as a marker of predisposition to hypertension and diabetic nephropathy in NIDDM. Diabetes Care 1994; 17:977–982.
26. Trevisan R, Viberti G. Sodium-hydrogen antiporter: its possible role in the genesis of diabetic nephropathy. Nephrol Dial Transplant 1997; 12:643–645.
27. Weidmann P, Beretta-Piccoli C, Trost BN. Pressor factors and responsiveness in hypertension accompanying diabetes mellitus. Hypertension 1985; 7:II33–II42.
28. Roland JM, O'Hare JP, Walters G, Corrall RJ. Sodium retention in response to saline infusion in uncomplicated diabetes mellitus. Diabetes Res 1986; 3:213–215.
29. Weidmann P, Ferrari P. Central role of sodium in hypertension in diabetic subjects. Diabetes Care 1991; 14:220–232.
30. Christlieb AR, Kaldany A, D'Elia JA. Plasma renin activity and hypertension in diabetes mellitus. Diabetes 1976; 25:969–974.
31. Price DA, De'Oliveira JM, Fisher ND, Williams GH, Hollenberg NK. The state and responsiveness of the renin-angiotensin-aldosterone system in patients with type II diabetes mellitus. Am J Hypertens 1999; 12:348–355.
32. Feman SS, Mericle RA, Reed GW, May JM, Workman RJ. Serum angiotensin converting enzyme in diabetic patients. Am J Med Sci 1993; 305:280–284.
33. Marre M, Bernadet P, Gallois Y, Savagner F, Guyene TT, Hallab M, Cambien F, Passa P, Alhenc-Gelas F. Relationships between angiotensin I converting enzyme

gene polymorphism, plasma levels, and diabetic retinal and re ial complications. Diabetes 1994; 43:384–388.

34. Opocher G, Mantero F, Rocco S, Trevisan R, Fioretto P, Semplicini A, Morocutti A, Zanette G, Donadon V, Perico N et al. Atrial natriuretic factor in hypertensive and normotensive insulin-dependent diabetics. J Hypertens 1989; 7:S236–S237.

35. Fioretto P, Muollo B, Faronato PP, Opocher G, Trevisan R, Mantero F, Remuzzi G, Crepaldi G, Nosadini R. Relationships among natriuresis, atrial natriuretic peptide and insulin in insulin-dependent diabetes. Kidney Int 1992; 41:813–821.

36. Pollare T, Lithell H, Berne C. Insulin resistance is a characteristic feature of primary hypertension independent of obesity. Metabolism 1990; 39:167–174.

37. DeFronzo RA; The effect of insulin on renal sodium metabolism. A review with clinical implications. Diabetologia 1981; 21:165–171.

38. Rowe JW, Young JB, Minaker KL, Stevens AL, Pallotta J, Landsberg L. Effect of insulin and glucose infusions on sympathetic nervous system activity in normal man. Diabetes 1981; 30:219–225.

39. Julius S. Autonomic nervous dysfunction in essential hypertension. Diabetes Care 1991; 14:249–259.

40. Lembo G, Iaccarino G, Vecchione C, Vecchione C, Rendina V, Parrella L, Trimarco B. Insulin modulation of β-adrenergic vasodilator pathway in human forearm. Circulation 1996; 93:1403–1410.

41. Moore RD. Stimulation of Na:H exchange by insulin. Biophys J 1981; 33:203–210.

42. Lever AF. Slow pressor mechanisms in hypertension: a role for hypertrophy of resistance vessels? J Hypertens 1986; 4:515–524.

43. Turner ST, Rebbeck TR, Sing CF. Sodium-lithium countertransport and probability of hypertension in Caucasians 47 to 89 years old. Hypertension 1992; 20:841–850.

44. Rebbeck TR, Turner ST, Sing CF. Sodium-lithium countertransport genotype and the probability of hypertension in adults. Hypertension 1993; 22:560–568.

45. Krolewski AS, Canessa M, Warram JH, Laffel LM, Christ ieb AR, Knowler WC, Rand LI. Predisposition to hypertension and susceptibility to renal disease in insulin-dependent diabetes mellitus. N Engl J Med 1988; 318:140–145.

46. Trevisan R, Nosadini R, Fioretto P, Semplicini A, Donadon V, Doria A, Nicolosi G, Zanuttini D, Cipollina MR, Lusiani L, Avogaro A, Crepa di G, Viberti GC. Clustering of risk factors in hypertensive insulin-dependent diabetics with high sodium-lithium countertransport. Kidney Int 1992; 41:855–861.

47. Giordano M, Castellino P, Solini A, Canessa ML, DeFronzo RA. Na /Li and Na$^+$/H$^+$ countertransport activity in hypertensive non-insulin-dependent diabetic patients: role of insulin resistance and antihypertensive treatment. Metabolism 1997; 46:1316–1323.

48. Sowers JR, Epstein M. Diabetes mellitus and associated hypertension, vascular disease, and nephropathy. An update. Hypertension 1995; 26:869–879.

49. Schneider DJ, Nordt TK, Sobel BE. Attenuated fibrinolysis and accelerated atherogenesis in type II diabetic patients. Diabetes 1993; 42:1–7

50. Carmassi F, Morale M, Pucetti R, De Negri F, Monzani F, Navalesi R, Mariani G. Coagulation and fibrinolytic system impairment in insulin dependent diabetes mellitus. Thromb Res 1992; 67:643–654.

51. Vukovich T, Proidl S, Knobl P, Teufelsbauer H, Schnack C, Schernthaner G. The

effect of insulin treatment on the balance between tissue plasminogen activator and plasminogen activator inhibitor-1 in type 2 diabetic patients. Thromb Haemost 1992; 68:253–256.

52. Landin K, Tengborn L, Smith U. Elevated fibrinogen and plasminogen activator inhibitor (PAI-1) in hypertension are related to metabolic risk factors for cardiovascular disease. J Intern Med 1990; 227:273–278.

53. Epstein M. Diabetes and hypertension: the bad companions. J Hypertens 1997; 15(suppl 2):S55–S62.

54. Tesfamariam B, Brown ML, Cohen RA. Elevated glucose impairs endothelium-dependent relaxation by activating protein kinase C. J Clin Invest 1991; 87:1643–1648.

55. Cagliero E, Roth T, Roy S, Lorenzi M. Characteristics and mechanisms of high-glucose-induced overexpression of basement membrane components in cultured human endothelial cells. Diabetes 1991; 40:102–110.

56. Dohi Y, Hahn AWA, Boulanger CM, Buhler FR, Luscher TF. Endothelin stimulated by angiotensin II augments contractility of spontaneously hypertensive rat resistance arteries. Hypertension 1992; 19:131–137.

57. Kawaguchi H, Sawa H, Yasuda H. Endothelin stimulates angiotensin I to angiotensin II conversion in cultured pulmonary artery endothelial cells. J Mol Cell Cardiol 1990; 22:839–842.

58. Zhang H, Schmeisser A, Garlichs CD, Plotze K, Damme U, Mugge A, Daniel WG. Angiotensin II-induced superoxide anion generation in human vascular endothelial cells: role of membrane-bound NADH-/NADPH-oxidases. Cardivasc Res 1999; 44: 215–222.

59. Feener EP, Northrup JM, Aiello LP, King GL. Angiotensin II induces plasminogen activator inhibitor-1 and -2 expression in vascular endothelial and smooth muscle cells. J Clin Invest 1995; 95:1353–1362.

60. Galatius-Jensen S, Wroblewski H, Emmeluh C, Bie P, Haunso S, Kastrup J. Plasma endothelin in congestive heart failure: effect of the ACE inhibitor, fosinopril. Cardiovasc Res 1996; 32:1148–1154.

61. Di Pasquale P, Valdes L, Albano V, Bucca V, Scalzo S, Pieri D, Maringhini G, Paterna S. Early captopril treatment reduces plasma endothelin concentrations in the acute and subacute phases of myocardial infarction: a pilot study. J Cardiovasc Pharmacol 1997; 29:202–208.

62. Vaughan DE, Rouleau JL, Ridker PM, Arnold JM, Menapace FJ, Pfeffer MA. Effects of ramipril on plasma fibrinolytic balance in patients with acute myocardial infarction. Circulation 1997; 96:442–447.

63. Oshima S, Ogawa H, Mizuno Y, Yamashita S, Noda K, Saito T, Sumida H, Suefuji H, Kaikita K, Soejima H, Yasue H. The effects of the angiotensin-converting enzyme inhibitor imidapril on plasma plasminogen activator inhibitor activity in patients with acute myocardial infarction. Am Heart J 1997; 134:961–966.

64. Mancini GBJ, Henry GC, Macaya C, O'Neill BJ, Pucillo AL, Carere RG, Wargovich TJ, Mudra H, Luscher TF, Klibaner MI, Haber HE, Uprichard ACG, Pepine CJ, Pitt B. Angiotensin-converting enzyme inhibition with quinapril improves endothelial vasomotor dysfunction in patients with coronary artery disease. Circulation 1996; 94:258–265.

65. O'Driscoll G, Green D, Rankin J, Stanton K, Taylor R. Improvement in endothelial function by angiotensin converting enzyme inhibition in insu in-dependent diabetes mellitus. J Clin Invest 1997; 100:678–684.

66. Curb JD, Pressel SL, Cutler JA, Savage PJ, Applegate WB, Black H, Camel G, Davis BR, Frost PH, Gonzalez N, Guthrie G, Oberman A, Rutan GH, Stamler J. Effect of diuretic-based antihypertensive treatment on cardiovascular disease risk in older diabetic patients with isolated systolic hypertension. Systolic Hypertension in the Elderly Program Cooperative Research Group. JAMA 1996; 276:1886–1892.

67. Tuomiletho J, Rastenyte D, Birkenhager WH, Thijs L, Ant kainen R, Bulpitt CJ, Fletcher AE, Forette F, Goldhaber A, Palatini P, Sarti C, Fagard R, for The Systolic Hypertension in Europe Trial Investigators. Effect of calcium-channel blockade in older patients with diabetes and systolic hypertension. N Engl J Med 1999; 340: 677–684.

68. UK Prospective Diabetes Study Group. Tight blood pressure control and risk of macrovascular and microvascular complications in type 2 diabetes: UKPDS 38. BMJ 1998; 317:703–713.

69. UK Prospective Diabetes Study (UKPDS) Group. Intensive blood-glucose control with sulphonylureas or insulin compared with conventional treatment and risk of complications in patients with type 2 diabetes (UKPDS 33). Lancet 1998; 352:837–853.

70. UK Prospective Diabetes Study Group. Efficacy of atenolol and captopril in reducing risk of macrovascular and microvascular complications in type 2 diabetes: UKPDS 39. Br Med J 1998; 317:713–720.

71. Hansson L, Zanchetti A, Carruthers SG, Dahlof B, Elmfeldt D, Julius S, Menard J, Rahn KH, Wedel H, Westerling S for the HOT Study Group. Effects of intensive blood-pressure lowering and low-dose aspirin in patients with hypertension: principal results of the Hypertension Optimal Treatment (HOT) randomised trial. Lancet 1998; 351:1755–1762.

72. Heart Outcomes Prevention Evaluation (HOPE) Study Investigators. Effects of ramipril on cardiovascular and microvascular outcomes in people with diabetes mellitus: results of the HOPE study and MICRO-HOPE substudy. Lancet 2000; 355:253–259.

73. Estacio RO, Jeffers BW, Hiatt WR, Biggerstaff SL, Gifford N, Schrier RW. The effect of nisoldipine as compared with enalapril on cardiovascular outcomes in patients with non-insulin-dependent diabetes and hypertension. N Engl J Med 1998; 338:645–652.

74. Estacio RO, Jeffers BW, Gifford N, Schrier RW. Effect of blood pressure control on diabetic microvascular complications in patients with hypertension and type 2 diabetes. Diabetes Care 2000; 23(suppl 2):B54–B64.

75. Schrier RW, Estacio R, Ester A, Mehler P. Effects of aggressive blood pressure control in normotensive type 2 diabetic patients on albuminuria, retinopathy and strokes. Kidney Int (in press).

76. Tatti P, Pahor M, Byington RP, Di Mauro P, Guarisco R, Strollo G, Strollo F. Outcome results of the Fosinopril Versus Amlodipine Cardiovascular Events Random-

ized Trial (FACET) in patients with hypertension and NIDDM. Diabetes Care 1998; 21:597–603.

77. Hansson L, Lindholm LH, Niskanen L, Lanke J, Hedner T, Niklason A, Luomanmaki K, Dahlof B, de Faire U, Morlin C, Karlberg BE, Wester PO, Bjorck J-E, for the Captopril Prevention Project (CAPPP) study group. Effect of angiotensin-converting-enzyme inhibition compared with conventional therapy on cardiovascular morbidity and mortality in hypertension: the Captopril Prevention Project (CAPPP) randomised trial. Lancet 1999; 353:611–616.

78. Hansson L, Lindholm LH, Ekbom T, Dahlof B, Lanke J, Schersten B, Wester P-O, Hedner T, de Faire U, for the STOP-Hypertension-2 Study Group. Randomised trial of old and new antihypertensive drugs in elderly patients: cardiovascular mortality and morbidity in the Swedish Trial in Old Patients with Hypertension-2 study. Lancet 1999; 354:1751–1756.

79. Lindholm LH, Hansson L, Ekbom T, Dahlof B, Lanke J, Linjer E, Schersten B, Wester P-O, Hedner T, de Faire U, for the STOP Hypertension-2 Study Group. Comparison of antihypertensive treatments in preventing cardiovascular events in elderly diabetic patients: results from the Swedish Trial in Old Patients with Hypertension-2. J Hypertens 2000; 18:1671–1675.

80. Schrier RW, Estacio RO, Jeffers BW, Biggerstaff S, Krinsky E, Pincus JR, Bedigian MP. ABCD-2V: Appropriate Blood Pressure Control in Diabetes-Part 2 With Valsartan. Am J Hypertens 1999; 12:141A.

81. Davis BR, Cutler JA, Gordon DJ, Furberg CD, Wright JT Jr, Cushman WC, Grimm RH, LaRosa J, Whelton PK, Perry HM, Alderman MH, Ford CE, Oparil S, Francis C, Proschan M, Pressel S, Black HR, Hawkins CM. Rationale and design for the Antihypertensive and Lipid Lowering Treatment to Prevent Heart Attack Trial (ALLHAT). Am J Hypertens 1996; 9:342–360.

82. Mogensen CE. Long-term antihypertensive treatment inhibiting progression of diabetic nephropathy. Br Med J 1982; 285:685–688.

83. Parving HH, Andersen AR, Smidt UM, Svendsen PA. Early aggressive antihypertensive treatment reduces rate of decline in kidney function in diabetic nephropathy. Lancet 1983; 1:1175–1178.

84. Chaturvedi N, Sjolie A-K, Stephenson JM, Abrahamian H, Keipes M, Castellarin A, Rogulja-Pepeonik Z, Fuller JH, and the EUCLID Study Group. Effect of lisinopril on progression of retinopathy in normotensive people with type 1 diabetes. Lancet 1998; 351:28–31.

85. The Joint National Committee on Prevention, Detection, Evaluation, and Treatment of High Blood Pressure and the National High Blood Pressure Education Program Coordinating Committee. The Sixth Report of the Joint National Committee on Prevention, Detection, Evaluation, and Treatment of High Blood Pressure. Arch Intern Med 1997; 157:2413–2446.

86. 1999 World Health Organization-International Society of Hypertension guidelines for the management of hypertension. J Hypertens 1999; 17:151–183.

87. American Diabetes Association. Standards of medical care for patients with diabetes mellitus. Diabetes Care 2000; 23:S32–S42.

88. Elliott WJ, Weir DR, Black HR. Cost-effectiveness of the lower treatment goal

(of JNC VI) for diabetic hypertensive patients. Arch Intern Med 2000; 160:1277–1283.

89. Modulation of the renin-angiotensin system and retinopathy. Heart 2000; 84(suppl 1):i29–i31.

90. Sheinfeld GR, Bakris GL. Benefits of combination angiotensin-converting enzyme inhibitor and calcium antagonist therapy for diabetic patients. Am J Hypertens 1999; 12:80S–85S.

91. Bakris GL, Weir MR, Sowers JR. Therapeutic challenges in the obese diabetic patient with hypertension. Am J Med 1996; 101:33S–46S.

5

Hyperlipidemia, Diabetes, and the Heart

Henry N. Ginsberg
Columbia University College of Physicians and Surgeons, New York, New York

I. INTRODUCTION

There can be no doubt that patients with diabetes mellitus (DM) are at very high risk of developing and dying from atherosclerotic cardiovascular disease (ASCVD). Numerous prospective cohort studies have indicated that DM is associated with a three- to fourfold increase in risk for coronary artery disease (CHD). The increase in risk is particularly evident in both younger age groups and women. Females with type 2 DM appear to lose most of the protection from ASCVD that characterizes nondiabetic females. When a diabetic patient has a myocardial infarction, in-hospital mortality of patients with DM is 50% greater than that of the general population. Furthermore, diabetics have a twofold increased rate of death within 2 years of surviving a myocardial infarction. Overall, CHD is the leading cause of death in individuals with DM who are over the age of 35 years.

What is the pathophysiological basis for this marked increased in ASCVD-associated morbidity and mortality in the diabetic population? Clearly, a significant portion of this increased risk is associated with the presence of well-characterized risk factors for CHD that can be found in nondiabetics as well. However, a significant proportion remains unexplained. For example, patients with DM, particularly those with type 2 DM, have abnormalities of plasma lipids and lipoprotein concentrations that are less commonly present in nondiabetics. Additionally, patients with poorly controlled type 1 DM can also have a dyslipidemic pattern that is relatively unique compared to nondiabetics. In order

85

to better understand the abnormalities in lipids and lipoproteins commonly seen in patients with DM, and thereby develop optimal therapeutic approaches, we must first review briefly what is known about normal lipid and lipoprotein physiology.

II. LIPOPROTEINS

In the bloodstream, all the cholesterol and triglycerides are carried in spherical macromolecular complexes called lipoproteins. The development of the lipoprotein system, from an evolutionary standpoint, was necessary because the major lipids in our blood, esterified cholesterol (cholesterol linked to a fatty acid) and triglyceride, are insoluble in plasma, which is an aqueous media. By covering the cholesteryl esters and triglyceride with a coating of phospholipid (which are both lipid-soluble and water-soluble molecules) and proteins, the lipoprotein system allows the water-insoluble core lipids to be transported through an aqueous circulatory system. The different lipoproteins have been defined by their physicochemical characteristics, particularly by their flotation characteristics during very high-speed ultracentrifugation. Although lipoprotein particles actually form a continuum, varying in composition, size, density, and function, they have been separated into major groupings related to their overall composition and/or function (Table 1). Hundreds to thousands of triglyceride and cholesteryl ester molecules are carried in the core of different lipoproteins.

As noted above, the surface of the lipoproteins contains phospholipids and proteins, called apolipoproteins. The apolipoproteins not only help to solubilize the core lipids, but also play critical roles in the regulation of plasma lipid and lipoprotein transport. The major apolipoproteins are described in Table 2. Apolipoprotein (apo) B is a key protein on several of the lipoproteins. Apo B100 (so

Table 1 Physicochemical Characteristics of the Major Lipoprotein Classes

Lipoprotein	Density	MW	Diam	Lipid (%)		
				TG	CHOL	PL
Chylomicrons	0.95	400×10^6	75–1200	80–95	2–7	3–9
VLDL	0.95–1.006	$10–80 \times 10^6$	30–80	55–80	5–15	10–20
IDL	1.006–1.019	$5–10 \times 10^6$	25–35	20–50	20–40	15–25
LDL	1.019–1.063	2.3×10^6	18–25	5–15	40–50	20–25
HDL	1.063–1.21	$1.7–3.6 \times 10^6$	5–12	5–10	15–25	20–30

Density: g/dL; MW: daltons; diameter: nm; lipid (%): percent composition of lipids; apolipoproteins make up the rest.

Table 2 Characteristics of the Major Apolipoproteins

Apolipoprotein	MW	Lipoproteins	Metabolic functions
apo A-1	28,016	HDL, chylomicrons	Structural component of HDL; LCAT activator
apo A-II	17,414	HDL, chylomicrons	Unknown
apo A-IV	46,465	HDL, chylomicrons	Unknown; possibly facilitates transfer of apos between HDL and chylomicrons
apo B-48	264,000	chylomicrons	Necessary for assembly and secretion of chylomicrons from the small intestine
apo B-100	514,000	VLDL, IDL, LDL	Necessary for the assembly and secretion of VLDL from the liver; structural protein of VLDL, IDL and LDL; ligand for the LDL receptor
apo C-I	6,630	chylomicrons, VLDL, IDL, HDL	May inhibit hepatic uptake of chylomicrons VLDL remnants
apo C-II	8,900	chylomicrons, VLDL, IDL, HDL	Activator of lipoprotein lipase
apo C-III	8,800	chylomicrons, VLDL, IDL, HDL	Inhibitor of lipoprotein lipase; inhibits hepatic uptake of chylomicron and VLDL remnants
apo E	34,145	chylomicrons, VLDL, IDL, HDL	Ligand for binding of several lipoproteins to the LDL receptor, LRP, and proteoglycans
apo(a)	250,000–800,000	Lp(a)	Composed of LDL apo B linked covalently to apo(a); function unknown, but is an independent predictor of coronary artery disease

named because it is the full-length protein made from the messenger RNA) is synthesized in the liver, as is required for the secretion of liver-derived very-low-density lipoproteins (VLDL), intermediate-density lipoproteins (IDL), and low-density lipoproteins (LDL). Apo B48 is a truncated form of apo B100 (it is made from the first half of the messenger RNA for apo B100) that is made in the small intestine and is required for secretion of chylomicrons after ingestion of a meal. Apo A-I is the major structural protein in high-density lipoproteins (HDL) and plays a key role in reverse cholesterol transport. Other apolipoproteins will be discussed in the context of their roles in lipoprotein metabolism.

III. LIPOPROTEIN METABOLISM

A. Intestinal Lipoproteins and Transport of Dietary Lipids in Diabetes Mellitus

Chylomicrons are assembled in the enterocytes of the small intestine after ingestion of dietary fat (triglyceride) and cholesterol. In the lymph and the blood,
chylomicrons acquire several apolipoproteins, including apo C-II, apo C-III, and
apo E. In the capillary beds of adipose tissue and muscle, chylomicrons interact
with the enzyme lipoprotein lipase (LPL), which is activated by apo C-II, and
the chylomicron core triglyceride is hydrolyzed. The lipolytic products, free fatty
acids, can be taken up by fat cells where they are converted back into triglyceride,
or by muscle cells, where they can be used for energy. Apo C-III can inhibit
lipolysis, and the balance of apo C-II and apo C-III determines, in part, the effi-
ciency with which LPL hydrolyzes chylomicron triglyceride. The product of this
lipolytic process is the chylomicron remnant, which has only about 25% of the
original chylomicron triglyceride remaining. Importantly, the chylomicron remnants are relatively enriched in cholesteryl esters; they have not lost any of the
dietary cholesterol first incorporated into the chylomicron in the enterocyte, and
they have accumulated cholesteryl esters transferred from HDL in the circulation
(see below). The cholesterol-rich chylomicron remnants are also enriched in apo
E and interact with several receptor pathways on hepatocytes that rapidly remove
them from the circulation. Uptake of chylomicron remnants involves binding
to the LDL receptor, the LDL receptor-related protein (LRP), and cell-surface
proteoglycans; apo E appears to play a crucial role in each of these processes.

In patients with diabetes, chylomicron and chylomicron-remnant metabolism can be altered significantly. Thus, in patients with poorly controlled type 1
DM, LPL, which is regulated at both the level of gene transcription and cellular
processing by insulin, can be low, leading to inefficient lipolysis of the chylomicron triglyceride. As a result, postprandial triglyceride levels can be increased
in poorly treated type 1 diabetics. Insulin therapy rapidly reverses this condition
resulting in the clearance of chylomicron triglycerides from plasma. However,
in well-controlled type 1 DM, LPL measured in postheparin plasma (heparin
releases LPL from the surface of endothelial cells where it is usually found), as
well as adipose tissue LPL can be normal or increased, and chylomicron triglyceride clearance can be normal.

Defective metabolism of chylomicrons has also been observed in type 2
DM, although LPL is normal or only slightly reduced in this group. Confounding
a full understanding of postprandial lipemia in patients with type 2 DM is the
underlying insulin resistance and the associated dyslipidemia. Since fasting hypertriglyceridemia is characteristic of patients with type 2 DM, and is correlated
with increased postprandial triglyceride levels, it is difficult to identify a direct
effect of type 2 DM on chylomicron metabolism. For example, chylomicrons

and VLDL compete for the same supply of LPL. If LPL is limited or VLDL secretion from the liver is very high, lipolysis of chylomicron triglyceride is likely to be impaired.

Once the chylomicron has undergone adequate lipolysis, it becomes the chylomicron remnant. As noted above, apo E is thought to play a critical role in the hepatic uptake of chylomicron remnants, and some studies have indicated a role for the apo E2 phenotype in the hyperlipidemia of diabetes. Apo E2 is an allelic form of apo E that is found in about 10% of the population and is defective in binding to the LDL receptor. If a patient with DM has an apo E allele, this might impact negatively on the removal of chylomicron remnants in those patients. On the other hand, apo E2 appears to interact normally with LRP, the alternative receptor for remnants. Another possible reason for decreased remnant removal could be that apo E becomes glycated and that this modification of apo E causes a loss of affinity for either the LDL or the LRP receptors. Finally, hepatic triglyceride lipase (HTGL), which both hydrolyzes chylomicron- and VLDL-remnant triglycerides as well as acting as a bridge for those molecules to bind to the liver cell surface, might be reduced in patients with DM. However, several studies have indicated that HTGL is elevated in hypertriglyceridemic individuals with or without DM.

In summary, several studies have demonstrated increased postprandial lipemia in patients with DM. In untreated type 1 patients, reduced LPL is probably the key component of the problem and the lipemia can be reduced by good glycemic control. In patients with type 2 DM, the underlying fasting dyslipidemia is likely to be the major contributor to the postprandial lipemia, with LPL playing a minor role. Accumulation of atherogenic postprandial remnants is also commonly observed in patients with DM, but the basis for this abnormality is less well understood. Finally, the postprandial lipemia commonly present in type 2 DM may be an important contributor to low HDL cholesterol levels characteristic of patients with this disease (Table 3).

Table 3 Abnormalities in Postprandial Lipid Metabolism

Type of diabetes	Poorly controlled	Well controlled
Type 1	Decreased LPL	Normal or increased LPL
	Increased postprandial triglycerides	Normal postprandial triglycerides
	Impaired remnant removal	Impaired remnant removal
Type 2	Moderately reduced LPL	Normal or slightly reduced LPL
	Increased postprandial triglycerides	Increased postprandial triglycerides
	Impaired remant removal	Impaired remnant removal

B. Hepatic Lipoproteins and Transport of Endogenous Lipids in Diabetes Mellitus

1. Very-Low-Density Lipoproteins

VLDL are assembled in the endoplasmic reticulum of hepatocytes when the core lipids, triglycerides and cholesterol, are the core lipids associate with apo B-100 and phospholipids. Although some apo C-I, apo C-II, apo C-III, and apo E may be present on the nascent VLDL particles as they are secreted from the hepatocyte, the majority of these molecules are probably added to VLDL after their entry into plasma. Recent studies in cultured liver cells indicate that a significant proportion of newly synthesized apo B100 may be degraded before association with lipid and secretion, and that this degradation can be inhibited by higher rates of triglyceride and possibly cholesteryl ester synthesis by the liver. If this occurs in vivo, high free fatty acid flux to the liver that is common in patients with insulin resistance and type 2 DM, and which should stimulate synthesis of triglycerides and cholesteryl esters, may drive high secretion rates of VLDL.

Once in the plasma, VLDL triglyceride is hydrolyzed by LPL (activated by apo C-II and inhibited by apo C-III), generating smaller and denser VLDL remnants, and, subsequently IDL. VLDL remnants and IDL particles are similar to chylomicron remnants but, unlike chylomicron remnants not all IDL are removed by the liver. Thus, in addition to removal by hepatic LDL and possibly LRP receptors, IDL particles can also undergo further catabolism to become LDL. Some LPL activity appears necessary for normal functioning of the metabolic cascade from VLDL to IDL to LDL. It also appears that apo E and HTGL play important roles in the generation of LDL. Apo C-I can inhibit VLDL remnant and IDL removal by the liver. Apo B100 is essentially the sole protein on the surface of LDL, and the lifetime of plasma LDL appears to be determined mainly by the availability of LDL receptors. Approximately 60 to 70% of LDL catabolism from plasma occurs via the LDL receptor pathway. The remaining tissue uptake is by nonreceptor or alternative receptor pathways, such as pathways that recognize glycosylated and/or oxidatively modified lipoproteins. Of note, these modified lipoproteins can be present in increased amounts in the blood of patients with DM.

Hypertriglyceridemia, with increased VLDL levels, is a characteristic lipid abnormality in patients with type 2 DM. In type 1 DM, triglyceride levels correlated closely with glycemic control, and marked hypertriglyceridemia can be found in ketotic diabetics with severe insulin deficiency. In these cases, decreased LPL activity is usually the basis for the severe lipemia, which is composed of both VLDL and chylomicrons. On the other hand, the basis for increased VLDL levels in poorly controlled but nonketotic type 1 DM subjects is usually overproduction of these lipoproteins. When patients with type 1 DM are very tightly controlled in terms of glycemia and receive multiple doses of insulin daily, plasma triglycerides can actually be "low normal," and lower than average production rates of VLDL have been observed in such instances.

In patients with type 2 DM, overproduction of VLDL, with increased secretion of both triglyceride and apo B100, seems to be the common etiology of increased plasma VLDL levels. Increased assembly and secretion of VLDL are probably a direct result of the insulin resistance and increased free fatty acid flux characteristic of type 2 DM. Although LPL levels have been reported to be reduced in some type 2 diabetic patients, that is probably only a significant contributor in the minority of cases. Because obesity and insulin resistance are common in type 2 DM, full delineation of the pathophysiology underlying the hypertriglyceridemia has been difficult. The complex interaction between the determinants also makes therapy less effective (see below). For example, in contrast to type 1 DM, where intensive insulin therapy normalizes (or even "supernormalizes") VLDL levels and metabolism, therapy of type 2 DM with either insulin or oral agents only partly corrects VLDL abnormalities in the majority of patients.

2. Low-Density Lipoproteins

In general, LDL cholesterol levels and LDL metabolism are usually normal in patients with DM. Indeed, intensive insulin treatment has been found to cause LDL production rates to fall concomitant with reduced VLDL production. However, LDL receptor gene expression is regulated, at least in part, by insulin, and severe insulin deficiency may lead to reduced catabolism of LDL. In poorly controlled patients, glycosylated LDL can increase, and reduced catabolism of LDL via the LDL receptor pathway has been observed in some, but not all, in vitro studies using diabetic LDL and cultured fibroblasts. Heavily glycosylated LDL is removed more slowly than normal LDL in humans.

Regulation of plasma levels of LDL in patients with type 2 DM, like that of its precursor VLDL, is complex. When hypertriglyceridemia is present, dense, triglyceride-enriched and cholesteryl ester LDL are present. This is the result of an exchange of triglyceride for cholesteryl ester between VLDL (or chylomicrons) and LDL; the exchange is mediated by a protein called cholesteryl ester transfer protein (CETP). Thus individuals with type 2 DM and mild-to-moderate hypertriglyceridemia may have the pattern B profile of LDL described by Austin and Krauss. Overproduction of LDL apo B100 has been demonstrated in type 2 DM patients, particularly if there is concomitant elevation of VLDL.

Fractional removal of LDL, mainly via LDL receptor pathways, can be increased, normal, or reduced in type 2 DM. Increased LDL fractional catabolism is often seen in nondiabetics with significant hypertriglyceridemia, and the same abnormality probably exists in type 2 DM patients. As noted above, insulin is needed for normal LDL receptor gene expression, and reduced LDL fractional removal from plasma has been observed in more severe patients with type 2 DM.

Glycosylation of LDL can also occur in type 2 DM patients, and these multiple potential impacts on LDL metabolism make it difficult to predict what level of LDL will be present in any individual with type 2 DM; overall, LDL elevations are not more commonly present in people with type 2 DM than they are in nondiabetics. Of note, women with type 2 DM seem to have higher LDL cholesterol levels than nondiabetic women, while diabetic and nondiabetic men have similar plasma concentrations of LDL cholesterol. This may be one reason why DM affects the risk for ASCVD to a greater degree in women than in men.

In summary, type 1 DM may be associated with elevations of VLDL triglyceride and LDL cholesterol if diabetic control is very poor or if the patient is actually ketotic. In contrast, type 2 DM is usually associated with lipid abnormalities, most common of which is a combination of high triglycerides, increased numbers of cholesteryl-enriched remnants, and reduced HDL cholesterol levels (see below). This combination of abnormalities is called the dyslipidemia of insulin resistance/diabetic. Despite a focus on the latter abnormalities, and although LDL concentrations are either unchanged or slightly higher in patients with DM, studies indicate that glycosylated LDL can be taken up by macrophage scavenger receptors and contribute to foam cell formation. Furthermore, other studies indicate that LDL from patients with diabetes, particularly small, dense LDL, may be more susceptible to oxidative modification and catabolism via macrophage-scavenger receptors. Thus, the health care team needs to focus on the entire lipid profile of the patient with DM, considering the various atherogenic components in toto, and choosing therapeutic goals consistent with the risk of the patient and the clinical trial evidence indicating that risk can be reduced.

C. High-Density Lipoproteins and Reverse Cholesterol Transport in Diabetes Mellitus

Of all the lipoproteins, the regulation of HDL levels may be the most complex. HDL is the most heterogeneous lipoprotein class, with many subclasses varying in size, density, lipid composition, and apolipoprotein components. To make matters more confusing, several methods have been used to isolate these subclasses and so several overlap in terms of structure and/or function. The majority of HDL are formed by the apparent coalescence of individual phospholipid-apolipoprotein disks containing apo A-I, apo A-II, apo A-VI, and possibly apo E. The exact mechanisms regulating these "mergers" are not known, although two plasma proteins, lecithin cholesterol acyltransferase (LCAT) and CETP are clearly involved. The small intestine does secrete some spherical HDL directly.

Nascent HDL was usually classified as HDL_3 and was considered to be the main acceptor of cell membrane-free cholesterol. Recent studies have identified even more primitive HDL forms called pre-beta and pre-alpha HDL. These disk-like HDLs, consisting of apo A-I and phospholipid, appear to be the best acceptors of membrane free cholesterol and are considered to be the initial HDL particles involved in reverse cholesterol transport (RCT). Very recent and exciting findings suggest that a cell protein called ABC1 is required for efficient transfer of cellular free cholesterol to the primitive HDL apo A-I disks. It is likely that all of these HDL subtypes can initiate RCT, which is thought to be the way we collect cholesterol that is accumulating all over our bodies (including, potentially, the artery wall) and send it to the liver for excretion as biliary cholesterol or bile acids. When LCAT generates cholesteryl ester from the free cholesterol acquired, the apo A-I disks are converted to spherical lipoproteins and can continue to accept free cholesterol. After adequate free cholesterol conversion to cholesteryl ester, HDL_3 become HDL_2. It appears that HDL_2 can deliver cholesteryl ester to the liver via a process called selective uptake (the cholesteryl ester enters the cells without uptake of the entire particle) or transfer cholesteryl esters to triglyceride-rich lipoproteins. The selective uptake of cholesteryl esters from HDL to several organs, including the liver, was demonstrated to be the result of HDL interaction with a receptor called scavenger receptor B-1 (SRB-1). It is not known if either ABC1 or SRB-1 are affected by diabetes, but their discovery has accelerated the pace of research focused on the role of HDL in protection from ASCVD and CHD.

CETP-mediated transfer of cholesteryl ester from HDL to triglyceride-rich lipoproteins appears to be another major pathway for movement of cholesteryl ester out of HDL_2. The cholesteryl esters can then be taken up by the liver, or other peripheral tissues, as chylomicron remnants, VLDL remnants, or IDL, and finally LDL are removed from plasma. If hepatic uptake of apo B lipoproteins is rapid and efficient, then CETP-mediated movement of cholesteryl esters from HDL to VLDL and chylomicrons may be antiatherogenic, serving as a parallel or alternative system to that centered upon HDL and SRB1. On the other hand, if the apo B lipoproteins, after having become cholesteryl-ester enriched, are not efficiently removed by the liver, they have the potential of delivering themselves (and their cholesteryl esters) back to peripheral tissues, including the artery wall.

Patients with type 1 DM usually have normal HDL cholesterol levels, and studies of the relationship between HDL cholesterol levels and degree of glycemic control in these patients have been inconsistent. HDL levels may actually be increased in individuals receiving intensive insulin therapy, and this may be linked to increased LPL activity and/or reduced HTGL activity. There do not appear to be differences in apo A-I metabolism between patients with type 1 DM and nondiabetics matched for a wide range of HDL cholesterol concentrations.

In patients with type 2 DM, the lower levels of plasma HDL cholesterol do not seem to be related to control or mode of treatment in patients with type 2 DM. However, as it was for the apo B lipoproteins, our understanding of the metabolism of HDL in type 2 DM is complicated by the common presence of obesity and insulin resistance–associated dyslipidemia in this group. An inverse relationship between plasma insulin (or C-peptide), measures of insulin resistance, and HDL cholesterol levels has been identified consistently. Fractional catabolism of apo A-I is increased in type 2 DM with low HDL, but that is no different from what is seen in nondiabetics with similar lipoprotein profiles. While Apo A-I levels are reduced consistently, correction of hypertriglyceridemia does not usually alter apo A-I levels.

In summary, HDL levels are normal or even elevated in tightly controlled, well-insulinized patients with type 1 DM, whereas low HDL cholesterol concentrations are a hallmark of type 2 DM. The latter abnormality has several defined components, including increased fractional removal of apo A-I from plasma and increased CETP-mediated transfer of HDL cholesteryl esters to apo B lipoproteins. Defective apo A-I lipoprotein-mediated efflux of cellular free cholesterol (possibly related to defects in ABC1), defective LCAT activity, increased selective delivery of HDL_2 cholesteryl ester to hepatocytes via SRB1 (although this might be antiatherogenic), and possible effects of glycosylation of HDL apo C-II, apo C-III, and apo E are other potential key players (Table 4).

Table 4 Abnormalities in Fasting Lipid Metabolism

Type of diabetes	Poorly controlled	Well controlled
Type 1	Increased VLDL secretion	Normal or low VLDL secretion
	Decreased LPL	Normal or increased LPL
	Increased fasting triglycerides	Normal of low fasting triglycerides
	Decreased remnant removal	Normal remnant removal
	Decreased LDL receptors	Normal LDL receptors
	High glycosylated LDL	Minimal glycosylated LDL
	Increased LDL cholesterol	Normal or low LDL cholesterol
	Lower HDL cholesterol	Normal or high HDL cholesterol
Type 2	Increased VLDL secretion	Increased VLDL secretion
	Moderately decreased LPL	Normal or slightly low LPL
	Increased fasting triglycerides	Increased fasting triglycerides
	Variable remnant removal	Variable remnant removal
	Normal LDL receptors	Normal LDL receptors
	Higher glycosylated LDL	Minimal glycosylated LDL
	Variable LDL cholesterol	Variable LDL cholesterol
	Low HDL cholesterol	Low HDL cholesterol
	Low apoA-I	Low apoA-I

IV. TREATMENT OF DIABETIC DYSLIPIDEMIA

A. Nonpharmacological Therapy

Weight loss, diet, and exercise are the mainstays of therapy for the treatment of diabetes. The presence of dyslipidemia increases the rationale for intensive diet intervention. Importantly, improvements in plasma lipids can be observed even in the absence of weight loss. Reductions in dietary saturated fat and cholesterol intake can improve the lipid profile even if caloric intake is unchanged.

Weight cannot only improve glycemic control and insulin sensitivity, but can positively affect lipoprotein patterns as well. Numerous studies have demonstrated that when weight reduction is achieved and maintained in type 2 DM patients, there is a sustained decrease in triglyceride levels. Most, but not all, studies show an increase in HDL cholesterol, as well as an improvement in the ratio of total to HDL cholesterol in type 2 DM patients who lose weight.

There is some controversy concerning the optimal weight loss diet in diabetics. The need for significant reductions in total calories implies that there must be a restriction in all nutrients (i.e., fat, carbohydrate, and protein). Since fats are more calories per gram than carbohydrates or proteins, a high-carbohydrate (high soluble fiber) low-fat diet would be a sound first approach. However, if this approach proved deleterious, with development of poor glycemic control and higher blood levels of triglycerides, a diet higher in fat (but low in saturated fats) can then be attempted. A sustained, gradual weight loss is widely accepted as the best way to prevent loss of muscle mass and precipitation of gallstones. Very-low-calorie diets of about 600 kcal/day may be a reasonable short-term approach in patients who are morbidly obese and/or severely hypertriglyceridemic.

From the mid-1970s until recently, the ADA recommendations were essentially in agreement with those of the American Heart Association (AHA). The Step 1 AHA diet indicates that up to 55 to 60% of total daily energy should be in the form of carbohydrates (mostly complex, high-fiber carbohydrates); no more than 30% in the form of fat; and no more than 10% in the form of saturated fat. The remainder of the energy from fat should be derived from monounsaturated and polyunsaturated fats. Less than 300 mg of cholesterol should be taken in on a daily basis, while protein consumption should account for 10 to 15% of calories.

During the past decade, some investigators have advocated higher fat and lower carbohydrate diets for patients with DM, particularly the type 2 DM with dyslipidemia. The basis for this shift is evidence from small clinical studies and from epidemiological studies. In the clinical studies, higher carbohydrate diets were found to be associated with higher triglycerides; in the epidemiological studies, higher fat diets (low in saturated fats) were associated with lower rates of ASCVD. On the other hand, there is no evidence that low-fat diets cause deterioration of diabetic control in patients with type 1 DM. Additionally, there are other studies demonstrating that diets high in carbohydrates can improve diabetic control and glucose tolerance in patients with type 2 DM. Importantly, inclusion of large quantities of soluble fiber in the high-carbohydrate diet abrogates many of the potential adverse effects of increased carbohydrate on diabetic control and dyslipidemia. Not all patients with type 2 DM may benefit by increased dietary fiber, and there are certainly those patients who may not be able to tolerate high-fiber diets, especially if they have gastroparesis.

Based on all of the above information, the ADA modified its dietary recommendations recently by focusing on reductions of dietary saturated fat and cholesterol, and allowing for individualization of diet in terms of the optimal replacement for saturated fat. Fiber is stressed as an important component of carbohydrate-containing foods. At the present time, it seems reasonable to recommend the diet approved by both the ADA and the AHA as a first approach for all diabetics regardless of their plasma lipid concentrations. If an adverse response to the recommended diet occurs, such as worsening diabetic control or hypertriglyceridemia, a diet higher in monounsaturated fat (or polyunsaturated fat) could then be substituted. A cautionary note relevant to the use of high monounsaturated fat diet: fat has more than twice the caloric density of carbohydrates (9 kcal/g vs. 4 kcal/g). The use of high-fat diets may, therefore, predispose to weight gain.

B. Exercise

Exercise is an excellent approach to improving cardiovascular fitness. However, exercise alone, without concomitant weight loss, did not improve either the abnormal response to an oral glucose load or insulin sensitivity in obese glucose-intolerant subjects. In additional, exercise alone without weight loss was ineffective in improving lipid profiles in type 2 diabetics. Of course, exercise is almost obligatory if one is to maintain weight loss achieved through caloric restriction.

C. Glycemic Control: Effects on Lipids

Treatment of type 2 DM with hypoglycemic agents has a variable, drug-dependent, effect on plasma lipid levels (Table 5). Sulfonylureas have little or no effects on plasma lipids. Insulin treatment can be associated with lower triglycerides, probably as the result of better glycemic control. Recent additions to the therapeutic choices available for type 2 DM, metformin and the thiazolidinediones, can lower plasma triglyceride concentrations 5 to 15% and 5 to 25%, respectively. In particular, the thiazolidinediones, which improve peripheral insulin sensitivity, possibly lower triglycerides by causing plasma levels of free fatty acids. Insulin treatment tends to lower LDL, while sulfonylurea therapy has little or no effect. Metformin has been observed to reduce LDL 5 to 10%, while thiazolidinediones

Table 5 Effects of Hypoglycemic Agents on Plasma Lipids and Lipoproteins

Agent	Effects on triglycerides	Effects on LDL cholesterol	Effects on HDL cholesterol
Insulin	If patient in poor glycemic control: ↓ 10–15%	If patient in poor glycemic control: ↓ 5–10%	If patient in poor glycemic control: ↑ 10–15%
Sulfonylurea	Little or no effect unless patient in poor glycemic control ↓ 10–15%	Little or no effect	Little or no effect
Metformin	↓ 5–15%	Little or no effect	Little or no effect (↑ < 5%)
TZDs[a]	↓ 5–25%; possible variability by specific agent	↑ 5–15%; possible variability by specific agent	↑ 10–15%

[a] TZDs = thiazolidinediones.

usually raise LDL cholesterol by a similar degree. The metabolic basis for these latter changes has not been fully defined.

Although control of hyperglycemia does not correlate well with HDL cholesterol levels in patients with type 2 DM, intensive insulin therapy has been shown to increase total HDL and HDL_2 levels in some, but not all, studies of patients with type 1 DM. Therapy with sulfonylureas does not seem to increase HDL cholesterol concentrations. On the other hand, modest increases in HDL levels, concomitant with modest decreases in triglyceride concentrations, have been observed with metformin therapy. More recently, the thiazoladinediones have been shown to moderately raise HDL cholesterol levels in patients with type 2 DM.

D. Lipid-Lowering Drugs

1. Introduction

Drug therapy should be initiated for the treatment of dyslipidemia only after an adequate trial of diabetic control, diet, weight loss, and exercise (Table 6). The initial presentation of the patient, the severity of the dyslipidemia, and the presence of other risk factors for CHD or CHD itself determine how long nonpharmacological approaches should be tried. It is clear that lipid-lowering agents will be less efficacious, or actually ineffective, if these related factors are not optimally approached first. On the other hand, severely dyslipidemic patients, and those

Table 6 Effects of Lipid-Altering Drugs

Drug	Triglycerides	LDL cholesterol	HDL cholesterol
Statins	Depending on patient initial triglyceride and degree of LDL lowering: triglycerides ↓ 10–30%	Depending on which statin used and dose: ↓ 20–55%	In general: ↑ 5–10%
Fibrates	↓ 25–45%	Variable depending on patient initial LDL level and degree of triglyceride lowering: ↑ 10–30%, no change, or ↓ 10–20%	Depending on patient initial triglyceride level and degree of triglyceride drop; ↑ 10–25%
Niacin	↓ 20–35%	↓ 10–20%	↑ 10–20%
Resins	↑ 0–20% (may be higher if initial triglyceride >300 mg/dL)	↓ 15–25%	Variable; ↑ 0–5%
Estrogen[a]	↑ 10–20% (may be higher if initial triglyceride >300 mg/dL)	↓ 10–20%	↑ 10–20%

[a] The effects of estrogen therapy may be modulated by the addition of progestins, some of which may reduce the effect of estrogen on HDL cholesterol.

who have very high risk for development of CHD, require earlier initiation of pharmacotherapy. If the patient already has clinically significant CHD or other vascular disease, then drug treatment may be indicated concomitant with other interventions. Furthermore, the severity of the dyslipidemia, independent of glycemic control, is an indicator of the presence of genetic causes of the dyslipidemia that are independent of the DM. This can also be taken into account when considering initiation of specific lipid-lowering therapy. Health professionals cannot wait: the length of time taken in an attempt to have the patient make these lifestyle changes should depend on "forever" to control the plasma glucose or achieve weight loss before moving on to specific lipid-altering treatment.

2. HMG-CoA Reductase Inhibitors

The treatment of hypercholesterolemia has undergone a revolution during the past 12 years with the availability of potent, safe HMG-CoA reductase inhibitors, also known as statins. Lovastatin, pravastatin, fluvastatin, simvastatin, atorva-statin, and cerivastatin are available drugs in this category in the United States. They inhibit HMG-CoA reductase, the rate-limiting enzyme in cholesterol syn-thesis. This results in both decreased hepatic production of apo B-containing lipoproteins and upregulation of LDL receptors. The combination of these effects, fewer apoprotein B lipoproteins entering the blood stream, and more efficient removal of those lipoproteins back into the liver have the overall effect of dramat-ically lowering plasma levels of LDL cholesterol. VLDL triglyceride concentra-tions are also reduced in many subjects with moderate hypertriglyceridemia. Tri-glyceride reductions are directly related to both the initial triglyceride level and the reduction of LDL cholesterol achieved. The most potent statins (simvastatin and atorvastatin), at the highest doses, can lower LDL cholesterol by up to 45 to 55%, and decrease triglycerides 20 to 45%. Reductase inhibitors can raise HDL cholesterol by up to 10%, but should not be considered as first-line agents in individuals with very low HDL levels.

The statins are very safe and effective medications. The main side effect associated with statin therapy is a myositis, characterized by diffuse, severe mus-cle tenderness and weakness, and elevated levels of CPK (usually greater than 10 times the upper limit of normal). In severe cases, rhabdomyolysis and concom-itant myoglobinemia can place patients at risk for renal failure due to myoglobin-uria. This is particularly a risk in diabetics who have preexisting proteinurea. However, the incidence of myositis when statins are used as monotherapy is only about 1 in 500 patients. If the patient receives careful instructions about the signs and symptoms, with advice to stop the medication and consume large volumes of liquids, serious outcomes should be avoidable. Statins can also cause non-clinically significant elevations in liver function tests in 1 to 2% of patients, and only at the higher doses of each agent. The statins do not appear to have any effects on diabetic control. Most importantly, results from several clinical trials have demonstrated reductions in CHD events and deaths in type 2 diabetic pa-tients treated with statins. Therefore, the statins are the first-line therapeutic agents for diabetic patients with isolated high levels of LDL cholesterol, with combined hyperlipidemia, or with moderate hypertriglyceridemia and an LDL cholesterol level above NCEP goal. Statins can also be used in conjunction with other hypolipidemic agents under some circumstances.

3. Fibric Acid Derivatives

This class of agents has a proven track record for lowering plasma triglycerides and raising HDL cholesterol levels. The fibrates are, therefore, important drugs in the treatment of diabetic dyslipidemia. Fenofibrate and gemfibrozil are the agents presently available in the United States. The use of fibrates in patients with type 2 DM results in lowering of triglyceride from 35 to 45% and increases in HDL cholesterol from 10 to 20%. These agents appear to work by both decreasing hepatic VLDL production, as well as increasing the activity of LPL. Unfortunately, fibrates have modest and variable effects on LDL cholesterol in most patients with DM. Indeed, they may even raise LDL levels in patients with hypertriglyceridemia; this increase is often from a very low level, however. The usual dose is 600 mg twice daily of gemfibrozil, and 200 mg once-daily for micronized fenofibrate. These agents are contraindicated in patients with gallstones and, because they are tightly bound to plasma proteins, levels of other drugs (e.g. coumadin) should be monitored carefully. Fibrates do not significantly affect glycemic control.

Although fibrate treatment may be associated with a rise in LDL cholesterol concentrations, clinical trials of fibrate therapy that included patients with DM have shown their efficacy in preventing CHD events. In the Helsinki Heart Study, the two groups with hypertriglyceridemia (with and without concomitant elevations in LDL cholesterol) had increases or no changes in LDL cholesterol levels during gemfibrozil therapy and yet achieved the same reduction in CHD events as did the group with isolated LDL elevations in whom LDL cholesterol levels fell 10 to 12% with treatment. In the Veterans Administration HDL Intervention Trial, gemfibrozil was efficacious in a group of men who had CHD and an LDL cholesterol that was low (111 mg/dL) at baseline and did not change during the trial. In both of these trials, gemfibrozil treatment was associated with modest increases in HDL cholesterol and approximately 25% decreases in triglyceride levels.

Compared to fibrates, statin therapy of patients with type 2 DM produces much greater reductions in LDL. On the other hand, fibrate treatment results in greater reductions in triglycerides and increases in HDL. When type 2 DM patients have been treated with the combination of statin and fibrate, there have been powerful, positive effects on the entire dyslipidemic pattern. In view of the very high risk for CHD in patients with type 2 DM, and the characteristic dyslipidemia that they have, combination therapy may be necessary in a significant proportion of patients. Of note, the combination of statins and fibrates increases the risk of myositis to about 1 to 2%.

4. Nicotinic Acid (Niacin)

As noted above in detail, the most common lipid abnormalities present in patients with DM are elevated triglycerides and low HDL cholesterol levels. Importantly, however, LDL cholesterol levels are increased above ideal levels in these high-risk patients and so an agent that affected all three lipid classes would be highly effective. The availability of such a drug might reduce the need for combination therapy with statins and fibrates. Niacin (1–3 g/day) has the ability to potently lower triglycerides (25–40%) and raise HDL cholesterol (10–25%). Niacin also lowers LDL cholesterol (15–20%) and this adds to its potential efficacy in a high-risk population. Niacin has several side effects, however, that limit its utility in nondiabetics. Although usually harmless, niacin produces a prostaglandin-mediated vasodilatation that in turn causes flushing and pruritus. These can occur about 30 min after ingestion and can last as long as 1 h; patients turn red and feel hot. Niacin can cause gastric irritation and exacerbate peptic ulcer disease. Its use has also been associated with hyperuricemia and gout. Of potential importance, niacin causes an elevation of hepatic transaminases in about 5% of patients. Rarely, niacin can also cause a clinically significant hepatitis. Of particular relevance to patients with type 2 DM, some studies have demonstrated that niacin therapy worsens diabetic control, likely by inducing insulin resistance. Not all investigators believe that niacin is contraindicated in patients with diabetes and the recent publication of the ADMIT study indicated that, with modifications of hypoglycemic therapy, regular niacin can be used effectively in patients with type 2 DM. In addition, the availability of an intermediate-release form of niacin (Niaspan) has rekindled interest in its potential in this population.

5. Bile Acid Binding Resins

Bile acid binding resins, which interrupt the enterohepatic recirculation of those molecules within the small intestine, can lead to increased conversion of liver cholesterol to bile acids. As a secondary outcome, hepatic LDL receptors increase and LDL cholesterol levels in blood fall. Three bile acid sequestering agents are now available. The original two drugs, cholestyramine and colestipol have proven records for safety and efficacy. Usual doses are 8 to 24 g/day for cholestyramine and 10 to 30 g/day for colestipol. Colestipol is also available in 1-g tablets. Colesevalem is a much more potent sequestrant that has recently become available. It is used at a dose of 3.6 g/day. Bile acid binding resins are not absorbed and, therefore, have no systemic toxicities. A drawback to the use of older bile acid binding resins in diabetics is the increase in hepatic VLDL triglyceride production and plasma triglyceride levels commonly associated with their use; this may not be as common with colesevalem. Additional major side effects of these agents include bloating and constipation, which may pose a significant problem in the diabetic with gastroparesis, and interference with the absorption of other oral medications. These also may not be as much of a problem with colesevalem. Bile acid resins are typically used as adjuncts to statins (or when patients cannot take statins) in diabetics with pure elevations of total and LDL cholesterol.

6. Hormone Replacement Therapy

In prospective observational studies of mostly nondiabetic women, estrogen replacement therapy has been associated with a 44% decrease in risk for CHD. About 30% of the beneficial effects of hormones in these studies have been estimated to be caused by changes in lipid levels, specifically LDL cholesterol-lowering and HDL cholesterol-elevating effects. Another potential benefit relates to the ability of estrogen to lower Lp(a) levels about 20%. A potentially negative effect of estrogen administration is the increase in plasma triglycerides that occurs via increased hepatic secretion of VLDL. Severe hyperlipidemia and pancreatitis have been observed in women with preexisting hypertriglyceridemia who were receiving oral estrogen treatment.

There were no published studies on the effects of hormone replacement therapy in women with diabetes mellitus prior to 2 years ago. Early oral contraceptives containing relatively large amounts of estrogen were associated with worsened glucose tolerance and increased risk of myocardial infarction and stroke. In additional, as noted above, estrogen is known to increase triglyceride levels and diabetic women often have hypertriglyceridemia. Recent studies in the past 2 years have demonstrated that estrogen replacement therapy in women with type 2 DM for periods of 6 to 12 weeks lowered blood glucose levels and glycosylated hemoglobin levels without causing insulin resistance. Furthermore, estrogen treatment lowered LDL and raised HDL cholesterol levels, and did not significantly affect plasma triglycerides.

The efficacy of estrogen replacement therapy has been called into question by the results of the HERS study. That placebo-controlled trial showed no benefit in women with prior myocardial infarction who received combined equine conjugated estrogens (Premarin) plus continuous low-dose medroxyprogesterone (Provera). These surprising results may derive from the use of medroxyprogesterone, a synthetic progestin that can lower HDL cholesterol and is less protective against vasospasm compared to natural molecules such as micronized progesterone. Micronized progesterone has recently become commercially available (Prometrium) and cyclic micronized progesterone with continuous conjugated estrogen may be an optimal form of hormone replacement therapy. Further studies, particularly in postmenopausal women without prior CHD events, are needed.

V. SUMMARY

The diabetic patient with hyperlipidemia can be treated with both lifestyle interventions and pharmacotherapy. A variety of options are available to improve plasma lipids and thus reduce risk of CHD.

The physician has effective and safe lipid-altering agents from which to choose. The typical patient with type 2 DM has an LDL cholesterol of 130 to 150 mg/dL, a triglyceride of 175 to 250 mg/dL, and an HDL cholesterol of less than 40 mg/dL for a man or less than 45 mg/dL for a woman. If maximal nonpharmacological therapy fails to cause significant improvement, this patient will benefit from initiation of statin therapy. For the diabetic patient with isolated hypertriglyceridemia and low HDL cholesterol (with LDL cholesterol <120 mg/dL), fibric acid derivatives appear to be the first choice in most cases. In many cases, this will be all that is necessary. If LDL cholesterol rises during fibrate therapy and requires treatment, there are several alternatives. First, a bile acid binding resin could be added to the fibrate: this would lower LDL cholesterol without significantly affecting triglyceride levels. The second alternative would be to either switch to an HMG-CoA reductase inhibitor: this would be the logical choice if the triglyceride elevation (before or during fibrate treatment) was only moderate (less than 250 mg/dL). The third choice would be to add the reductase inhibitor to the fibrate. The latter combination is very effective in correcting severe combined hyperlipidemia, but carries an increased risk of myositis. This combination can be used successfully, particularly if the patient knows clearly the symptoms of myositis. The final choice, nicotinic acid, could be used in patients with severe, combined hyperlipidemia. Although recent studies suggest better efficacy and safety than previously believed, the use of niacin should be limited to specialists, and may best be reserved for those diabetics already on insulin with significant combined hyperlipidemia.

In those patients who present with elevations of both LDL cholesterol and plasma triglycerides, an HMG-CoA reductase inhibitor is probably the most effective single agent. Again, niacin could also be used as a sole drug, with caution taken as described above. A fibric acid derivative can be added if triglycerides are not sufficiently reduced by either of those drugs alone. Alternatively, fibrates could be used initially with bile acid binding resins.

Therapy for the diabetic patient with an isolated reduction in HDL cholesterol, where LDL cholesterol is below the guidelines for drug therapy (<130 mg/dL) and triglycerides are less than 150 to 200 mg/dL, is not clearly defined. Fibrates have not been demonstrated to be very effective in raising HDL cholesterol levels in nondiabetics with isolated reductions in HDL, although no similar studies have been carried out in diabetics. Niacin may be more effective in elevating HDL cholesterol concentrations when they are low in the absence of hypertriglyceridemia, but all of the caveats of niacin use in diabetes mellitus would apply here as well. An alternative to raising HDL in these subjects would be to treat more aggressively LDL cholesterol levels, with the goal of reducing them to <100 mg/dL. It must be clear, however, that there are no endpoint trials supporting any approach to isolated reductions in HDL cholesterol either in nondiabetics or diabetics.

SUGGESTED READING

1. Haffner SM. Management of dyslipidemia in adults with diabetes (technical review). Diabetes Care 1998; 21:160–178.

2. Ginsberg HN. Lipoprotein physiology in nondiabetic and diabetic states: relationship to atherogenesis. Diabetes Care 1991; 14:839–855.

3. American Diabetes Association. Management of dyslipidemia in adults with diabetes (position statement). Diabetes Care 1999; 22:S56–S59.

4. National Cholesterol Education Program. Second report of the expert panel on detection, evaluation, and treatment of high blood cholesterol in adults. Circulation 1994; 89:1333–1445.

5. Ginsberg HN. Effects of statins on triglyceride metabolism. Am J Cardiol 1998; 81(4A):32B–35B.

6. Pyorala K, Pedersen TR, Kjekshus J, Faegerman O, Olsson AG, Thorgeirsson G. Cholesterol lowering with simvastatin improves prognosis of diabetic patients with coronary artery disease. A subgroup analysis of the Scandanavian Simvastatin Survival Study. Diabetes Care 1997; 20:614–620.

7. Goldberg RB, Mellies MJ, Sacks FM, et al. Cardiovascular events and their reduction with pravastatin in diabetic and glucose intolerant myocardial infarction survivors with average cholesterol levels: subgroup analysis in the cholesterol and recurrent events (CARE) trial. Circulation 1998; 98:2513–2519.

9. Tikkanen MJ, Laakso M, Ilmonen M, et al. Treatment of hypercholesterolemia and combined hyperlipidemia with simvastatin and gemfibrozil in patients with NIDDM. A multicenter comparison study. Diabetes Care 1998; 21:477–481.

10. Hulley S, Grady D, Bush T, et al. Randomized trial of estrogen plus progestin for secondary prevention of coronary heart disease in postmenopausal women. Heart and Estrogen/progestin Replacement Study Research Group. JAMA 1998; 280:605–613.

11. Andersson B, Mattsson L-A, Hahn L, et al. Estrogen replacement therapy decreases hyerpandrogenicity and improves glucose homeostasis and plasma lipids in postmenopausal women with noninsulin-dependent diabetes mellitus. J Clin Endocrinol Metab 1997; 82:638–643.

12. Brussaard HE, Gevers Leuven JA, Kluft C, et al. Effect of 17beta-estradiol on plasma lipids and LDL oxidation in postmenopausal women with type II diabetes mellitus. Arterioscler Thromb Vasc Biol 1997; 17:324–330.

13. Ginsberg HN, Plutzky J, Sobel BE. A review of metabolic and cardiovascular effects of oral antidiabetic agents: Beyond glucose lowering. J Cardiovasc Risk 1999; 6:337–347.

14. Trigatti B, Rigotti A, Krieger M. The role of the high-density lipoprotein receptor SR-BI in cholesterol metabolism. Curr Opin Lipidol 2000; 11:123–131.

15. Howard BV. Diabetes and plasma lipoproteins in Native Americans. Studies of the Pima Indians. Diabetes Care 1993; 16:284–291.

16. Tuck CH, Holleran S, Berglund L. Hormonal regulation of lipoprotein(a) levels: effects of estrogen replacement therapy on lipoprotein(a) and acute phase reactants in postmenopausal women. Arterioscler Thromb Vasc Biol 1997; 17:1822–1829.

6

The Coagulation and Fibrinolytic Systems, Diabetes, and the Heart: Therapeutic Implications for Patients with Type 2 Diabetes

David J. Schneider and Burton E. Sobel
University of Vermont, Burlington, Vermont

An understanding of the propensity for patients with diabetes to sustain acute coronary syndromes is potentiated by consideration of the roles of thrombosis, platelet activation, and fibrinolysis in their genesis and derangements in all three systems associated with diabetes. In this selective review, we shall highlight several recent observations and concepts pertinent to clinical practice and particularly to medical management of patients with diabetes. We hope the information presented will be useful in selecting and implementing specific therapeutic approaches likely to reduce the risk of acute coronary events in patients with type 2 diabetes.

I. THROMBOSIS, ATHEROSCLEROSIS, AND ACUTE CORONARY SYNDROMES

Thrombosis appears to be a major contributor to atherogenesis. Early in the evolution of atherosclerosis, microthrombi present on the luminal surface of vessels can potentiate progression of atherosclerosis by exposing the vessel wall to clot-associated mitogens. In later stages, mural thrombi are associated with gradual growth of atherosclerotic plaques and explosive consequences of plaque rupture including coronary occlusion responsible for acute coronary syndromes.

The classical view that acute coronary syndromes are attributable to high-grade occlusive, stenotic coronary lesions comprising final steps in a continuum that begins with fatty streaks and culminates in high-grade stenosis has been modified. Thrombotic occlusion is, in fact, frequently the result of thrombus induced by rupture of vulnerable plaques that were themselves not highly obstructive. Thus, as many as two-thirds of lesions responsible for acute coronary syndromes are minimally obstructive (less than 50% stenotic) immediately before plaque rupture. Conversely, asymptomatic disruption of lipid-rich plaques associated with limited, nonocclusive thrombosis appears to be responsible for intermittent, often clinically silent, plaque growth.

Thrombi can contribute to plaque growth by direct incorporation. Exposure of vessel wall constituents to clot-associated mitogens and cytokines can accelerate neointimalization and proliferation of vascular smooth muscle cells. Mural accumulation of fibrin and fibrin degradation products promotes the migration of vascular smooth muscle cells and monocytes into the neointima. Thrombin itself and growth factors released from platelet alpha granules such as platelet-derived growth factor and transforming growth factor beta activate smooth muscle cells potentiating their migration and proliferation.

The extent of thrombosis in response to plaque rupture depends upon factors potentiating thrombosis (prothrombotic factors), platelet reactivity, factors limiting thrombosis (antithrombotic factors), and the local capacity of the fibrinolytic system reflecting a balance between activity of plasminogen activators and their primary physiological inhibitor, plasminogen activator inhibitor type 2. Activity of plasminogen activators leads to the generation of plasmin, an active serine proteinase, from plasminogen, an enzymatically inert circulating zymogen present in high concentration ($\sim$2 μM) in blood. The activity of plasmin is limited by inhibitors such as α_2-antiplasmin and α_2-macroglobulin.

When thrombosis is limited because of plasmin-dependent fibrinolysis at the time of rupture of a plaque, plaque growth may be clinically silent. When thrombosis is exuberant because of factors such as limited fibrinolysis, the thrombus may become occlusive and precipitate an acute coronary syndrome (acute myocardial infarction, unstable angina, or sudden cardiac death).

The rupture of an atherosclerotic plaque initiates coagulation and adhesion of platelets because of exposure to blood of luminal surfaces denuded of endothelium and hence to constituents such as collagen. The coagulation cascade in arterial thrombotic events is initiated by tissue factor, a cell-membrane-bound glycoprotein that binds circulating coagulation factor VII/VIIa to form the coagulation factor "tenase" complex that activates both circulating coagulation factors IX and X expressed on activated macrophages and monocytes as well as fibroblasts and endothelium in response to cytokines at the site of plaque rupture. Initiation of thrombin-generating activity may reflect release of platelet coagulation factor V/Va, contained in alpha granules, which is a cofactor for coagulation factor Xa. Subsequent assembly of the "prothrombinase" complex comprising prothrombin, coagulation factors Xa and Va, calcium, and membrane surface on platelet and other phospholipid membranes leads to generation of thrombin. Thrombin in turn cleaves fibrinogen to form fibrin. The generation of thrombin is amplified initially by its activation of circulating coagulation factors VIII (a cofactor for activated coagulation factor IX) and V (a cofactor for factor X) with consequent activation of the so-called intrinsic pathway of the coagulation cascade. Thrombin generation is sustained by activation by thrombin of other components in the intrinsic pathway including factor XI with consequent activation of coagulation factor IX. Platelets are activated by thrombin. Activated platelets markedly amplify generation of thrombin by releasing procoagulants and providing a potentiating surface replete with coagulation factor Va and Xa binding proteins.

A complex feedback system limits generation of thrombin. The tissue factor (extrinsic) pathway becomes inhibited by tissue factor pathway inhibitor (TFPI) previously called lipoprotein-associated coagulation inhibitor (LACI). Paradoxically, high concentrations of thrombin attenuate coagulation by binding to thrombomodulin on the surface of endothelial cells. This complex activates protein C (to yield protein Ca) that, in combination with protein S, cleaves (inactivates) coagulation factors Va and VIIIa.

Exposure of platelets to the subendothelium as a result of plaque rupture leads to adherence mediated by collagen and von Willebrand factor multimers within the vessel wall. The exposure of platelets to agonists including collagen, von Willebrand factor, ADP (released by damaged red blood cells and activated platelets), and thrombin leads to accelerated activation of platelets. Activation is a complex process. It entails shape change (pseudopod extension that increases the surface area of the platelet); activation of surface glycoprotein IIb/IIIa; release of products from dense granules such as calcium, ADP, and serotonin and from alpha granules such as fibrinogen, factor V/Va, growth factors, and platelet factor 4, which inhibits heparin; and a change in the conformation of the platelet membrane that promotes binding of coagulation factors to phospholipids and their assembly.

Activation of surface glycoprotein IIb/IIIa entails a conformational change that exposes a binding site for fibrinogen on the activated conformer. Each molecule of fibrinogen can bind two platelets, thereby leading to aggregation. After activation, the plasma membranes of platelets express negatively charged phospholipids on the outer surface that facilitate the assembly of protein constituents and subsequent activity of the tenase and prothrombinase complexes. Thus, platelets participate in thrombosis by: (1) forming a hemostatic plug (shape change, adherence to the vascular wall, and aggregation); (2) supplying coagulation factors and calcium (release of alpha and dense granule contents); and (3) providing a surface for the assembly of coagulation factor complexes. In addition, activation leads to vasoconstriction mediated by release of thromboxane and other vasoactive substances.

Both local and systemic factors can influence the extent of thrombosis occurring in association with plaque rupture. Local factors involve the morphology and biochemical composition of the plaque. Atheromatous plaques with substantial lipid content are particularly prone to initiate thrombosis. The severity of vascular injury and the extent of plaque rupture influence the extent to which blood is exposed to the subendothelium and consequently thrombogenicity.

II. THE COAGULATION SYSTEM AND DIABETES MELLITUS

The final common pathway resulting from activation of the coagulation system is generation of thrombin and thrombin-mediated formation of fibrin from fibrinogen. Generation of thrombin depends on activation of procoagulant factors and is limited by antithrombotic factors and inhibitors. A marker of thrombin activity is fibrinopeptide A (FPA), released when fibrinogen is cleaved by thrombin. This peptide has a very short half-life in the circulation because it is cleared promptly by the kidneys. Elevated concentrations in blood are, therefore, indicative of thrombin activity in vivo. Subjects with diabetes mellitus (both types 1 and 2) have increased concentrations of FPA in blood and in urine compared with those in nondiabetic subjects.

The increased concentrations of FPA seen in association with diabetes reflect an altered balance between prothrombotic and antithrombotic phenomena in subjects with diabetes mellitus favoring thrombosis. Patients with diabetes mellitus have increased concentrations in blood of the prothrombotic factors fibrinogen, von Willebrand factor, and factor VIIa coagulant activity. Among them, elevated concentrations of fibrinogen have been most strongly associated with an increased risk of development of cardiovascular disease. Although the mechanisms responsible for increased concentrations of fibrinogen and von Willebrand factor have not yet been fully elucidated, elevated concentrations in blood of insulin and proinsulin may be determinants in subjects with type 2 diabetes. This possibility is suggested by the close correlation between elevated concentrations of fibrinogen and hyperinsulinemia and hyperproinsulinemia in otherwise healthy subjects. Prediabetic subjects and patients in early stages of type 2 diabetes have marked insulin resistance reflected by a compensatory increase in the concentrations in blood of insulin and proinsulin. Thus, hyper(pro)insulinemia has been implicated in the evolution of concomitantly increased concentrations of fibrinogen. Improvement in metabolic control per se (euglycemia and amelioration of hyperlipidemia) has not been associated with normalization of the increased concentrations in blood of fibrinogen, von Willebrand factor, or factor VII coagulant activity.

First-degree nondiabetic relatives of subjects with type 2 diabetes exhibit increased concentrations of fibrinogen and factor VIIa coagulant activity in blood compared with values in age-matched controls. These are associated with other features indicative of insulin resistance. Thus, increased concentrations of prothrombotic factors seen typically in subjects with type 2 diabetes mellitus appear to be dependent on insulin resistance and hyperinsulinemia rather than to reflect the metabolic derangements typical of the diabetic state. Accordingly, hormonal abnormalities, particularly insulin resistance and hyper(pro)insulinemia, have been implicated as determinants of the prothrombotic state.

Decreased activity of antithrombotic factors in blood can potentiate thrombosis. Of note, concentrations in blood of protein C and activity of antithrombin are decreased in diabetic subjects. Unlike changes in concentrations of prothrombotic factors, altered concentrations and activity of antithrombotic factors appear to be reflections of the metabolic state typical of diabetes such as hyperglycemia, regardless of whether type 1 or type 2 diabetes is responsible. In fact, decreased antithrombotic activity has been associated with nonenzymatic glycation of antithrombin.

To recapitulate, functional activity of the prothrombinase complex and of thrombin itself are increased consistently in blood of subjects with diabetes. The increased activity is likely to be a reflection of increased procoagulant activity of platelets and monocytes in association with increased concentrations of fibrinogen, von Willebrand factor, and factor VII. Diminished activity in blood of antithrombotic factors secondary to glycation of antithrombin (and also of protein C) may contribute to the prothrombotic state. To date, no anticoagulant pharmacological regimen has been identified that unequivocally decreases the intensity of the prothrombotic state in subjects with diabetes. To the extent that glycation of proteins contributes to a prothrombotic state, optimal glycemic control should attenuate it. Accordingly, an important approach to attenuation of a prothrombotic state is normalization of the metabolic abnormalities typical of diabetes. Results in the DCCT trial are consistent with this interpretation. Despite the fact that the trial focused on microvascular complications of diabetes, known to be influenced by hyperglycemia, a trend toward reduction of macrovascular events was seen with stringent glycemic control.

The potential value of improving metabolic control with specific regimens that are insulin sensitizing rather than insulin providing, thereby limiting hyper(pro)insulinemia while achieving metabolic (glycemic and lipidemic) control, has been recognized. With respect to cardiovascular events, this concept will be evaluated in the BARI 2D trial. BARI 2D is a study of patients with diabetes and cardiovascular disease, all of whom will be treated with an objective of optimal metabolic control (HbA1C $\leq$ 7.0%). However, the approaches will differ. Thus, patients will be assigned randomly to diverse regimens designed to achieve metabolic control with either insulin-providing or insulin-sensitizing agents.

III. PLATELET FUNCTION AND DIABETES MELLITUS

Patients with diabetes, particularly those with macrovascular disease, have an increased circulating platelet mass secondary to increased ploidy of megakaryocytes. In addition, platelets isolated from the blood of subjects with diabetes exhibit impaired capacity to mediate vasodilatation, apparently because of release of a short-acting platelet-derived substance(s) that interferes with the ADP-induced dilatory response seen in normal vessels with intact endothelium.

Platelets from diabetic subjects demonstrate increased reactivity. They exhibit increased degranulation and increased aggregation in response to diverse stimuli. In addition, the procoagulant capacity of platelets from subjects with diabetes mellitus is increased. Thus, the generation of coagulation factor Xa and of thrombin is increased by three- to sevenfold in samples of blood containing platelets from diabetic as opposed to nondiabetic subjects.

One potential mechanism responsible for the increased platelet reactivity associated with diabetes is decreased membrane fluidity, potentially reflecting increased glycation of platelet membrane proteins. A reduction in membrane fluidity occurs when platelets from normal subjects are incubated in media containing concentrations of glucose similar to those seen in blood from subjects with poorly controlled diabetes. Because membrane fluidity is likely to alter membrane receptor accessibility by ligands, reduced membrane fluidity may contribute to the predisposition to activation of platelets. Accordingly, improved glycemic control and consequently decreased glycation of membrane proteins may increase membrane fluidity and decrease hyperreactivity. In fact, we have found that treatment with insulin is associated with an increased risk of high platelet reactivity. Accordingly, it appears that both metabolic control and a focus on optimal hormonal balance modification of insulin resistance and diminution of the often associated hyper(pro)insulinemia are needed to attenuate increased platelet reactivity.

IV. FIBRINOLYSIS AND DIABETES

Decreased fibrinolytic system capacity is observed consistently as judged from analysis of blood from patients with diabetes mellitus, particularly those with type 2 diabetes. We have found that impaired fibrinolysis in subjects with type 2 diabetes mellitus, not only under baseline conditions but also in response to physiological (transitory venous occlusion) challenge, is attributable to augmented concentrations in blood of circulating plasminogen activator inhibitor type-1 (PAI-1). Increased PAI-1 is seen also in blood from patients with other insulin-resistant states such as obesity, hypertension, and the polycystic ovarian syndrome.

Increased expression of PAI-1 is a marker of increased risk of acute myocardial infarction as judged from its presence in relatively young, long-term survivors of acute myocardial infarction compared with age-matched subjects who had not experienced any manifestations of overt coronary artery disease. Because the endogenous fibrinolytic system influences the evolution and persistence of thrombosis and the rapidity and extent of lysis of thrombi associated with vascular damage and its repair, overexpression of PAI-1 is likely to exacerbate both development and persistence of thrombi. Results of laboratory studies of transgenic mice deficient in PAI-1 compared with wild-type animals are consistent with this hypothesis. Twenty-four hours after arterial injury, persistence of thrombosis and the residual thrombus burden are greater in wild-type mice that are not deficient in PAI-1. Analogous observations are seen in analyses of human tissues after fatal pulmonary embolism. Increased expression of PAI-1 in association with pulmonary thromboembolism is evident. Thus, increased expression of PAI-1 typical of that seen in type 2 diabetes is likely to be a determinant of increased and persistent thrombosis.

Increased expression of PAI-1 in diabetes is likely to be multifactorial. A direct effect of insulin and of proinsulin on the expression of PAI-1 has been suggested by positive correlations between the concentrations of both with those of PAI-1 in vivo. Glucose, triglycerides, and circulating free fatty acids as well as those liberated by hydrolysis of triglycerides appear to contribute to the overexpression of PAI-1. Insulin and its precursors directly augment expression of PAI-1 in vitro. Insulin and triglycerides in combination exert a synergistic increase in accumulation of PAI-1 in conditioned media of diverse cells in culture when both are present in pathophysiological concentrations. Thus, the combination of hyperinsulinemia, hyperglycemia, and hypertriglyceridemia appears to be a major determinant of the increased PAI-1 in blood in vivo in subjects with diabetes. Accordingly, it is not surprising that experimentally induced hyperinsulinemia combined with hypertriglyceridemia and hyperglycemia increases the concentration of PAI-1 in blood in normal subjects. Both phenomena, hormonal (hyperinsulinemia) and metabolic (hyperglycemia and hypertriglyceridemia) derangements typical of type 2 diabetes mellitus contribute together to elevations of the concentration of PAI-1 in blood. Other constituents known to be capable of increasing PAI-1 expression include glycated LDL and oxidized LDL, both of which are often increased in blood in patients with insulin resistance and type 2 diabetes. In addition to potentiating elevation of PAI-1 in blood, insulin increases expression of PAI-1 in vessel walls. We have shown that pathophysiological concentrations of insulin increase the expression of PAI-1 by human arteries in vitro, an effect seen both in segments that appear to be grossly normal and in those that exhibit atherosclerotic changes. The increased PAI-1 expression is seen in arterial segments from subjects with or without insulin-resistant states in vivo. Augmented expression of PAI-1 is seen in response to insulin with vascular smooth muscle cells in culture and with cocultured endothelial cells and smooth muscle cells. The insulin-dependent increase in vessel wall PAI-1 may alter the evolution of atherosclerotic plaques favoring development of vulnerable as opposed to relatively stable plaques as discussed below. It may also contribute to elevation of PAI-1 in blood via release of PAI-1 from the vascular smooth muscle and endothelial cells themselves. Vulnerable, as opposed to relatively stable, atherosclerotic plaques are characterized by large lipid cores within thin relatively acellular fibrous caps. Increased expression of PAI-1 in the vessel wall may potentiate the development of such atherosclerotic plaques n the setting of any atherogenic stimulus. Stable plaques are characterized by a high ratio of vascular smooth muscle cells to lipid and thicker caps rendering them less prone to rupture. Falk and Davies demonstrated that lethal acute coronary syndromes are generally associated with vulnerable rather than stable plaques. We have hypothesized that migration of vascular smooth muscle cells into the neointima during the evolution of plaques is one factor contributing to their stability. Migration depends on cell surface expression and activity of plasminogen activators, particularly urokinase. Accordingly, in diabetes, the overexpression of PAI-1 by vascular smooth muscle cells may limit their migration and hence promote formation of vulnerable plaques that are relatively acellular and particularly prone to rupture.

Therapy designed to reduce insulin resistance and the often-associated hyperinsulinemia reduces concentrations of PAI-1 in blood. Thus, treatment of women with polycystic ovarian syndrome with metformin or with troglitazone decreases both blood insulin and PAI-1. Changes in the concentration of PAI-1 in blood correlate significantly with those of insulin. The concordance supports the view that hyperinsulinemia contributes to the increased PAI-1 expression in vivo. The changes in PAI-1 expression are likely to be secondary at least in part to the decrease in concentrations of insulin in blood rather than the direct effects of the pharmacological agents used to reduce them on PAI-1 expression per se. Thus, troglitazone decreases PAI-1 expression in vascular smooth muscle and endothelial cells in vitro, yet lowers PAI-1 in blood in vivo in diabetic and obese nondiabetic subjects with pretreatment hyperinsulinemia. Metformin, not itself an insulin sensitizer, decreases hepatic gluconeogenesis and hence concentrations of insulin in vivo. PAI-1 decreases as well.

The exposure of human hepatoma cells to gemfibrozil decreases basal and insulin-stimulated secretion of PAI-1. This inhibitory effect is seen in vitro. However, gemfibrozil does not lower PAI-1 in blood in vivo despite reducing the concentration of triglycerides in blood by 50 to 60%. No changes in insulin sensitivity or plasma concentrations of insulin are seen after treatment of patients with gemfibrozil. Thus, unlike therapy with agents that reduce insulin resistance and lower concentrations of insulin, therapy with gemfibrozil that reduces triglycerides without affecting concentrations of insulin does not lower PAI-1 in vivo. These observations support the likelihood that insulin per se is a critical determinant of altered expression of PAI-1 in subjects with insulin resistance such as those with type 2 diabetes mellitus. As judged from results in studies in which human hepatoma cells were exposed to insulin and triglycerides in vitro, modest elevations in the concentration of triglycerides and free fatty acids in the setting of hyperinsulinemia may be sufficient to augment expression of PAI-1. Thus, although the concentration of triglycerides in blood in patients treated with gemfibrozil was decreased by 50%, the prevailing concentration of triglycerides may have been sufficient to lead to persistent elevation of PAI-1 in blood in the setting of hyperinsulinemia. Recent results in studies with several statins, including atorvastatin, fail to show reduction of PAI-1 in blood, despite diminution of concentrations of triglycerides consistent with this possibility.

V. THERAPEUTIC IMPLICATIONS

Consideration of the known derangements in platelet function, the coagulation system, and the fibrinolytic system and their probable contributions to exacerbation of macrovascular disease in type 2 diabetes give rise to several therapeutic considerations. Stringent glycemic control is an imperative to protect patients against microvascular complications including nephropathy, retinopathy, and neuropathy. However, we believe it should be achieved under conditions in which prevailing concentrations of insulin in blood are minimized. Furthermore, adjunctive measures are likely to be helpful. Empirical use of aspirin (160 to 325 mg/day in a single dose) seems appropriate in view of the high likelihood that covert coronary artery disease is present even in asymptomatic subjects with type 2 diabetes and the compelling evidence that prophylactic aspirin reduces the risk of heart attack when coronary disease is present. Reduction of angiotensin-II and IV levels, known to stimulate PAI-1 expression, is desirable and can be achieved with the use of ACE inhibitors to lower blood pressure to 130/85 mmHg and protect against nephropathy. Because many of the derangements contributing to a prothrombotic state in diabetes are caused by hyperglycemia, reduction of hemoglobin A1c levels to 7% is desirable. Accordingly, the use of diet, exercise, oral hypoglycemic agents, insulin sensitizers, and, if necessary, insulin is appropriate. However, because other derangements contributing to an imbalance between thrombosis and fibrinolysis as well as perhaps to evolution of vulnerable plaques such as attenuation of fibrinolysis by PAI-1 secondary to insulin resistance and hyperinsulinemia, the use of insulin sensitizers should be emphasized along with insulin or with other oral hypoglycemic agents if they are needed is likely to be beneficial.

Prophylactic administration of anticoagulants or of fibrinolytic drugs has not been shown to be indicated in the treatment of patients with diabetes mellitus. However, the use of potent antiplatelet agents is warranted in their treatment when symptomatic coronary artery disease is present. Beneficial effects of glycoprotein IIb/IIIa inhibitors are striking in diabetic subjects who require percutaneous coronary interventions (PCI). Analysis of results in diabetic subjects with acute coronary syndromes demonstrates that treatment of diabetic patients with acute coronary syndromes undergoing PCI with tirofiban reduces the 30-day incidence of death or myocardial infarction from 15.5 to 4.7%. Similarly, treatment with abciximab during elective percutaneous coronary intervention reduces the mortality rate after 1 year from 4.5 to 2.5%. Accordingly, GP IIb/IIIa inhibitors should be used aggressively in the treatment of diabetic subjects with acute coronary syndromes (unstable angina and non-ST-elevation myocardial infarction) and uniformly in association with percutaneous coronary intervention.

As noted above, hypertension should be treated vigorously, generally with ACE inhibitors, because of their demonstrated renal protective effects and normalization of the imbalance in the fibrinolytic system of diabetic subjects. Treatment with ACE-inhibitors is associated with a reduced rate of recurrent coronary thrombosis. Results both in vitro and in vivo demonstrate that ACE inhibition, by decreasing formation of angiotensin-II and angiotensin-IV, decreases expression of PAI-1. Thus, ACE-inhibitor therapy is likely to reduce cardiovascular events through diverse mechanisms, including its effect on the decreased fibrinolytic capacity in diabetes.

VI. CONCLUSIONS AND IMPLICATIONS FOR PRACTICE

Subjects with diabetes mellitus have a high prevalence and rapid progression of cardiovascular, peripheral vascular, and cerebral vascular disease secondary and in part attributable to: (1) increased platelet reactivity; (2) increased prothrombotic activity reflecting increased concentrations and activity of coagulation factors and decreased activity of antithrombotic factors; and (3) decreased fibrinolytic system capacity resulting from overexpression of PAI- by hepatic, arterial, and adipose tissue in response to hyperinsulinemia, hypertriglyceridemia, and hyperglycemia. The macrovascular disease appears to be accelerated by an insulin-dependent imbalance between concentrations of plasminogen activators and PAI-1 in blood and in vessel walls. Therapy designed to reduce insulin resistance decreases concentrations in blood not only of insulin but also of PAI-1. Thus, the treatment of subjects with diabetes, and particularly type 2 diabetes, should be designed to achieve stringent metabolic control while at the same time reducing insulin resistance and hyperinsulinemia. Treatment designed to attenuate both the hormonal and metabolic abnormalities is likely to reduce hyperactivity of platelets, decrease the intensity of the prothrombotic state, and normalize activity of the fibrinolytic system in blood and in vessel walls, thereby reducing the rate of progression of macrovascular disease and its sequelae.

SUGGESTED READING

1. Jones RL. Fibrinopeptide-A in diabetes mellitus. Relation to levels of blood glucose, fibrinogen disappearance, and hemodynamic changes. Diabetes 1985; 34:836–843.
2. Mansfield MW, Heywood DM, Grant PJ. Circulating levels of factor VII, fibrinogen, and von Willebrand factor and features of insulin resistance in first-degree relatives of patients with NIDDM. Circulation 1996; 94:2171–2176.
3. Lupu C, Calb M, Ionescu M, Lupu F. Enhanced prothrombin and intrinsic factor X activation on blood platelets from diabetic patients. Thromb Haemost 1993; 70:579–583.
4. McGill JB, Schneider DJ, Arfken CL, Lucore CL, Sobel BE. Factors responsible for impaired fibrinolysis in obese subjects and NIDDM patients. Diabetes 1994; 43:104–109.
5. Sobel BE. Increased plasminogen activator inhibitor-1 and vasculopathy. A reconcilable paradox. Circulation 1999; 99:2496–2498.
6. Calles-Escandon J, Mirza S, Sobel BE, Schneider DJ. Induction of hyperinsulinemia combined with hyperglycemia and hypertriglyceridemia increases plasminogen activator inhibitor type-1 (PAI-1) in blood in normal human subjects. Diabetes 1998; 47: 290–293.
7. Theroux P, Alexander J Jr, Pharand C, Barr E, Snapinn S, Ghannam AF, Sax FL. Glycoprotein IIb/IIIa receptor blockade improves outcomes in diabetic patients presenting with unstable angina/non-ST-elevation myocardial infarction: results from the platelet receptor inhibition in ischemic syndrome management in patients limited by unstable signs and symptoms (PRISM-PLUS) study. Circulation 2000; 102:2466–2472.
8. Bhatt DL, Marso SP, Lincoff AM, Wolski KE, Ellis SG, Topol EJ. Abciximab reduces mortality in diabetics following percutaneous coronary intervention. J Am Coll Cardiol 2000; 35:922–928.
9. Ridker PM, Vaughan DE. Potential antithrombotic and fibrinolytic properties of the angiotensin converting enzyme inhibitors. J Thromb Thrombolysis 1995; 1:251–257.

7

Insulin Resistance, Compensatory Hyperinsulinemia, and Coronary Heart Disease: Syndrome X

Gerald M. Reaven
Stanford University School of Medicine, Stanford, California

I. INTRODUCTION

The goal of this chapter will be to provide evidence for the importance of insulin resistance and compensatory hyperinsulinemia, and the manifestations of insulin resistance/compensatory hyperinsulinemia (syndrome X), in the genesis of coronary heart disease (CHD) in nondiabetic individuals. Although insulin resistance, and the body's response to this defect, are central to the development of CHD in patients with type 2 diabetes, the pathophysiological characteristics of type 2 diabetes and syndrome X are sufficiently different so as to preclude a thoughtful discussion of both syndromes within the constraints of this chapter. On the other hand, discussion of the relationship between insulin resistance, compensatory hyperinsulinemia, and CHD in those with syndrome X will be of considerable relevance to patients with type 2 diabetes.

II. WHAT IS INSULIN RESISTANCE?

The ability of insulin to stimulate muscle glucose disposal varies approximately tenfold in the population at large. Insulin-resistant individuals develop type 2 diabetes when they can no longer secrete enough insulin to maintain the degree of compensatory hyperinsulinemia necessary to maintain euglycemia. However, the vast majority of individuals that demonstrate muscle insulin resistance are able to sustain the magnitude of compensatory hyperinsulinemia needed to prevent gross decompensation of glucose tolerance.

As commonly used, the phrase "insulin resistance" refers to a decrease in the ability of a defined amount of insulin to stimulate glucose disposal by muscle. However, there is no accepted criterion that permits a precise definition of the magnitude of the defect in insulin-stimulated glucose disposal by muscle that provides the means to designate a person as "insulin sensitive" or "insulin resistant." Instead, as shown in Figure 1, insulin-stimulated glucose disposal rates in nondiabetic individuals vary continuously from the most insulin-sensitive to the most insulin-resistant individual, and the best we can do is to understand that the more insulin-resistant an individual, the more at risk they are of developing one or more of the manifestations of syndrome X. The variability of insulin-stimulated glucose disposal is 490 healthy volunteers is shown in Figure 1. These measurements were made with the insulin suppression test, an approach to quantify insulin-mediated glucose disposal by determining the steady-state plasma insulin (SSPI) and steady-state plasma glucose (SSPG) concentrations achieved during the last 30 min of a continuous infusion of octreotide, insulin, and glucose. The octreotide infusion suppresses endogenous insulin secretion, and the exogenous insulin infusion produces a steady-state level of physiological hyperinsulinemia. Because the SSPI concentration is similar for all subjects, the SSPG concentration provides a direct measure of the ability of insulin to mediate disposal of an infused glucose load; the higher the SSPG concentration, the more insulin resistant the individual.

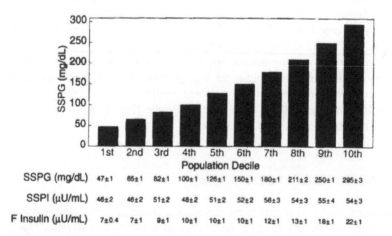

Figure 1 SSPG concentrations of 490 volunteers divided into deciles. The mean (±SEM) SSPG, SSPI, and fasting (F) insulin concentration of each decile are shown below each bar. (Reproduced from Ref. 20 with permission of the author and publisher.)

Each of the bars in Figure 1 represents the mean SSPG concentration for 49 individuals. It is apparent that there is an enormous spread of SSPG concentrations in the 490 volunteers (i.e., the degree of insulin resistance varies dramatically in the population at large). Indeed, there is an approximate tenfold difference between the most insulin-sensitive and insulin-resistant individuals. It should also be noted from Figure 1 that the fasting (F) insulin concentrations increase in parallel with the SSPG concentrations.

Based upon the results of prospective studies, it has been estimated that the upper 25 to 33% of the nondiabetic population (i.e., the upper three deciles in terms of SSPG concentration) are at greatly increased risk of presenting with one or more of the manifestations of syndrome X.

If 25 to 33% of the population at large is sufficiently insulin resistant to be at increased risk of syndrome X and/or type 2 diabetes, it is of obvious interest to know what determines the ability of insulin to stimulate muscle glucose disposal. At one level, this question is easy to answer. Differences in degree of obesity and physical activity are the two most important lifestyle variables that modulate insulin action, and they explain approximately 25% each of the variations in insulin action from person to person. By inference, it can then be argued that differences in genetic background account for the remaining 50% of the variability in insulin resistance. Although the actual numerical values may not be entirely accurate, they represent reasonable approximations. The crucial thing to remember is that variations in body weight and level of physical activity are *modulators* of insulin action; they are not the primary *cause* of insulin resistance.

A second point that must be appreciated is that although the ability of insulin to mediate glucose disposal by muscle is the conventional way of assessing insulin resistance, adipose tissue appears to be as resistant to regulation by insulin as muscle. The belated recognition of adipose tissue insulin resistance is easily understood if both the techniques usually used to assess resistance to insulin-mediated glucose disposal and the differences in the dose-response characteristics of insulin action on adipose tissue versus muscle are taken into account. For example, a plasma insulin concentration of ~20 μU/mL will suppress by approximately 50% the release of free fatty acids (FFA) by adipose tissue; a circulating insulin concentration that has relatively little effect on stimulating glucose disposal by muscle. The infusion techniques conventionally used to quantify insulin resistance (i.e., the ability of insulin to stimulate glucose disposal by muscle) are almost uniformly performed by maintaining steady-state plasma insulin concentrations at least fourfold greater than the level needed to half-maximally suppress adipose tissue lipolysis. As a result, plasma FFA levels are maximally suppressed in all subjects, and differences in adipose tissue resistance to insulin cannot be discerned. It is now clear that the degree of insulin resistance in muscle and in adipose tissue is highly correlated, and that both defects contribute to the manifestations of syndrome X.

If not for this difference in tissue dose-response curve, the increase in plasma FFA concentrations would be proportionate to the degree of hyperinsulinemia in subjects with syndrome X. However, because of the enhanced sensitivity of the adipose tissue to insulin, plasma FFA concentrations are only marginally increased as long as hyperinsulinemia is maintained. On the other hand, the fact that there is a less dramatic increase in plasma FFA concentration should not obscure the fact that adipose tissue insulin resistance contributes substantially to the development of syndrome X.

Although attention has been focused on the parallel abnormalities that exist in muscle and adipose tissue to their regulation by insulin, it is important to understand that many of the manifestations of syndrome X are due to the effects of the compensatory hyperinsulinemia on tissues that remain insulin sensitive, despite the presence of muscle and adipose tissue insulin resistance in the same individual. There are several examples of this phenomenon. For example, there is evidence that the sympathetic nervous system (SNS) remains normally responsive to insulin stimulation in individuals with muscle insulin resistance. Thus, the compensatory hyperinsulinemia present in insulin-resistant individuals leads to enhanced SNS activity and a series of changes that helps explain why insulin-resistant/hyperinsulinemic individuals are at increased risk to develop hypertension.

There is also substantial evidence that the liver does not share in the insulin resistance present in muscle and adipose tissue. For example, muscle insulin resistance leads to higher insulin levels (to prevent the development of type 2 diabetes), and higher FFA concentrations occur because of adipose tissue insulin resistance. In contrast, the liver is functionally normal, and its response to the higher insulin and FFA levels is to enhance its synthesis and secretion of triglyceride (TG)-rich lipoproteins, leading to hypertriglyceridemia.

Another major organ that retains normal insulin sensitivity, despite muscle and adipose tissue insulin resistance, is the kidney, and there are two features of syndrome X that are likely to be dependent on the retention of normal insulin action on the kidney—hyperuricemia and salt-sensitive hypertension—both of which will be discussed in greater detail subsequently.

III. WHY IS INSULIN RESISTANCE IMPORTANT?

As shown in Figure 2, insulin-resistant individuals are at increased risk of developing either type 2 diabetes or one or more of the cluster of abnormalities subsumed under the general heading of syndrome X. Although these two syndromes have been separated for pedagogic purposes, it should be emphasized that they share many attributes not the least of which is increased risk of CHD, and that a finite proportion of individuals initially designated as syndrome X will eventually develop type 2 diabetes.

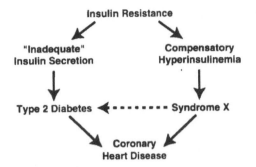

Figure 2 A schematic description of the relationship between insulin resistance, insulin secretory response, type 2 diabetes, and syndrome X and coronary heart disease (CHD).

The relationship between insulin resistance and type 2 diabetes has been defined as the consequence of multiple prospective, population-based studies published over the past 30 years. There seems to be little doubt that insulin resistance and/or hyperinsulinemia (a surrogate measure of insulin resistance in nondiabetic individuals) are the most powerful predictors of the development of type 2 diabetes. The role of an impairment of insulin secretory function is less well understood, and the phrase "inadequate insulin secretion," as seen in Figure 2, is a euphemism that should not obscure the fact that absolute plasma insulin concentrations throughout the day are, on the average, higher in absolute terms in the majority of patients with type 2 diabetes as compared to normoglycemic individuals.

As emphasized earlier, most insulin-resistant individuals remain in the right limb of Figure 2; they secrete enough insulin to avoid becoming sufficiently hyperglycemic to merit the diagnosis of type 2 diabetes. However, this victory is a hollow one, and in 1988 a relationship between insulin resistance, compensatory hyperinsulinemia, and a cluster of related abnormalities, all of which increase risk of CHD, was identified and designated as syndrome X. In the remainder of this section, the evidence linking insulin resistance and compensatory hyperinsulinemia to all the abnormalities now presumed to comprise syndrome X will be reviewed (Table 1).

A. Glucose Metabolism

Within the population satisfying the criteria for normal glucose tolerance, the greater their degree of insulin resistance, the higher their plasma glucose concentration. In a smaller subset of insulin-resistant individuals, the degree of compensatory hyperinsulinemia is not sufficient to maintain normal glucose tolerance, and they are classified as having either impaired fasting glucose or impaired glu-

Table 1 Manifestations of Insulin Resistance/
Compensatory Hyperinsulinemia (Syndrome X)

A. Glucose Metabolism
   1. Impaired fasting glucose
   2. Impaired glucose tolerance
B. Uric Acid Metabolism
   1. ↑ Plasma uric acid concentration
   2. ↓ Plasma renal uric acid clearance
C. Dyslipidemia
   1. ↑ Triglyceride concentration
   2. ↑ Postprandial lipemia
   3. ↓ HDL cholesterol concentration
   4. ↓ LDL particle diameter
D. Blood Pressure
   1. ↑ Blood pressure
   2. ↑ Sympathetic nervous system activity
   3. ↑ Renal sodium retention
E. Procoagulant Activity
   1. ↑ Plasminogen activator inhibitor-1
   2. ↑ Fibrinogen
F. Reproductive System
   1. Polycystic ovary syndrome

---

cose tolerance. In an even smaller number of insulin-resistant individuals, insulin secretory function fails to the degree that permits manifest hyperglycemia to develop. Such individuals have type 2 diabetes. Syndrome X and type 2 diabetes share insulin resistance as a basic metabolic defect, but the designation of syndrome X should be limited to individuals who have maintained sufficient insulin secretory function to remain nondiabetic.

B. Uric Acid Metabolism

An association between increases in plasma uric acid concentration and increased CHD risk has been known for many years. Hyperuricemia is commonly seen in individuals with glucose intolerance, dyslipidemia, and hypertension. Significant correlations exist between plasma uric acid concentration and both insulin resistance and the plasma insulin response to an oral glucose challenge in healthy volunteers, and individuals with asymptomatic hyperuricemia have higher plasma insulin responses to oral glucose; higher TG and lower high-density lipoprotein (HDL) cholesterol concentrations; and higher blood pressure when compared to volunteers with normal serum uric acid concentrations.

The increase in plasma uric concentrations in insulin-resistant, nondiabetic individuals appears to result from a decrease in renal uric acid clearance secondary to the effect of compensatory hyperinsulinemia on the handling of uric acid by the kidney. This is one of several instances in which a manifestation of syndrome X occurs because one organ system remains sensitive to insulin action, in this case the kidney, whereas the muscle in the same individual is insulin resistant.

C. Dyslipidemia

The most central feature of syndrome X is hypertriglyceridemia. However, there are several other abnormalities that rarely occur in the absence of an increase in plasma TG concentration and belong to the cluster of CHD risk factors that make up syndrome X.

1. Hypertriglyceridemia

A direct relationship exists between insulin resistance, compensatory hyperinsulinemia, and plasma TG concentration, and this association is seen in both hypertriglyceridemic and normotriglyceridemic subjects. Since hepatic very-low-density lipoprotein (VLDL)–TG synthesis and secretion are highly correlated with plasma VLDL–TG concentrations, it can be concluded that the more insulin resistant an individual, and the higher the resultant plasma insulin concentration, the greater will be the increase in hepatic VLDL–TG synthesis and secretion, and the more elevated the plasma TG concentration. The increase in hepatic VLDL–TG secretion in syndrome X results from the effect of the ambient hyperinsulinemia, enhancing the hepatic conversion of FFA to TG, and an increase in FFA flux to the liver as a result of resistance to the antilipolytic effect of insulin at the level of the adipose tissue. As discussed above, the liver is responding normally to the day-long hyperinsulinemia in the presence of muscle and adipose tissue insulin resistance.

2. Postprandial Lipemia

Once fasting hypertriglyceridemia develops in insulin-resistant individuals, there will be an accentuation of postprandial lipemia, and the accumulation of TG-rich lipoproteins throughout the day. Both insulin resistance and compensatory hyperinsulinemia, significantly and independently, predict the postprandial accumulation of TG-rich lipoproteins in nondiabetic individuals. Thus, elevations in postprandial lipemia are highly correlated with insulin resistance and compensatory hyperinsulinemia, directly by unknown mechanisms, and indirectly by the ability of insulin resistance and/or compensatory hyperinsulinemia to stimulate hepatic VLDL–TG secretion and increase the fasting TG pool size.

3. HDL Cholesterol

The association of low-HDL cholesterol concentrations with hypertriglyceridemia is at least partly due to the exchange of cholesteryl ester from HDL to VLDL, modulated by cholesteryl ester transfer protein, with the reciprocal movement of TG from VLDL to HDL. As a consequence, HDL cholesterol concentrations fall and HDL–TG concentrations increase. In addition, the fractional catabolic rate (FCR) of apoprotein A-1 (the major apoprotein of HDL) is increased in situations characterized by insulin resistance/hyperinsulinemia, and the faster the FCR of apoprotein A-1, the lower the HDL cholesterol concentration. Thus, insulin resistance and compensatory hyperinsulinemia contribute to a low-HDL cholesterol concentration, indirectly by being responsible for the increase in VLDL pool-size, and directly by increasing the FCR of apoprotein A-1.

4. Low-Density-Lipoprotein Particle Diameter

LDL particle size in most individuals can be characterized by a predominance of either larger LDL (diameter > 255 Å, pattern A) or smaller LDL (≤ 255Å, pattern B) particles. Individuals with pattern B have higher plasma TG and lower HDL cholesterol concentrations, and are at increased risk of CHD. Healthy volunteers with small, dense LDL particles (pattern B) are also relatively insulin resistant, glucose intolerant, hyperinsulinemic, hypertensive, and hypertriglyceridemic, and have a lower HDL cholesterol concentration. Thus, this change in LDL composition is part of the cluster of abnormalities constituting syndrome X.

D. Blood Pressure

Hypertension can occur for a variety of reasons, and essential hypertension represents a heterogeneous group of disorders. However, it is likely that ~50% patients with essential hypertension are insulin resistant and hyperinsulinemic. Furthermore, insulin resistance/hyperinsulinemia is a powerful predictor of the development of high blood pressure, and normotensive, first-degree relatives of patients with high blood pressure, as a group, have been shown to be insulin resistant and hyperinsulinemic. However, not all insulin-resistant/hyperinsulinemic individuals have elevated blood pressure; therefore, the abnormalities in insulin metabolism simply lead to physiological changes that place an individual at increased risk of developing hypertension. The two most prominent of these changes involve enhanced sympathetic nervous system activity and renal sodium retention.

1. Sympathetic Nervous System (SNS) Activity

Resting heart rate is higher in patients with high blood pressure, as well as being a predictor of hypertension. This association could be secondary to enhanced

SNS activity in insulin-resistant and hyperinsulinemic subjects, and injection of insulin acutely stimulates SNS discharge. Insulin resistance/hyperinsulinemia are significantly correlated with heart rate in normotensive, healthy volunteers; another example in which the compensatory hyperinsulinemia associated with muscle insulin resistance increases activity of a tissue that remains normally insulin sensitive. An increase in SNS activity, secondary to insulin resistance/hyperinsulinemia, provides an explanation for why resistance to insulin-mediated glucose disposal and/or hyperinsulinemia, and an increase in heart rate, have been shown to predict development of hypertension. Furthermore, enhanced SNS activity certainly could increase risk of hypertension, both directly, by its action on vascular tone, and indirectly, by increasing renal sodium reabsorption.

2. Sodium Retention

Acute infusions of insulin increase renal sodium retention in both normal individuals and patients with high blood pressure, and insulin-induced retention of sodium by the kidney is independent of the ability of insulin to stimulate muscle glucose disposal (i.e., another instance in which tissue sensitivity to an action of insulin is maintained despite a loss of muscle and adipose tissue insulin sensitivity). Since hyperinsulinemia enhances renal sodium retention, it should not be surprising that insulin-resistant individuals are also salt-sensitive, and that salt and water retention in response to a high salt intake is markedly accentuated in those patients with hypertension who are also insulin resistant and hyperinsulinemic.

E. Procoagulant Activity

There is evidence that impaired fibrinolysis and a hypercoaguable state are associated with insulin resistance/hyperinsulinemia.

1. Plasminogen Activator Inhibitor-1 (PAI-1)

PAI concentrations are higher in patients with hypertriglyceridemia, hypertension, and CHD, suggesting that PAI-1 concentrations are related to insulin resistance and/or compensatory hyperinsulinemia. Epidemiological evidence in support of this view comes from the European Concerted Action on Thrombosis and Disabilities Angina Pectoris Study, indicating that PAI-1 concentrations were significantly associated with hyperinsulinemia, hypertriglyceridemia, and hypertension in 1500 patients with angina pectoris. Furthermore, insulin-resistant/hyperinsulinemic women have a higher PAI-1 concentrations, associated with higher TG and lower HDL cholesterol concentrations, than insulin-sensitive women matched for age, body mass index, and abdominal obesity. Thus, high concentrations of PAI-1 are another manifestation of syndrome X.

2. Fibrinogen

Elevated fibrinogen levels have also been postulated to be part of the syndrome X cluster, but the evidence is not as strong as the case of PAI-1. Although insulin resistance and fibrinogen levels have been shown to be correlated, the relationship, in this case, may not be an independent one, but rather the manifestation of an acute phase reaction in patients with CHD.

F. Reproductive System

Polycystic ovary syndrome (PCOS) is the most common endocrine abnormality in premenopausal women, and insulin resistance and compensatory hyperinsulinemia play a fundamental role in the etiology of this syndrome. This is another example of an organ, in this case the ovary, responding normally to hyperinsulinemia by increasing testosterone secretion in the face of muscle and adipose tissue insulin resistance. Indeed, in this instance, the ovary may be supersensitive to insulin stimulation. In any event, the primary clinical manifestations of PCOS (hirsutism, abnormal menstruation, and difficulty in conceiving) are secondary to increased insulin-stimulated testosterone secretion by the ovary. Women with PCOS are at increased risk to develop both type 2 diabetes and the dyslipidemia of syndrome X. Both of these changes suggest that insulin-resistant and hyperinsulinemic women with PCOS will be at increased risk of CHD, and there is now evidence of enhanced atherogenesis in middle-aged women with PCOS.

IV. SYNDROME X AND CHD

Definition of risk factors for any clinical syndrome have historically relied upon the combination of results from population-based studies of the natural history of the condition being examined, as well as placebo-controlled intervention studies in which a specific risk factor is decreased, and the clinical impact assessed. This process works very well when the role of a single risk factor is being evaluated. For example, there is no longer any question that a high-LDL cholesterol concentration increases risk of CHD, or that lowering it will reduce the incidence of CHD. Unfortunately, the situation becomes much more complicated when a cluster of potentially powerful CHD risk factors may exist in the same individual (i.e., syndrome X).

Before attempting to briefly summarize the data linking the individual manifestation of syndrome X to CHD risk, it is essential to explicitly emphasize the difficulties inherent in this task. Results are now available from multiple epidemiological studies documenting statistically significant relationships between the various manifestations of syndrome X and CHD. The confusion begins when these data are utilized in multiple regression models in an effort to discern which of the abnormalities associated with syndrome X are "independent" predictors of CHD. Although these conventional statistical approaches are widely used, it is necessary to question their appropriateness in this situation. To begin with, many of the reports attempting to define the CHD risk of the cluster of abnormalities that make up syndrome X are retrospective, using data collected before the current definition of syndrome X as described in Table 1, and without having experimental values for variables that might be important links between insulin resistance/compensatory hyperinsulinemia and CHD.

In addition, even if all the relevant variables have been measured, several conditions must be satisfied before conclusions based on multivariate analyses can be considered to be valid. In particular, considerable caution must be exercised when multiple variables, all closely related, are entered into the same multiple regression model. At a minimum, it is necessary that the intra- and interindividual variability of all variables tested in the model be similar: a criterion that is rarely, or ever, even considered, let alone met. Furthermore, when two very closely related variables are entered into the same multivariate analysis, it is not at all unlikely that the conclusion may be that *neither* contributes to CHD risk. This issue will be addressed in greater detail when discussing the relationship between CHD and the dyslipidemia of syndrome X.

Finally, it must be realized that all population-based, prospective, epidemiological studies base their analysis and conclusions on the value of a putative CHD risk factor, measured at baseline, and assumed to be relatively stable over the several-year period of the study in question. Is there any reason to assume that this is the case? Is the stability of all potential CHD risk factors the same over time? For all these reasons, it is difficult to provide accurate estimates of the power of syndrome X as a CHD risk factor, and to decide which one of its manifestations is the major culprit.

Given these caveats, in this section an attempt will be made to briefly comment upon the evidence linking the manifestations of syndrome X to CHD.

A. Glucose Metabolism

Although there is epidemiological evidence linking hyperglycemia to CHD, it is not clear that hyperglycemia, per se, increases risk of CHD. For example, CHD risk in patients with impaired glucose tolerance is increased to almost the same degree as is the case in patients with type 2 diabetes. Thus, it seems more likely that the relationship between plasma glucose concentration and CHD is related to the fact that individuals with even minor elevations in plasma glucose concentration are likely to exhibit many of the manifestations of syndrome X (i.e., hyperinsulinemia, dyslipidemia, etc.) and it is these changes that are responsible for the accelerated atherogenesis.

B. Uric Acid Metabolism

Multiple epidemiological studies have identified an increased prevalence of hyperuricemia in patients with CHD. There are also more recent publications suggesting that an increase in uric acid concentration is an independent predictor of CHD. On the other hand, there is abundant evidence of a direct relationship between insulin resistance/compensatory hyperinsulinemia and uric acid concentration, and that hyperuricemia is associated with an increase in the prevalence of hypertension, the dyslipidemic changes characteristic of syndrome X, and a procoagulant state. Thus, although the possibility that a high uric acid level directly increases CHD risk cannot be ruled out, it seems most likely that the epidemiological link represents an epiphenomenon, and it is the presence of other manifestations of syndrome X that accounts for the relationship between uric acid concentration and CHD risk.

C. Dyslipidemia

The association between the changes in lipoprotein metabolism that occur in association with insulin resistance/hyperinsulinemia is the most difficult to discuss due to the close relationship between the dyslipidemic manifestations of syndrome X listed in Table 1. Perhaps the best way to approach this issue is to focus initially on the association between hypertriglyceridemia and CHD—the link between syndrome X and atherogenesis with the longest history.

The existence of an association between hypertriglyceridemia and CHD has been known for more than 40 years, and the majority of studies aimed at defining the risk factors involved in the development of CHD have demonstrated a highly statistically significant relationship between plasma TG concentration and risk of CHD. However, when more sophisticated statistical methods are used to evaluate the relative impact of a number of individual factors that might be related to CHD, the relation between plasma TG concentration and CHD frequently loses its statistical significance. For example, when attempts are made to differentiate between the risk factor status of changes in concentration of total and/or LDL cholesterol, HDL cholesterol, and TG, it is often concluded that an increase in plasma TG concentration is not an "independent" risk factor for CHD. More specifically, when both HDL cholesterol and TG concentrations have been measured and multivariate analysis is used, a low-HDL cholesterol concentration almost always emerges as an independent risk factor for CHD, whereas a high-TG concentration often does not. The conclusion that hypertriglyceridemia is not an independent risk factor for CHD leads to the widely accepted view that increases in plasma TG concentration are only of clinical relevance when the magnitude of the change increases the risk of pancreatitis. However, the role of a low-HDL cholesterol concentration as increasing risk of CHD is widely accepted. Furthermore, although the notion that the postprandial accumulation of TG-rich lipoprotein was atherogenic was first discussed ~40 years, only in the last few years have publications appeared that clearly demonstrate that these particles are associated with increased CHD risk. Finally, there is increasing evidence that the presence of smaller and denser LDL particles is associated with increased CHD risk, particles that occur in individuals with high-TG and low-HDL cholesterol concentration.

All of these changes—hypertriglyceridemia, lower HDL cholesterol concentrations, enhanced postprandial lipemia, and small, dense LDL particles—comprise an extremely atherogenic lipoprotein profile. Efforts to differentiate between the "independence" of each of them do not seem particularly useful, particularly when the appropriateness of the statistical analyses used in this attempt is questionable. As discussed above, great care must be used when multiple regression analyses are employed in an attempt to define the "independence" of closely related variables. Questioning the attempt to differentiate between the "independence" of closely related CHD risk factors is particularly relevant in view of the close relationships between plasma TG concentration and (1) HDL cholesterol concentration; (2) LDL particle diameter; and (3) magnitude of postprandial lipemia. It is much more useful to understand that these changes are commonly seen in insulin-resistant/hyperinsulinemic individuals, and they are all likely to make a substantial contribution to the increased CHD risk associated with syndrome X.

D. Blood Pressure

As discussed previously, ~50% of patients with essential hypertension are insulin resistant/hyperinsulinemic, and display many of the other manifestations of syndrome X (i.e., glucose intolerance, dyslipidemia, and increased procoagulant activity). There is now evidence that strongly suggests that CHD risk is significantly greater in insulin-resistant/hyperinsulinemic patients with high blood pressure than in those who do not share this defect. The implication of these observations are twofold. CHD is the major cause of morbidity and mortality in patients with essential hypertension, yet clinical trials continue to indicate that lowering blood pressure is more effective in decreasing stroke than heart attack. The simplest conclusion from these findings is that CHD in patients with essential hypertension is not simply a matter of an increase in blood pressure. The fact that CHD risk in this population varies as a function of whether or not insulin resistance/hyperinsulinemia is present provides support for that point of view.

Second, and of greater pragmatic importance, is the notion that efforts to decrease CHD in patients with hypertension must focus not only on lowering blood pressure, but also on taking into account all the other CHD risk factors present in these individuals. In this context, attention to the manifestations of syndrome X must be paramount.

E. Procoagulant State

Plasma concentrations of PAI-1 and fibrinogen are increased in patients with CHD, and both of these changes are appreciated as being related to syndrome X. In contrast to the other manifestations of insulin resistance/hyperinsulinemia, these abnormalities are likely to have a larger role in increasing the risk of heart attack, rather than accelerating the process of atherogenesis. The association between insulin resistance/hyperinsulinemia and PAI-1 seems to be stronger than the link to fibrinogen. Regardless of ultimate understanding of the nature of the relationship between insulin resistance/hyperinsulinemia, PAI-1, and fibrinogen, there seems to be general agreement that these procoagulant changes contribute to the increased risk of CHD in insulin-resistant/hyperinsulinemic individuals.

F. Reproductive System

PCOS is the newest member of syndrome X, and understanding its relationship to CHD is evolving. It is quite clear that the prevalence of the manifestations of syndrome X are increased in patients with PCOS, and there is evidence from surrogate estimates that CHD risk is also increased. It is likely that the incidence of CHD will be increased in women with PCOS, secondary to the other manifestations of syndrome X, not to the characteristic signs and symptoms of the syndrome.

IV. DIAGNOSIS OF SYNDROME X

Since insulin resistance and compensatory hyperinsulinemia are the basic abnormalities leading to the manifestations of syndrome X, it would seem reasonable that these measurements should be central to its diagnosis. However, quantification of insulin resistance is not practical, and there is no gold standard for classifying an individual as hyperinsulinemic, or relating a given insulin concentration to a clinical outcome. Furthermore, use of various formulas based on fasting insulin concentrations or fasting insulin and glucose concentrations to quantify insulin resistance does not provide clinically relevant information. On the other hand, it is relatively simple and quite straightforward to simply determine what, if any, manifestations of syndrome X are present. For this purpose, measurement of: (1) plasma glucose concentrations, fasting and 120 min after a 75-g glucose challenge; (2) lipid and lipoprotein concentrations; and (3) blood pressure provide

Table 2 Diagnosis of Syndrome X

Variable	Unlikely	Likely
Glucose (fasting)	<90 mg/dL	>105 <126 mg/dL
Glucose (120 min)	<140 mg/dL	140–200 mg/dL
Triglyceride	<125 mg/dL	>200 mg/dL
HDL cholesterol		
Men	>45 mg/dL	<35 mg/dL
Women	>55 mg/dL	<45 mg/dL
Blood pressure	<130/80 mm/Hg	>140/90 mmHg

an effective and economical way to search for syndrome X. If all of these values are perfectly normal, it is highly *unlikely* that the individual is either insulin resistant or hyperinsulinemic. On the other hand, Table 2 presents values that make it quite *likely* that an abnormality associated with insulin resistance and compensatory hyperinsulinemia exists, and provides the information necessary to initiate rational treatment of syndrome X.

V. TREATMENT OF SYNDROME X

Muscle and adipose tissue insulin resistance are the basic abnormalities leading to the manifestations of syndrome X and, therefore, it would seem reasonable that efforts to enhance insulin sensitivity would be the most fundamental therapeutic approach. On the other hand, this goal is more easily stated than achieved. The major obstacle is that the only established approaches involve changing behavior, an intervention that is not always successful.

A. Enhancing Insulin Sensitivity

There is considerable evidence that obesity and sedentary behavior decrease insulin sensitivity, and that weight loss and increased physical fitness will enhance insulin sensitivity.

1. Weight Loss

Insulin sensitivity will improve in insulin-resistant individuals with weight loss of as little as 10 to 15 pounds. In addition, there will be an improvement in CHD risk factors associated with insulin resistance/compensatory hyperinsulinemia. However, it is important to realize that not all overweight individuals are insulin resistant, and perhaps as many as 25% of overweight/obese individuals are normally insulin sensitive, without any of the manifestations of syndrome X. In this latter instance, weight loss has essentially no effect on insulin-mediated glucose disposal or any CHD risk factors associated with syndrome X. The obvious implication is that efforts to achieve weight loss in overweight/obese individuals should be focused on the subset that will benefit substantially from the intervention.

2. Physical Activity

An improvement in physical fitness will also enhance insulin sensitivity, and aerobic exercise for ~30 min, 3 to 4 times per week, is approximately as powerful as 10 to 15 pounds of weight loss in improving insulin action in insulin-resistant individuals. On the other hand, and in contrast to weight loss, the benefits of exercise programs disappear quite quickly if they are discontinued. It is also important to stress the potential dangers if inappropriate exercise programs are initiated. For all of these reasons, weight loss is probably a more pragmatic approach to enhancing insulin sensitivity than is a program of intensive physical activity. However, even if it is difficult to maintain the level of exercise necessary to significantly affect insulin-mediated glucose disposal, any increase in physical activity will potentiate the ability to lose weight and keep it off.

3. Thiazolidenedione (TZD) Compounds

The last few years have seen the introduction of three drugs that enhance insulin-mediated glucose disposal in patients with type 2 diabetes. Two of these, rosiglitazone and pioglitazone, currently have FDA approval as antihyperglycemic agents, and it is likely that additional compounds of this class will be introduced. There is every reason to believe that TZD compounds would be of substantial clinical benefit in patients with syndrome X, and there is some evidence that several specific manifestations of syndrome X will improve with TZD therapy. However, whether the use of TZD compounds will eventually be shown to reduce CHD in patients with syndrome X awaits the results of the intervention studies necessary to evaluate this possibility. Until such time, the use of TZD compounds in nondiabetic subjects should be limited to approved research studies.

B. Overcoming the Manifestations of Syndrome X

Although therapeutic efforts aimed at enhancing insulin sensitivity may be limited, there is no reason to adopt a nihilistic approach to attenuating the CHD risk factors in patients with syndrome X. Indeed, there are both dietary and pharmacological interventions that can substantially reduce the manifestations of syndrome X.

1. Macronutrient Composition

As indicated earlier, weight loss will significantly improve insulin sensitivity in overweight, insulin-resistant individuals. However, not all overweight patients are able to lose weight, nor are all patients with syndrome X obese. In both of these situations, changes in macronutrient composition can be of substantial benefit.

Dietary recommendations to reduce CHD have until quite recently been based upon the principle that hypercholesterolemia (more specifically, an elevated LDL cholesterol level) is the only CHD risk factor that needs to be addressed. The result has been almost total emphasis on the use of low-fat–high-carbohydrate (CHO) diets. More to the point, advice to replace saturated fat (SF) with CHO in order to lower LDL cholesterol concentrations continues to be given, regardless of how insulin resistant the individual. Unfortunately, this dietary approach will make all of the manifestations of syndrome X worse. The greater the CHO content in an isocaloric diet, the more insulin must be secreted in order to maintain glucose homeostasis. This poses no danger to insulin-sensitive individuals, but low-SF/high-CHO diets will significantly increase the already high day-long plasma insulin concentrations in patients with syndrome X. As a consequence, fasting plasma TG concentrations will increase, as will the day-long postprandial accumulations of remnant lipoproteins. In addition, HDL cholesterol concentrations will further decrease, as will LDL particle diameter. In order to avoid this problem, SF should be replaced with monounsaturated (MUF) and polyunsaturated fat (PUF). This maneuver results in a fall in LDL cholesterol concentration as great as is seen with low-SF/high-CHO diets, without any untoward effects on the manifestations of syndrome X. Given this information, weight maintenance diets containing (as percent of total calories) approximately 15% protein, 40% fat (<10% SF, ~20% MUF, and the rest as PUF), and 45% CHO will decrease LDL cholesterol concentrations without accentuating the manifestations of syndrome X.

2. Pharmacological Agents

There are effective drugs to address the abnormalities of lipoprotein metabolism present in patients with syndrome X, as well as to lower blood pressure when hypertension is one of the manifestations of syndrome X.

Dyslipidemia. The characteristic abnormality of lipoprotein metabolism in patients with syndrome X is hypertriglyceridemia, usually associated with a low-HDL cholesterol concentration, increased postprandial lipemia, and small, dense LDL particles. The use of fibric acid derivatives in patients with syndrome X will significantly lower plasma TG concentrations, as well as improve all of the abnormalities associated with hypertriglyceridemia. In addition, there is now evidence that the use of this class of drugs will decrease CHD risk in patients with the dyslipidemia associated with syndrome X.

Hypertension. Approximately 50% of patients with syndrome X have high blood pressure, and, as discussed previously, the risk of CHD is greatly increased in individuals when high blood pressure is one of the manifestations of syndrome X. Consequently, attention should be given to the choice of antihypertensive drugs in these individuals. Specifically, it seems reasonable to avoid the use of antihypertensive agents that will accentuate insulin resistance and/or its manifestations. However, it should be noted that low-dose thiazide diuretic therapy (12.5 mg of hydrochlorthiazide) is effective in lowering blood pressure, without untoward side effects on glucose or lipid metabolism, and that use of β-receptor antagonists is indicated in patients with a history of prior myocardial infarction.

Hypercholesterolemia. Although a high-LDL cholesterol concentration is not part of syndrome X, patients can have combined dyslipidemia (a high-TG and low-HDL concentration *plus* a high-LDL cholesterol concentration). These individuals are most at risk for CHD. As such, the need to lower LDL cholesterol concentration should not be ignored, and treatment with HMG CoA reductase inhibitors should be initiated if diet alone does not control LDL cholesterol concentrations in patients with syndrome X.

VI. CONCLUSION

The ability of insulin to stimulate glucose uptake varies widely from person to person. In an effort to maintain glucose homeostasis, the pancreatic β-cell will do its best to secrete whatever amount of insulin is required to accomplish this goal. If the β-cell cannot sustain this compensatory effort, type 2 diabetes supervenes. Although the pathophysiological consequences of the combination of insulin resistance and failing β-cell secretory function are clearly disastrous, the ability of insulin-resistant individuals to maintain normal or near-normal glucose tolerance by secreting large amounts of insulin is hardly benign. Specifically, it appears that the combination of insulin resistance and compensatory hyperinsulinemia predisposes individuals to develop the cluster of abnormalities described in this chapter—all of which increase risk of CHD. At this point, it is impossible to know if insulin resistance *per se*, or its downstream effects, are primarily responsible for accelerating the process of atherogenesis. Even more difficult is to try to separate the pathophysiological roles of insulin resistance versus hyperinsulinemia in this syndrome because the two phenomena are so closely linked physiologically. On the other hand, it is not difficult to suggest that the cluster of abnormalities associated with insulin resistance should be added to the list of traditional factors that increase risk of CHD. Indeed, even our view of traditional risk factors must be modified in view of recent evidence that smoking is associated with insulin resistance, hyperinsulinemia, and an increase in plasma TG and a decrease in HDL cholesterol concentrations. It should also be noted that the importance of insulin resistance and its consequence in the pathogenesis of CHD may be of particular relevance in individuals of non-European ancestry. For example, Asian Indians living in the U.K. have substantially more CHD than do individuals of European ancestry, associated with insulin resistance, hyperinsulinemia, increased plasma TG, and decreased HDL cholesterol concentrations.

In this chapter an effort has been made to explain what insulin resistance is, what the manifestations of insulin resistance/compensatory hyperinsulinemia are, and how they increase risk of CHD. In addition, a guide has been provided to the diagnosis, as well as to the outlines of a therapeutic approach for overcoming the CHD risk factors associated with syndrome X. Not until the fundamental role of insulin resistance in the genesis of both type 2 diabetes and CHD is recognized will it be possible both to stop the epidemic of type 2 diabetes and to more effectively decrease the prevalence of CHD.

SUGGESTED READING

1. Reaven GM. Role of insulin resistance in human disease. Diabetes 1998; 37:1595–1607.
2. Facchini F, Chen YD-I, Hollenbeck C, Reaven GM. Relationship between resistance to insulin-mediated glucose uptake, urinary uric acid clearance, and plasma uric acid concentration. JAMA 1991; 266:3008–3011.
3. Laws A, Reaven GM. Evidence for an independent relationship between insulin resistance and fasting plasma HDL-cholesterol, triglyceride and insulin concentrations. J Intern Med 1992; 231:25–30.
4. Reaven GM, Chen Y-DI, Jeppesen J, Maheux P, Krauss RM. Insulin resistance and hyperinsulinemia in individuals with small, dense, low density lipoprotein particles. J Clin Invest 1993; 92:141–146.
5. Juhan-Vague I, Thompson SG, Jespersen J, on behalf of the ECAT Angina Pectoris Study Group: Involvement of the hemostatic system in the insulin resistance syndrome. Arterioscler Thromb 1993; 13:1865–1873.
6. Reaven GM. Pathophysiology of insulin resistance in human disease. Physiol Rev 1995; 75:473–486.
7. Reaven GM. Hypertriglyceridemia: The central feature of Syndrome X. Cardiovasc Risk Factors 1996; 6:29–35.
8. Reaven GM, Lithell H, Landsberg L. Hypertension and associated metabolic abnormalities—the role of insulin resistance and the sympathoadrenal system. N Engl J Med 1996; 334:374–381.
9. Chen YD-I, Reaven GM. Insulin resistance and atherosclerosis. Diabetes Rev 1997; 5:331–342.

10. Reaven GM. The kidney: an unwilling accomplice in syndrome X. Am J Kidney Dis 1997; 30:928–931.

11. Reaven GM. Do high carbohydrate diets prevent the development or attenuate the manifestations (or both) of syndrome X? A viewpoint strongly against. Curr Opin Lipidol 1997; 8:23–27.

12. Yip J, Facchini FS, Reaven GM. Resistance to insulin-mediated glucose disposal as a predictor of cardiovascular disease. J Clin Endocrinol Metab 1998; 83:2773–2776.

13. Reaven GM. Insulin resistance and human disease: a short history. Clin Physiol Pharmacol 1998; 9:387–406.

14. Jeppesen J, Facchini FS, Reaven GM. Individuals with high total cholesterol/HDL cholesterol ratios are insulin resistant. J Intern Med 1998; 243:293–298.

15. Abbasi F, McLaughlin T, Lamendola C, Yeni-Komshian H, Tanaka A, Wang T, Nakajima K, Reaven GM. Fasting remnant lipoprotein cholesterol and triglyceride concentrations are elevated in nondiabetic, insulin-resistant, female volunteers. J Clin Endocrinol Metab 1999; 84:3903–3906.

16. Abbasi F, McLaughlin T, Lamendola C, Lipinska I, Tofler G, Reaven GM. Comparison of plasminogen activator inhibitor-1 concentration in insulin-resistant versus insulin-sensitive healthy women. Arterioscler Thromb Vasc Biol 1999; 19:2818–2821.

17. Chen N-G, Holmes M, Reaven GM. Relationship between insulin resistance, soluble adhesion molecules, and mononuclear cell binding in healthy volunteers. J Clin Endocrinol Metab 1999; 84:3485–3489.

18. Chen N-G, Abbasi F, Lamendola C, McLaughlin T, Cooke JP, Tsao PS, Reaven GM. Mononuclear cell adherence to cultured endothelium is enhanced by hypertension and insulin resistance in healthy nondiabetic volunteers. Circulation 1999; 100:940–943.

19. Abbasi F, McLaughlin T, Lamendola C, Kim H-S, Tanaka A, Wang T, Nakajima K, Reaven GM. High carbohydrate diets, triglyceride-rich lipoproteins, and coronary heart disease risk. Am J Cardiol 2000; 85:45–48.

20. Yeni-Komshian H, Carantoni M, Abbasi F, Reaven GM. Relationship between several surrogate estimates of insulin resistance and quantification of insulin-mediated glucose disposal in 490 healthy, nondiabetic volunteers. Diabetes Care 2000; 23:171–175.

8

Detection and Diagnosis of Syndromes of Insulin Resistance and of Diabetes Mellitus

Edward S. Horton
Joslin Diabetes Center, Harvard Medical School, Boston, Massachusetts

I. INTRODUCTION

In clinical practice, insulin resistance is defined as a state in which endogenously secreted or exogenously administered insulin has decreased effectiveness in regulating blood glucose. In this sense, "insulin resistance" is the opposite of "insulin sensitivity." Although insulin has many effects on cellular metabolism and on cell growth and differentiation that are mediated by distinct intracellular signaling pathways, it is a decreased sensitivity and responsiveness to insulin's action to stimulate glucose uptake in insulin-sensitive tissues such as skeletal muscle and adipose tissue and an impairment of its ability to decrease hepatic glucose output through inhibition of glycogenolysis and gluconeogenesis that constitute the clinical condition of insulin resistance. These effects are mediated by a cascade of phosphorylation reactions involving the insulin receptor, insulin receptor substrates (IRS-1 and IRS-2), and activation of the phosphoinositol 3' kinase (PI-3'-K) pathway. On the other hand, cell growth and differentiation are regulated primarily by the SHC, GRB-2, and the MAP-kinase pathways, which may or may not be resistant to insulin action and may actually exhibit increased activity as a result of compensatory hyperinsulinemia in insulin-resistant individuals. Thus, differential insulin resistance may exist with decreased insulin action on glucose uptake and metabolism and increased effects of insulin on cell growth and differentiation occurring simultaneously.

II. CAUSES OF INSULIN RESISTANCE

Insulin resistance may be caused by rare genetic defects that alter insulin binding to its cellular receptors or cause defects in receptor or postreceptor signal transduction (1). Recently, defects in the nuclear receptor, PPARγ, have also been linked to syndromes of severe insulin resistance (2). In addition, some endocrine-metabolic syndromes, such as Cushing's syndrome, acromegaly, and polycystic ovary syndrome, are associated with insulin resistance because of the hormonal imbalances associated with these conditions. However, in the most common forms of insulin resistance, single gene defects have not been identified and the development of insulin resistance represents a complex interaction among a poorly understood array of predisposing genetic factors and acquired environmental factors that modify insulin sensitivity. Among the latter, the most prominent are obesity (particularly intra-abdominal obesity), physical inactivity, and increasing age. It is also now well documented that metabolic abnormalities such as chronic elevations of plasma glucose or free fatty acids (FFA), as well as increases in tissue triglycerides, can lead to insulin resistance (3,4). This has led to the concepts of glucotoxicity and lipotoxicity, both of which are reversible with improved metabolic status. Although the mechanism by which chronic elevation of glucose results in insulin resistance is not fully understood, it is most likely related to changes in glucose transporter number and function as well as to changes in the activity of the PI-3'-K signaling pathway in insulin-sensitive tissues. Chronic elevation of FFAs, on the other hand, has multiple metabolic effects that both inhibit glucose utilization in peripheral tissues and increase hepatic glucose production through enhanced gluconeogenesis. In addition, intracellular triglyceride accumulation is associated with decreased insulin action in insulin-sensitive tissues. Yet another mechanism by which increased body fat accumulation may cause insulin resistance is through increased production of adipose tissue hormones such as TNF-α (5), which has an inhibitory effect on insulin action. Finally, various medications may cause insulin resistance. These include treatment with hormones such as glucocorticoids, growth hormone, progestational agents, high doses of androgens and anabolic steroids, or commonly used agents such as beta-adrenergic agonists or nicotinic acid.

III. INSULIN RESISTANCE AND GLUCOSE METABOLISM

When insulin resistance is present, fasting and postprandial blood glucose concentrations are maintained in the normal range by a compensatory increase in insulin secretion and the development of hyperinsulinemia. As long as the pancreatic beta cell is able to compensate adequately, glucose tolerance remains normal. However, if beta-cell function is inadequate, impaired glucose tolerance (IGT) may develop. This is characterized by the maintenance of a normal fasting blood glucose concentration but a value that is intermediate between normal and the diabetic range 2 h after a 75-g oral glucose load. With further impairment of beta-cell function, both fasting and postprandial blood glucose concentrations increase and overt diabetes mellitus develops. This sequence of events has been demonstrated in prospective studies of insulin resistance and beta-cell function in several populations, including studies of Pima Indians who have either progressed sequentially from normal glucose tolerance to IGT and then to diabetes or who have maintained normal glucose tolerance (NGT) over several years (6). In those who progressed to diabetes, there was only a modest increase in insulin resistance over time, whereas a marked decrease in beta-cell function occurred. In contrast, those who did not progress maintained adequate beta-cell function to compensate for their worsening insulin resistance.

It is now clear from the United Kingdom Prospective Diabetes Study (UKPDS) that once type 2 diabetes is established, it becomes progressively more difficult to control over time, often requiring combinations of oral antidiabetic agents and/or insulin therapy (7,8). This is due largely to a progressive loss of beta-cell function, which is insufficient to overcome the underlying insulin resistance. Thus, insulin resistance is a fundamental underpinning of an entire spectrum of glucose intolerance from NGT with compensatory hyperinsulinemia, to IGT or full-blown type 2 diabetes with progressive loss of pancreatic beta-cell function.

IV. THE INSULIN RESISTANCE SYNDROME

Insulin resistance and hyperinsulinemia are frequently associated with a cluster of clinical and biochemical abnormalities that have been described with increasing detail and given a variety of names including deadly quartet, syndrome X, insulin resistance syndrome, metabolic syndrome, and cardiovascular dysmetabolic syndrome (9–13). Many prefer to call it insulin resistance syndrome because insulin resistance and the resulting hyperinsulinemia appear to be the underlying abnormalities from which the other features of the syndrome are derived (see Chap. 7). The hallmarks of insulin resistance syndrome are obesity, particularly central or intra-abdominal obesity, glucose intolerance, or type 2 diabetes mellitus, hypertension, a dyslipidemia characterized by elevated triglycerides, low HDL cholesterol and small dense LDL cholesterol, a hypercoagulable state characterized by alterations in both thrombosis and fibrinolysis and increased atherosclerosis manifesting as coronary artery disease, peripheral vascular disease, or stroke (14–25). More recently, the polycystic ovary syndrome (PCOS) has been added to the list of characteristic features of the insulin resistance syndrome in women (25). From a clinical viewpoint, the syndrome should be suspected in anyone who has a personal or a family history of obesity, type 2 diabetes mellitus, hypertension, dyslipidemia, or premature cardiovascular disease. It should also be looked for in women with a history of gestational diabetes mellitus (GDM) or PCOS and members of various ethnic and racial groups that have increased risk for obesity and type 2 diabetes.

One of the most common manifestations of insulin resistance syndrome is the combination of obesity and type 2 diabetes mellitus. In the United States, approximately 80% of people with type 2 diabetes mellitus are overweight, defined as a body mass index (BMI) > 27 kg/m^2, and the current rapid rate of increase in the prevalence of type 2 diabetes mellitus is closely linked to the increasing prevalence of obesity and physical inactivity in our society (26). It is estimated that there are now approximately 16 million people in the United States with type 2 diabetes mellitus, about 5 million of whom are undiagnosed, and another 10 million adults who have IGT and are at high risk for developing diabetes. The prevalence of type 2 diabetes mellitus is increasing at all ages from adolescence to the elderly, with the most rapid rates of increase being observed in the younger age groups. In addition to obesity and physical inactivity as risk factors for diabetes, genetic factors also clearly play an important role, making a detailed family history an important part of the assessment. It is now well established that various racial-ethnic groups are at increased risk of developing type 2 diabetes, including African Americans, Hispanic Americans, Native Americans, Asian Americans, and Pacific Islanders, all of whom have significantly higher rates of developing type 2 diabetes than the Caucasian population (27–30). As noted above, women who have a history of gestational diabetes (GDM) or who have polycystic ovary syndrome (PCOS) often have insulin resistance and are at increased risk for developing type 2 diabetes mellitus (25).

In addition to evaluating patients for their state of glucose homeostasis (see below), one should also look for the other manifestations of insulin resistance syndrome, including acanthosis nigricans, mild-to-moderate hypertension, dyslipidemia, and evidence of premature atherosclerosis and cardiovascular disease.

A cluster of biochemical abnormalities is frequently associated with insulin resistance syndrome. These include a characteristic dyslipidemia consisting of elevated serum triglycerides and very-low-density lipoproteins (VLDL), a decrease in high-density-lipoprotein cholesterol (HDL-C), and a pattern of small, dense, low-density-lipoprotein (LDL) particles (31–34). Serum uric acid is often increased and, if measured, plasma FFA may be high. Fasting plasma glucose may be normal, intermediate (impaired fasting glucose), or in the diabetic range, but fasting insulin and C-peptide concentrations are usually elevated in relation to the degree of glycemia.

The insulin resistance syndrome is also associated with a hypercoagulable state characterized by a combination of procoagulant and antithrombolytic factors (35,36). Plasma fibrinogen is increased as is Von Willibrand factor (vWF) and plasminogen activity inhibitor 1 (PAI-1). Tissue plasminogen activator (tPA) is decreased and several studies have demonstrated impaired endothelial function and vascular reactivity in patients with insulin resistance syndrome (37,38).

While the mechanisms for the development of atherosclerosis in insulin resistance syndrome are complex and not yet fully understood, there is now substantial evidence that a chronic inflammatory process plays a significant role (39). Increases in endothelial cell–derived leukocyte adhesion molecules, such as intercellular adhesion molecule (ICAM) and vascular cell adhesion molecule (VCAM), are increased as are proinflammatory cytokines such as interleuken-6 (IL-6), TNF-α, and the acute phase-reactant C-reactive protein (CRP) (40,41).

Another commonly observed abnormality in insulin resistance syndrome is elevated serum homocystine, which may reflect altered oxidative stress mechanisms that may contribute to accelerated atherosclerosis (42). Finally, a possible role of insulin itself, particularly its effects on cell growth and differentiation, continues to be examined. The potential benefit of measuring any of the above so-called "nontraditional" risk factors for coronary artery disease in evaluating a patient with insulin resistance syndrome is still unclear. Many of the biochemical markers of these processes are not readily available (or standardized) in clinical laboratories and more research is needed to determine how useful they will be in clinical practice. However, studies of endothelial dysfunction, altered coagulation and fibrinolysis, chronic inflammation, or oxidative stress are providing many new insights into the pathobiology of the vascular disease associated with insulin resistance and diabetes.

V. DETECTION AND DIAGNOSIS OF ABNORMAL GLUCOSE METABOLISM IN INSULIN RESISTANCE SYNDROME

In 1997, the American Diabetes Association Expert Committee on the Diagnosis and Classification of Diabetes Mellitus established a new classification system and diagnostic criteria to define various states of abnormal glucose metabolism (43). Fasting plasma glucose was divided into three diagnostic categories: (1) normal < 110 mg/dL (6.1 mmol/L); (2) impaired fasting glucose (IFG) 110 to 125 mg/dL (6.1 to 6.9 mmol/L); and (3) diabetes mellitus ≥ 126 mg/dL (7.0 mmol/L). Likewise, the plasma glucose 2 h after a 75-g oral glucose load (OGTT) was used to define three diagnostic categories: (1) normal glucose tolerance < 140 mg/dL (7.8 mmol/L); (2) impaired glucose tolerance 140 to 199 mg/dL (7.8 to 11.1 mmol/L); and (3) diabetes mellitus ≥ 200 mg/dL (11.1 mmol/L). Diabetes can also be diagnosed by a casual plasma glucose ≥ 200 mg/dL (11.1 mmol/L) in conjunction with classic symptoms of diabetes, including polyuria, polydipsia, and unexplained weight loss. To establish a diagnosis of diabetes using either the fasting or 2-h OGTT plasma glucose criteria, the result must be confirmed by repeat testing on another day.

The rationale used for establishing these diagnostic categories is that several studies have demonstrated a close, although not perfect, association between a fasting plasma glucose concentration of 126 mg/dL and the 2-h OGTT value of 200 mg/dL and both of these levels correlate well with the appearance of microvascular complications of diabetes including retinopathy, nephropathy, and neuropathy. It is also recognized that IFG and IGT are both conditions that are associated with an increased risk of developing overt type 2 diabetes mellitus and an increased risk for cardiovascular disease. Although these criteria are based solely on measurements of plasma glucose, they do, in fact, reflect the interaction between insulin resistance and pancreatic beta-cell function as described previously. There is now great interest in examining the effects of lifestyle modifications that emphasize weight reduction and increased physical exercise or treatment with medications that decrease insulin resistance, enhance insulin secretion, or work through other mechanisms to prevent or delay progression from IGT to diabetes in high-risk individuals.

VI. MEASUREMENT OF INSULIN RESISTANCE

Several methods have been used to assess insulin resistance, but most are not readily available or practical for use in clinical practice. The easiest approach is to measure fasting plasma glucose and insulin concentrations or the glucose and insulin responses during an OGTT or test meal. The higher the insulin concentration in relation to the glucose level, the more insulin resistant the subject. One can also obtain similar information by measuring the C-peptide concentration in the fasting and stimulated states. Various methods have been developed to analyze glucose and insulin data, one of the most widely used being the homeostasis model (HOMA) that is most effectively used in large-population studies to assess insulin resistance and beta-cell function (44,45). A major drawback for using plasma insulin concentrations from individual patients is the wide range of normal values and lack of standardization of insulin assays used by clinical laboratories, both of which make interpretation of data difficult.

In a clinical research setting, insulin resistance is most commonly measured using the hyperinsulinemic glucose clamp technique (46) or the frequently sampled intravenous glucose tolerance test (FSIGT) using the minimal model method of Bergman (47–49). Both of these methods provide adequate measurements of insulin sensitivity in individual subjects, but they are both time consuming and difficult to perform and are not practical for routine clinical use. In the final analysis, the best way to identify patients with insulin resistance syndrome is to do so on the basis of the clinical features (i.e., the constellation of obesity, hypertension, dyslipidemia, IGT, or type 2 diabetes and accelerated atherosclerosis and cardiovascular disease).

VII. APPROACH TO TREATMENT

The most important thing to remember is that patients with insulin resistance syndrome are at increased risk for developing type 2 diabetes mellitus and accelerated atherosclerosis. Coronary artery disease (CAD) is the leading cause of death in patients with the insulin resistance syndrome, accounting for approximately 60% of mortality, and cerebrovascular and peripheral vascular disease also contribute significantly to mortality and morbidity. Therefore, the major goals of therapy are to prevent or treat diabetes and its complications and to reduce cardiovascular risk. Since obesity and physical inactivity are major contributing factors to insulin resistance, changes in lifestyle that emphasize weight reduction and regular exercise may be expected to reduce many features of the syndrome and should be a fundamental part of the treatment program.

Previous studies in China (50) and in Finland (51) have demonstrated that the incidence of progression from IGT to overt diabetes is significantly reduced by relatively modest decreases in body weight and increased physical activity and the recent announcement of the results of the NIH-sponsored Diabetes Prevention Program (DPP) (52) strongly supports the use of lifestyle modification to decrease the risk of developing diabetes in the U.S. population at risk by virtue of having IGT. In this study, a sustained weight loss of 10 to 15 pounds and an increase in exercise equivalent to brisk walking for 30 min 6 to 7 days a week reduced the risk of developing type 2 diabetes by 58% for at least 3 years. It is also encouraging that treatment with metformin also decreased the progression from IGT to type 2 diabetes mellitus by 31% in the DPP, although it was not as effective as weight reduction and increased physical activity. Several other studies are currently being conducted to determine if other medications, such as thiazolidenediones, insulin secretogues, or angiotensin receptor blockers may also be effective in treating insulin resistance syndrome, reducing cardiovascular risk, and preventing progression to overt diabetes.

It is also very important to keep in mind that, in addition to preventing and/or treating type 2 diabetes mellitus, all other aspects of insulin resistance syndrome should be treated aggressively to reduce the risk of cardiovascular disease. New targets for blood pressure and lipid (53) management have been established recently and it is recommended that, unless contraindicated, all patients with type 2 diabetes mellitus should be treated with aspirin to reduce the risk of myocardial infarction. Many studies have demonstrated that controlling blood pressure markedly decreases the risk of both micro- and macrovascular complications of type 2 diabetes mellitus (54) and a target blood pressure of

130/80 mmHg is now accepted for most patients. It is also clear that patients with diabetes respond well to lipid-lowering therapy with HMG CoA reductase inhibitors (statins) and fibric acid derivatives, often showing better reductions in cardiovascular events and death rates than patients without diabetes. Detailed approaches to treatment of diabetes and reduction in cardiovascular risk are presented in subsequent chapters and will not be discussed here.

VIII. SUMMARY

In summary, insulin resistance is the result of the interactions among multiple predisposing genetic factors that are not yet fully understood and a number of associated factors that decrease the effectiveness of insulin to regulate glucose uptake and metabolism in insulin-sensitive tissues such as skeletal muscle, adipose tissue, and the liver. Major factors contributing to insulin resistance are obesity, physical inactivity, and advancing age, although other conditions such as chronically elevated glucose and free fatty acids, increased intracellular triglycerides, and various endocrinopathies or medications may also play a role.

Insulin resistance must be differentiated from insulin resistance syndrome, which is characterized by a cluster of associated abnormalities that include hypertension, dyslipidemia, hyperuricemia, altered thrombosis and fibrinolysis, evidence of chronic inflammation, and accelerated atherosclerosis. Coronary artery disease and other macrovascular diseases are the major cause of mortality and morbidity in patients with insulin resistance syndrome, and cardiovascular risk reduction should be a major goal of therapy. Screening for and aggressive management of all aspects of insulin resistance syndrome are critical to reducing long-term micro- and macrovascular complications. Recent trials have also demonstrated the feasibility for preventative strategies based on lifestyle modification with emphasis on weight reduction and increased physical activity or the use of insulin-sensitizing medications.

REFERENCES

1. Kahn CR, Flier JS, Bar RS, Archer JA, Gordon P, Martin MM, Roth J. The syndromes of insulin resistance and acanthosis nigricans. N Engl J Med 1976; 294: 739–745.
2. Barroso I, Gurnell M, Crowley VEF, Agostini M, Schwabe JW, Soos MA, Maslen GL, Williams TDM, Lewis H, Schafer AH, Chatterjee VKK, O'Rahilly SO. Dominant negative mutations in human PPARγ associated with severe insulin resistance, diabetes mellitus and hypertension. A letter. Nature 1999; 402:880–883.
3. Henry RR. Glucose control and insulin resistance in non-insulin dependent diabetes mellitus. Ann Intern Med 1999; 124:97–103.

4. Boden G. Role of fatty acids in the pathogenesis of insulin resistance and NIDDM. Diabetes 1997; 46:3–10.
5. Hotamisligil GS, Shargill NS, Spiegelman BM. Adipose expression of tumor necrosis factor α: direct role in obesity-linked insulin resistance. Science 1993; 259: 87–91.
6. Weyer C, Bogardus C, Mott DM, Pratley RE. The natural history of insulin secretory dysfunction and insulin resistance in the pathogenesis of type 2 diabetes mellitus. J Clin Invest 1999; 104:787–794.
7. UK Prospective Diabetes Study Group. Intensive blood glucose control with sulphonylureas or insulin compared with conventional treatment and risk of complications in patients with type 2 diabetes (UKPDS 33). Lancet 1998; 352:837–853.
8. UK Prospective Diabetes Study Group. Effect of intensive blood glucose control with metformin on complications in overweight patients with type 2 diabetes (UKPDS 34). Lancet 1998; 352:854–865.
9. Reaven GM. Role of insulin resistance in human disease. Diabetes 1988; 37:1495–1607.
10. Opara JU, Levine JH. The deadly quartet—the insulin resistance syndrome. Southern Med J 1997; 90(12):1162–1168.
11. DeFronzo RA, Ferrannini E. Insulin resistance: a multifaceted syndrome responsible for NIDDM, obesity, hypertension, dyslipidemia, and atherosclerotic cardiovascular disease. Diabetes Care 1991; 14:173–194.
12. Liese AD, Mayer-Davis EJ, Troler HA, Davis CE, Keil U, Schmidt MI, Brancati FL, Heiss G. Familial components of the multiple metabolic syndrome: the ARIC Study. Diabetologia 1997; 40:963–970.
13. Fagan TC, Deedwania PC. The cardiovascular dysmetabolic syndrome. Am J Med 1998; 105:77S–82A.
14. Ferrannini E, Buzzigoli G, Bonadonna R, Giorico MA, Oleggini M, Graziadei L, Pedrinelli R, Brandi L, Bevilacqua S. Insulin resistance in essential hypertension. N Engl J Med 1987; 317:350–357.
15. Shen D-C, Shieh S-M, Fuh M, Wu D-A, Chen Y-DI, Reaven GM. Resistance to insulin-stimulated glucose uptake in patients with hypertension. J Clin Endocrinol Metab 1988; 66:580–583.
16. Reaven GM, Lithell H, Landsberg L. Hypertension and associated metabolic abnormalities: the role of insulin resistance and the sympathoadrenal system. N Engl J Med 1996; 334:374–381.
17. Chen Y-DI, Reaven G. Insulin resistance and atherosclerosis. Diabetes Rev 1997; 5(4):331–342.
18. Humphries DB, Stewart MW, Berrish TS, Barriocanal LA, Trajano LR, Ashworth LA, Brown MD, Miller M, Avery PJ, Alberti KGMM, Walker M. Multiple metabolic abnormalities in normal glucose tolerant relatives of NIDDM families. Diabetologia 1997; 40:1185–1190.
19. Haffner SM, Stern MP, Hazuda HP, Braxton DM, Patterson JK, Ferrannini E. Parental history of diabetes is associated with increased cardiovascular factors. Arteriosclerosis 1989; 9:928–933.
20. Haffner SM. The insulin resistance syndrome revisited. Diabetes Care 1996; 19: 275–277.

21. Olefsky JM, Kolterman OG, Scarlett JA. Insulin action and resistance in obesity and non-insulin dependent type 2 diabetes mellitus. Am J Physiol 1982; 243:E15–E30.

22. Gray RS, Fabsitz RR, Cowan LD, Lee ET, Howard BV, Savage PJ. Risk factor clustering in the insulin resistance syndrome: the Strong Heart Study. Am J Epidemiol 1998; 148:869–878.

23. Ferrannini E, Haffner SM, Mitchell BD, Stern MP. Hyperinsulinaemia: the key feature of a cardiovascular and metabolic syndrome. Diabetologia 1991; 34:416–422.

24. Juhan-Vague I, Thompson SG, Jespersen J. Involvement of the hemostatic system in the insulin resistance syndrome: a study of the 1,500 patients with angina pectoris. Arterioscler Thromb 1993; 13:1865–1873.

25. Dunaif A. Insulin resistance and the polycystic ovary syndrome: mechanism and implications for pathogenesis. Endocr Rev 1997; 18(6):774–800.

26. Mokdad AH, Ford ES, Bowman BA, Nelson DE, Engelgau, MM, Vinicor F, Marks JS. Diabetes trends in the US: 1990–1998. Diabetes Care 2000; 23:1278–1283.

27. Karter, AJ, Mayer-Davis EJ, Selby JV, D'Agostino Jr. RB, Haffner SM, Sholinsky P, Bergman R, Saad MF, Hamman RF. Insulin sensitivity and abdominal obesity in African-American, Hispanic, and non-Hispanic white men and women. The insulin resistance and atherosclerosis study. Diabetes 1996; 45:1547–1555.

28. Laws A, Jeppesen JL, Maheux PC, Schaaf P, Chen Y-DI, Reaven GM. Resistance to insulin stimulated glucose uptake and dyslipidemia in Asian Indians. Arterioscler Thromb 1994; 14:917–922.

29. Harris MI, Hadden WC, Knowler WC et al. Prevalence of diabetes mellitus and impaired glucose tolerance and plasma glucose levels in US population aged 20–74 years. Diabetes 1987; 36:523–534.

30. Haffner SM, Hazuda HP, Mitchell BD et al. Increased incidence of type 2 diabetes mellitus in Mexican Americans. Diabetes Care 1991; 14:102–108.

31. Reaven GM, Chen Y-DI, Jeppesen J, Maheux P, Krauss RM Insulin resistance and hyperinsulinemia in individuals with small, dense, low density lipoprotein particles. J Clin Invest 1993; 92:141–146.

32. American Diabetes Association. Consensus development conference on insulin resistance. Diabetes Care 1997; 21(2):310–314.

33. DeFronzo RA, Ferrannini E. Insulin resistance: a multifaceted syndrome responsible for NIDDM, obesity, hypertension, dyslipidemia, and atherosclerotic cardiovascular disease. Diabetes Care 1991; 14:173–194.

34. Haffner SM, Mykkanen L, Festa A, Burke JP, Stern MP. Insulin resistant prediabetic subjects have more atherogenic risk factors than insulin sensitive prediabetic subjects: implications for preventing coronary heart disease during the prediabetic state. Circulation 2000; 101:975–980.

35. Imperatore G, Riccardi G, Iovine C, Rivellese AA, Vaccaro O. Plasma fibrinogen: a new factor of the metabolic syndrome: a population-based study. Diabetes Care 1998; 21:649–654.

36. Juhan-Vague I, Alessel MC, Vague P. Increased plasma plasminogen activator inhibitor 1 levels: a possible link between insulin resistance and atherothrombosis. Diabetologia 1997; 34:457–462.

37. Caballero AE, Subodh A, Saouaf R, Lim SC, Smakowski P, Park JY, King GL,

LoGerfo FW, Horton ES, Veves A. Microvascular and macrovascular reactivity is reduced in subjects at risk for type 2 diabetes. Diabetes 1999; 48:1856–1862.

38. Balletshofer BM, Rittig K, Enderle MD, Volk A, Maerker E, Jacob S, Matthaei S, Rett K, Haring HU. Endothelial dysfunction is detectable in young normotensive first-degree relatives of subjects with type 2 diabetes in association with insulin resistance. Circulation 2000; 101:1780–1784.

39. Festa A, D'Agostino Jr R, Howard G, Mykkanen, L, Tracy RP, Haffner SM. Chronic subclinical inflammation as part of the insulin resistance syndrome. Circulation 2000; 102:42–47.

40. Pickup JC, Mattock MB, Chusny GD, Burt D. NIDDM as a disease of the innate immune system: association of acute-phase reactants and interleukin 6 with metabolic syndrome X. Diabetologia 1997; 40:1286–1292.

41. Frohlich M, Imhof A, Berg G, Hutchinson WL, Pepys MB, Boeing H, Muche R, Brenner H, Koenig W. Association between C-reactive protein and features of the metabolic syndrome. Diabetes Care 2000; 23:1835–1839.

42. Mallinow MR, Bostom AG, Krauss RM. Homocyst(e)ine, diet, and cardiovascular diseases. A statement for healthcare professionals from the Nutrition Committee, American Heart Association. Circulation 1999; 99:178–182.

43. The Expert Committee on the Diagnosis and Classification of Diabetes. Report of the Expert Committee on the Diagnosis and Classification of Diabetes Mellitus. Diabetes Care 2001; 24(1):S5–S20.

44. Matthews DR, Hosker JP, Rudenski AS, Naylor BA, Treacher DF, Turner RL, Homeostatis model assessment: insulin resistance and β cell function from fasting plasma glucose and insulin concentrations in man. Diabetologia 1985; 28:412–419.

45. Haffner SM, Miettinen H, Stern MP. The homeostasis model in the San Antonio Heart Study. Diabetes Care 1997; 20(7):1087–1092.

46. DeFronzo RA, Tobin JD, Andres R. Glucose clamp technique: a method for quantifying insulin secretion and resistance. Am J Physiol 1979; 237:E214–223.

47. Bergman RN, Phillips LS, Cobelli C. Physiologic evaluation of factors controlling glucose tolerance in men: measurement of insulin sensitivity and β cell glucose sensitivity from the response to intravenous glucose. J Clin Invest 1981; 68:1456–1467.

48. Bergman RN, Prager R, Volund A, Olefsky JM. Equivalence of the insulin sensitivity index in man derived by the minimal model method and the euglycemic glucose clamp. J Clin Invest 1987; 79:790–800.

49. Kahn SE, Prigeon RL, McCulloch DK, Boyko EJ, Bergman RN, Schwartz MW, Neifing JL, Ward WK, Beard JC, Palmer JP, Porte D. Quantification of the relationship between insulin sensitivity and β cell function in human subjects: evidence for a hyperbolic function. Diabetes 1993; 42:1663–1672.

50. Pan XR, Li GW, Hu YH, et al. Effects of diet and exercise in preventing NIDDM in people with impaired glucose tolerance: the Da Qing IGT and Diabetes Study. Diabetes Care 1997; 20:537–544.

51. Tuomilehto J, Lindstrom J, Eriksson JG, Valle TT, Hamalainen H, Ilanne-Parikka P, Keinanen-Kiukaanniemi S, Laakso M, Louheranta A, Rastas M, Salminen V, Uusitupa M. Prevention of type 2 diabetes mellitus by changes in lifestyle among subjects with impaired glucose tolerance. N Engl J Med 2001; 344:1343–1350.

52. The Diabetes Prevention Program Research Group. The Diabetes Prevention Pro-

gram: baseline characteristics of the randomized cohort. Diabetes Care 2000; 23: 1619–1629.

53. National Cholesterol Education Program Expert Panel. Third report on detection, evaluation and treatment of high blood cholesterol in adults (adult treatment panel 3). NIH publication 2000; 01–3670.

54. Adler AI, Stratton IM, Neil HAW, Yudkin JS, Matthews DR. Cull CA, et al. Association of systolic blood pressure with macrovascular and microvascular complications of type 2 diabetes (UKPDS) prospective observational study. Br Med J 2000; 321: 412–419.

9

Polycystic Ovary Syndrome, Insulin Resistance, and Cardiovascular Disease

Matthew C. Corcoran and David A. Ehrmann
University of Chicago Pritzker School of Medicine, Chicago, Illinois

I. INTRODUCTION

Polycystic ovary syndrome (PCOS) affects up to 10% of women of reproductive age (1,2), making it one of the most common endocrine disorders in this age group. Insulin resistance and hyperinsulinemia appear to be central to the pathogenesis of both the reproductive and metabolic aberrations that characterize the syndrome. This chapter focuses on the metabolic components of PCOS, particularly those which may impart risk for development of cardiovascular disease: obesity, impaired glucose tolerance and type 2 diabetes mellitus, hypertension, dyslipidemia, and obstructive sleep apnea.

II. OBESITY

Obesity is observed in 30 to 50% of women with PCOS (3,4) and was present in most of the patients originally described by Stein and Leventhal in 1935 (5). In addition, women with PCOS typically have an "android" pattern of obesity, indicative of a relative increase in visceral adiposity. The finding of an increased waist-to-hip ratio or other more sophisticated imaging measure of body fat distribution can serve as a surrogate measure of increased visceral fat depots. This pattern of distribution of body fat has been associated with elevated androgen levels as well as with abnormalities in glucose tolerance, insulin secretion, and lipoprotein profiles (6,7).

Obesity contributes to the insulin resistance in PCOS. However, the magnitude of insulin resistance exceeds that which would be predicted on the basis of total or even fat-free body mass (8). The cause of obesity in PCOS remains enigmatic. One possible explanation is that hyperinsulinemia exerts a lipogenic effect. Another possibility is that the anovulatory lack of progesterone predisposes to abdominal obesity and a change in muscle fiber type, both of which have deleterious metabolic consequences (9).

It has been reported that relative to controls matched for weight and body fat distribution, postprandial thermogenesis is reduced in women with PCOS and is associated with increased insulin resistance (10). However, the magnitude of the reduction in postprandial thermogenesis appears to be insufficient to account for the degree of the obesity in most PCOS patients. Insulin resistance has also been implicated in retarding the ability to reduce weight in response to a hypocaloric diet. A recent report (11), however, has documented that differences in insulin resistance do not predict weight loss in response to hypocaloric diets in healthy obese women. Whether this finding is applicable to women with PCOS remains unanswered.

Nonetheless, it has been clearly documented that attenuation of insulin resistance, whether by weight loss or pharmacologically with diazoxide, metformin, or troglitazone, ameliorates many of the metabolic aberrations in women with PCOS (12).

III. IMPAIRED GLUCOSE TOLERANCE AND TYPE 2 DIABETES

Obesity is a well-recognized risk-factor for development of type 2 diabetes, but alone is insufficient to cause glucose intolerance. Thus, while it is generally accepted that women with PCOS are predisposed to type 2 diabetes (13,14), the development of diabetes cannot be attributed solely to the obesity that typically accompanies PCOS.

Initial studies placed the prevalence of diabetes in PCOS at approximately 20% (8). More recent data have established that the prevalence of impaired glucose tolerance and type 2 diabetes mellitus among women with PCOS is even higher, with consistency across populations of varied ethnic and racial backgrounds (14,15). In two recent, large prospective studies, the prevalence of IGT was between 30 to 40% and that of type 2 diabetes between 5 to 10% (14,15). These prevalences approximate those in Pima Indians who have one of the highest rates of diabetes in the world (16). Evidence for an enhanced rate of development of diabetes is also evident from long-term follow-up of women with PCOS (17).

More recently, we have found a nearly five- to tenfold increase in the expected conversion rate from IGT to type 2 diabetes in PCOS (14,18). What factors underlie this predisposition to type 2 diabetes in PCOS? There is much to support a key role for insulin resistance. As noted, the magnitude of insulin resistance is greater in women with PCOS than in carefully matched controls (19–21). A distinct, and possibly selective (22), form of insulin resistance may account for these findings. Fibroblasts isolated from women with PCOS exhibit decreased insulin receptor autophosphorylation, both basally and in response to insulin stimulation (23). Phosphoaminoacid analysis has revealed a decrease in insulin-dependent receptor tyrosine phosphorylation and increased insulin-dependent receptor serine phosphorylation (23). The relative increase in serine phosphorylation could account, at least in part, for the post-receptor defect in insulin action since it has been shown that insulin receptor serine phosphorylation decreases the receptor's tyrosine kinase activity (24). In addition, it has been proposed that the presence of such defects in ex vivo cell culture of fibroblasts supports a genetic, rather than acquired, basis for insulin resistance (21).

Even though a substantial proportion of women with PCOS develop glucose intolerance, the majority do not, thus making it reasonable to ask whether the defects in insulin action described above are sufficient to account for the high prevalence of diabetes in this population. Specifically, what factors distinguish insulin-resistant women with PCOS who develop glucose intolerance from those who are able to maintain normoglycemia?

Insulin secretory defects play an important role in the propensity to develop diabetes in PCOS. Initial evidence for β-cell dysfunction in PCOS was derived from analyses of basal and postprandial insulin secretory responses in women with PCOS relative to weight-matched controls with normal androgen levels (25). The incremental insulin secretory response to meals was markedly reduced in women with PCOS, resulting from a reduction in the relative amplitude of meal-related secretory pulses rather than from a reduction in the number of pulses present. This pattern, which resembled that of type 2 diabetes more than that of simple obesity (26,27), was striking in that it was evident in these nondiabetic women with PCOS.

It was subsequently reported that women with PCOS had similar, or even exaggerated (28), acute insulin responses during a modified IVGTT, leading some to conclude that β-cell function was normal in PCOS. However, insulin secretion is most appropriately expressed in relation to the magnitude of ambient insulin resistance. The product of these measures can be quantitated (the so-called "disposition index") and related as a percentile to the hyperbolic relationship for these measures established in normal subjects (29). In so doing, we (13), as well as others (30), have found that a subset of PCOS subjects has β-cell secretory dysfunction. In absolute terms, women with PCOS had normal first-phase insulin secretion compared to controls. In contrast, when first-phase insulin secretion was analyzed in relation to the degree of insulin resistance, women with PCOS exhibited a significant impairment in β-cell function. This reduction was particularly marked in women with PCOS who had a first-degree relative with type 2 diabetes: the mean disposition index of women with PCOS and a family history of type 2 diabetes was in the eighth percentile, while that of those without such a family history was in the thirty-third percentile ($p < 0.05$). We have additionally quantitated β-cell function in PCOS by examining the insulin secretory response to a graded increase in plasma glucose and by the ability of the β-cell to adjust and respond to induced oscillations in the plasma glucose level (13). Results from both provocative stimuli were consistent: when expressed in relation to the degree of insulin resistance, insulin secretion was impaired in PCOS subjects with a family history of type 2 diabetes when compared to controls.

These results suggest that the risk imparted by insulin resistance to the development of type 2 diabetes in PCOS is enhanced by defects in insulin secretion. Further, a history of type 2 diabetes in a first-degree relative appears to define a subset of PCOS subjects with the most profound defects in β-cell function. Taken together, these findings are in accord with studies showing a high degree of heritability of β-cell function, particularly when examined in relation to insulin sensitivity (31), and among nondiabetic members of familial type 2 diabetic kindreds (32).

IV. HYPERTENSION

Women with PCOS would appear to be highly predisposed to the development of hypertension by virtue of their characteristic obesity and insulin resistance. However, the presence of systolic and/or diastolic elevations in blood pressure are not a uniform feature of PCOS during the reproductive years. In one study (33), women with PCOS and controls were compared using 24-h ambulatory blood pressure monitoring and echocardiography. Despite the fact that the PCOS women were significantly more insulin resistant than their matched controls, there was no difference in systolic or diastolic blood pressure levels or in left ventricular mass between groups. It is possible, however, that measurement of ambulatory blood pressures or left ventricular mass are not sufficiently sensitive to detect subtle effects, direct or indirect, of hyperinsulinemia upon the resistance vessels. With age, insulin resistance and secondary hyperinsulinemia may play a central role in the development of hypertension and atherosclerotic vascular disease. Data suggest that later in life sustained hypertension is three times more likely in women with PCOS compared to normal women (17,34).

The pathogenesis of hypertension in PCOS and other insulin-resistant states is complex. Insulin acts as a vasodilator through the induction of endothelial nitric oxide production (35). Nitric oxide, in turn, causes an increase in the concentration of cyclic GMP, which acts as a potent vasodilator. Thus, resistance to insulin action at the level of the vascular endothelium may contribute to the development of arterial hypertension. In both animals and normal humans, the infusion of insulin induces vasodilation. However, vasoconstriction predominates in the presence of insulin resistance. The hyperinsulinemia may also result in sustained hypertension via insulin's stimulatory effect on the sympathetic nervous system, resulting in an increased cardiac output, vasoconstriction, and increased sodium resorption by the kidneys. Additional effects of nitric oxide, including inhibition of growth and migration of vascular smooth muscle cells and attenuation of the vascular inflammatory reaction (36), may be decreased in the insulin-resistant state. Nitric oxide also inhibits thrombosis by preventing platelet adhesion and enhancing the ability of prostacyclin to inhibit platelet aggregation. Thus, the insulin-resistant state may mediate a cascade of events predisposing women with PCOS to hypertension and atherosclerosis.

V. MACROVASCULAR DISEASE AND THROMBOSIS: ROLE OF INHIBIN AND PAI-1 IN PCOS

Endogenous fibrinolysis is modulated intravascularly by endothelial cell–derived tissue plasminogen activator (tPA), resulting in the activation of plasminogen and subsequent plasmin formation. Plasminogen activator inhibitor-1(PAI-1) is a serine protease that is produced by liver and endothelial cells. It is capable of binding to tPA and neutralizing its activity. Over 90% of the immunoreactive PAI-1 in the bloodstream is stored in platelets; with platelet activation, PAI-1 is released along with other physiological mediators that inhibit the lysis of nascent clots (37). A homeostatic balance exists between the levels and activity of tPA and PAI-1, controlling net local fibrinolytic activity on the luminal surface of blood vessels. The homeostatic balance prevents the development of thrombosis and vascular occlusion, as PAI-1 regulates the removal of fibrin deposits from blood vessels. An imbalance favoring the relative excess of PAI-1 will result in decreased fibrinolytic activity and a predisposition to the formation of thrombus, placing patients at risk for recurrent thrombotic disease.

Many conditions that are associated with PCOS have been associated with decreased fibrinolytic activity, including obesity, diabetes, and hyperlipidemia (38). PAI-1 concentrations in PCOS may be as high, or even higher, than those typically seen in patients with type 2 diabetes (39). This increase in PAI-1 is likely to be one of several factors that place women with PCOS at risk for macrovascular disease (40–42). Consistently, the decreased fibrinolytic activity in these conditions has been associated with elevated PAI-1 protein and increased functional PAI-1 activity. Less consistently have there been altered concentrations of tPA protein in plasma. Several recent studies have documented elevated PAI-1 levels in women with PCOS. In one study (43), significantly higher PAI-1 levels were observed in lean women with polycystic ovaries and extreme menstrual disturbance compared to women with polycystic ovaries and normal menstrual cycles. This latter observation makes it tempting to speculate that a common factor, possibly hyperinsulinemia, could account for the ovulatory dysfunction and elevation in PAI-1 levels seen in PCOS.

Insulin and proinsulin both play a regulatory role in PAI-1 production by hepatic and endothelial cells (44) and a strong direct association between insulin levels and PAI-1 activity has been demonstrated in normals, obese women, and patients with type 2 diabetes (44). IGF-1 plays a synergistic role in the regulation of PAI-1 production (37).

Reduction in insulin levels by fasting, or the administration of either metformin (45,46) or troglitazone (39), results in lower PAI-1 levels/activity. Treatment of women with PCOS with troglitazone led to a 31% decrease in the concentration of PAI-1 protein in the blood and a 50% reduction in the functional activity of PAI-1 (39) that was significantly correlated with the decline in insulin levels during an oral glucose tolerance test. This finding is consistent with the proposed direct role of insulin in modulating expression of PAI-1. A modest reduction in tPA antigen levels (15%) was seen; however, fibrinolytic activity attributable to tPA in blood did not change after treatment with troglitazone. An improved fibrinolytic response to thrombosis might be anticipated as a result of the substantial decrease in the level and activity of PAI-1 after treatment with insulin-sensitizing agents.

VI. DYSLIPIDEMIA

Women with PCOS are frequently characterized as having hypertriglyceridemia, increased levels of VLDL and LDL, and a lower HDL cholesterol (47,48), a lipid pattern similar to that seen in patients with type 2 diabetes.

Various lipid subfractions may possess a greater atherogenic potential due to alterations in their lipid and apolipoprotein composition. Rajkhowa et al. (49) have reported that the HDL composition in obese PCOS subjects is modified by the depletion of lipid relative to protein, with significant reductions in both the HDL cholesterol and phospholipids to apoA-1. This suggests a reduced capacity for cholesterol removal from tissue with diminished antiatherogenic potential.

Both insulin resistance and hyperandrogenemia have been implicated in the pathogenesis of the lipid abnormalities in PCOS. Testosterone decreases lipoprotein lipase activity in abdominal fat cells, while insulin resistance impairs the ability of insulin to exert its antilipolytic effects and leads to altered activity of lipoprotein and hepatic lipases. These abnormalities are coupled with a decreased cholesterol ester transfer protein activity.

Evidence supporting an important role for insulin resistance in the pathogenesis of these lipid abnormalities includes the findings of Wild et al. (50), who noted that, among hyperandrogenic women, suppression of estradiol and testosterone levels with a GnRH agonist did not result in alteration of baseline lipid abnormalities. Rather, the lipid profiles remained aberrant and correlated with the degree of insulin resistance. Slowinska-Srzednicka (51) subsequently found that, after adjustment for age, BMI, and androgen levels, fasting insulin was a significant explanatory variable for triglyceride and apoA-1 levels in PCOS.

Although it is reasonable to predict that these lipid abnormalities in PCOS convey an increased risk for cardiovascular morbidity and mortality, little data exist to confirm this. Using a predictive, cohort model, Dahlgren and colleagues (34) have estimated that myocardial infarction would be seven times more common in women with PCOS than in the general population. The risk function was age-dependent, with an estimated risk ratio of 4.2 to develop ischemic heart disease for PCOS women 40 to 49 years of age, and a risk ratio of 11.0 for those 50 to 61 years of age as compared to age-matched referents. This calculated risk was not evident in a retrospective analysis of 30 years follow-up on 786 women diagnosed with PCOS between 1930 and 1979 (52). Of interest, there was a significant excess of deaths in which diabetes was listed as a contributing cause.

Finally, Wild and colleagues (53) evaluated 102 women presenting for coronary artery catheterization for the signs and symptoms of androgen excess, and found that hirsutism was more common in those women with confirmed coronary artery disease. In addition, women with polycystic ovaries by ultrasonography who were undergoing coronary arteriography have been found to have more extensive coronary artery disease compared to women with normal ovaries (54). Finally, carotid intima-media thickness was found to be significantly greater for women in their forties with a diagnosis of PCOS than for controls (55), suggesting an increased risk of subclinical atherosclerosis in women with PCOS.

VII. OBSTRUCTIVE SLEEP APNEA

Obese women with PCOS are at increased risk for obstructive sleep apnea (OSA) (56). Based on the increased prevalence of OSA in men, and recent evidence that androgens may play a role in the male predominance, overnight polysomnography was performed in obese women with PCOS and age/weight-matched controls (56). Women with PCOS had a significantly higher apnea-hypopnea index (AHI), and were more likely to suffer from symptomatic OSA syndrome. The AHI correlated with waist–hip ratio, as well as total and free testosterone levels. Vgontzas et al. (57) also reported that sleep-disordered breathing (SDB) and excessive daytime sleepiness are more frequent in women with PCOS than in premenopausal controls. Insulin resistance appeared to be a risk factor for SDB in women with PCOS.

Whether there is a causal relationship between OSA and cardiovascular morbidity and mortality is uncertain. However, recent evidence suggests that OSA may indirectly increase the risk of cardiovascular morbidity and mortality. The Wisconsin Sleep Cohort Study documented that an apnea index of five or more events per hour resulted in significantly higher systemic pressures than in snorers or normals (58). Lavie et al. (59) demonstrated a similar association between an increased apnea–hypopnea index and systolic and diastolic blood pressures during waketime hours. Furthermore, a 10% decrement in oxygen saturation during sleep was linearly associated with an increased risk of systemic hypertension (59). Several recent studies have demonstrated that OSA alone is not sufficient to cause persistently elevated pulmonary arterial pressures. Daytime hypoxia, resulting from obesity or underlying lung disease, is also necessary for the development of sustained pulmonary hypertension. The most common and significant cardiac rhythm abnormalities associated with OSA are severe bradycardia and ventricular asystole greater than 10 s (60). The physiological abnormalities associated with OSA, including hypoventilation, hypoxemia, respiratory acidosis, and vigorous inspiratory effort against a closed airway, result in parasympathetic stimulation and the resultant rhythm disturbances. Finally, there is little direct evidence to support the hypothesis that OSA contributes to vascular morbidity including myocardial infarction and stroke. It thus appears that obese women with PCOS are at increased risk for OSA, and that they should be questioned carefully regarding potential symptoms of sleep-disordered breathing. It remains speculative as to whether obstructive sleep apnea predisposes women with PCOS to a higher risk of systemic hypertension, and subsequent cardiovascular morbidity and mortality.

In conclusion, the metabolic alterations seen in PCOS appear to impart an increase in risk for the development of glucose intolerance and diabetes as well as lipid abnormalities and macrovascular disease. Advances in our understanding of the pathogenesis of the insulin resistance that underlies the development of these complications has provided the impetus for use of novel therapies, chief among them the insulin-lowering medications. The ultimate role of these agents in the treatment of PCOS and its metabolic sequelae remains to be determined.

VIII. CLINICAL AND THERAPEUTIC IMPLICATIONS

The evidence suggests that the metabolic syndrome of PCOS is placing young women at risk for premature macrovascular disease. Accordingly, management of PCOS in the future may shift from solely the control of symptoms to the primary prevention of chronic disease through management of cardiovascular risk factors. Women with PCOS should be carefully evaluated for the presence of obesity, hypertension, dyslipidemia, insulin resistance, and glucose intolerance. Some authorities advocate screening for impaired glucose tolerance and diabetes in all women with PCOS. It is probably prudent to utilize the standard oral glucose tolerance test in women with PCOS that are obese, display signs of insulin resistance (acanthosis nigricans), or have a significant family history of type 2 diabetes mellitus. Fasting plasma glucose levels do not correlate well with the results of glucose tolerance testing in this patient population. Therefore, they should not be relied upon for screening in women felt to be at significant risk for impaired glucose tolerance and diabetes. Screening for dyslipidemia is also important; fasting lipid subfractions, to include triglyceride levels, should be determined. A total cholesterol may be less sensitive for detecting atherogenic abnormalities that are common in women with PCOS. Women with PCOS should be counseled on lifestyle modification, including weight management, nutrition and exercise counseling, and smoking cessation, if appropriate. Weight reduction in obese women with PCOS should be encouraged. Adherence to necessary changes may result in a lessening of insulin resistance, insulin levels, and reverse some of the metabolic aberrations. Furthermore, moderate weight loss has been demonstrated to result in improvements in menstrual function and fertility.

Management of hypertension and cardiovascular risk factors might best follow the strategies utilized in diabetes management given the similar clinical determinants of cardiovascular risk. Due to cost and side-effect profiles, the physician must emphasize the protective benefits of antihypertensive therapy over the long term in those patients who require treatment. The selection of an antihypertensive agent may initially involve the use of an angiotensin converting enzyme inhibitor, which decreases the progression of microalbuminuria and nephropathy in patients with type 2 diabetes. Spironolactone is also a reasonable agent to utilize in hirsute patients that will benefit from androgenic receptor blockade. In considering other agents, thought should be given to the ability of the medication to adversely affect lipid profiles and/or insulin sensitivity.

There is no objective evidence that the daily use of aspirin therapy in women with PCOS has a beneficial role in retarding the evolution of macrovascular disease, although this prophylactic strategy is utilized by many physicians in the management of patients with type 2 diabetes. In a recent meta-analysis of 145 randomized assignment studies including 4500 patients with diabetes, aspirin use in moderate dosage reduced cardiovascular morbidity and mortality. With respect to the dyslipidemia and potential cardiovascular risk, many believe that women with PCOS should be considered similar to those with disorders of insulin resistance and diabetes. Accordingly, appropriate lifestyle and nutritional modifications, as well as pharmacological interventions, should be employed to achieve target values set forth by the NCEP. As current research unfolds, we may find that the quality, as well as the quantity, of certain lipoprotein subclasses should be addressed to achieve a healthier lipid profile.

Insulin-sensitizing agents, such as metformin and the thiazolidinediones, may gain a greater role in the management of these patients in the future. The insulin sensitizers have many potential beneficial effects on the metabolic profile and subsequent cardiovascular risk, including the attenuation of peripheral insulin resistance and a subsequent lowering of plasma insulin levels. Furthermore, they have beneficial effects on triglyceride and HDL subfractions, as well as PAI-1 levels. The ultimate role of these agents in the treatment of PCOS and its metabolic sequelae remains to be determined.

REFERENCES

1. Ehrmann DA, Barnes RB, Rosenfield RL. Polycystic ovary syndrome as a form of functional ovarian hyperandrogenism due to dysregulation of androgen secretion. Endocrin Rev 1995; 16:322–353.
2. Knochenhauer ES, Key TJ, Kahsar-Miller M, Waggoner W, Boots LR, Azziz R. Prevalence of the polycystic ovary syndrome in unselected black and white women of the southeastern United States: a prospective study. J Clin Endocrinol Metab 1998; 83:3078–3082.
3. Conway GS, Honour JW, Jacobs HS. Heterogeneity of the polycystic ovary syndrome: clinical, endocrine and ultrasound features in 556 patients. Clin Endocrinol 1989; 30:459–470.
4. Franks S. Polycystic ovary syndrome: a changing perspective Clin Endocrinol 1989; 31:87–120.
5. Stein IF, Leventhal ML. Amenorrhea associated with bilateral polycystic ovaries. Am J Obstet Gynecol 1935; 29:181–191.
6. Sonnenberg GE, Hoffman RG, Mueller RA, Kissebah AH. Splanchnic insulin dynamics and secretion pulsatilities in abdominal obesity. Diabetes 1994; 43:468–477.
7. Kissebah AH. Upper body obesity: abnormalities in the metabolic profile and the androgenic/estrogenic balance. In: Dunaif A, Givens J, Haseltine F, Merriam G, eds. Current Issues in Endocrinology and Metabolism: Polycystic Ovary Syndrome. Cambridge, MA: Blackwell Scientific, 1992:359–374.
8. Dunaif A, Segal KR, Futterweit W, Dobrjansky A. Profound peripheral insulin resistance, independent of obesity, in polycystic ovary syndrome. Diabetes 1989; 38: 1165–1174.
9. Björntorp P. Classification of obese patients and complications related to the distribution of surplus fat. Nutrition 1990; 6:131–137.
10. Robinson S, Chan S-P, Spacey S, Anyaoku V, Johnston DG Franks S. Postprandial thermogenesis is reduced in polycystic ovary syndrome and is associated with increased insulin resistance. Clin Endocrinol 1992; 36:537–543.
11. McLaughlin T, Abbasi F, Carantoni M, Schaaf P, Reaven G. Differences in insulin resistance do not predict weight loss in response to hypocaloric diets in healthy obese women. J Clin Endocrinol Metab 1999; 84:578–581.
12. Ehrmann DA. Insulin-lowering therapeutic modalities for polycystic ovary syndrome. Endocrinol Metab Clin North Am 1999; 28:423–438, viii.
13. Ehrmann DA, Jeppe S, Byrne M, Karrison T, Rosenfield RL, Polonsky K. Insulin

secretory defects in polycystic ovary syndrome. Relationship to insulin sensitivity and family history of non-insulin-dependent diabetes mellitus. J Clin Invest 1995; 96:520–527.

14. Ehrmann DA, Barnes RB, Rosenfield RL, Cavaghan MK, Imperial J. Prevalence of impaired glucose tolerance and diabetes in women with polycystic ovary syndrome. Diabetes Care 1999; 22:141–146.

15. Legro RS, Kunselman AR, Dodson WC, Dunaif A. Prevalence and predictors of risk for type 2 diabetes mellitus and impaired glucose tolerance in polycystic ovary syndrome: a prospective, controlled study in 254 affected women. J Clin Endocrinol Metab 1999; 84:165–169.

16. World Health Organization: Diabetes Mellitus: Report of a WHO Study Group. Geneva WHO, 1985 (Tech. Rep. Ser., no. 727).

17. Dahlgren E, Janson PO, Johansson A, Linstedt G, Oden A, Crona N, Knutsson F, Mattson L, Lundberg P. Women with polycystic ovary syndrome wedge resected in 1956 to 1965: a long-term follow-up focusing on natural history and circulating hormones. Fertil Steril 1992; 57:505–513.

18. Edelstein SL, Knowler WC, Bain RP, Andres R, Barrett-Connor EL, Dowse GK, Haffner SM, Pettitt DJ, Muller DC, Collins VR, Hamman RF. Predictors of progression from impaired glucose tolerance to NIDDM: an analysis of six prospective studies. Diabetes 1997; 46:701–710.

19. Dunaif A, Graf M, Mandeli J, Laumas V, Dobrjansky A. Characterization of groups of hyperandrogenic women with acanthosis nigricans, impaired glucose tolerance and/or hyperinsulinemia. J Clin Endocrinol Metab 1987; 65:499–507.

20. Dunaif A, Graf M. Insulin administration alters gonadal steroid metabolism independent of changes in gonadotropin secretion in insulin-resistant women with the polycystic ovary syndrome. J Clin Invest 1989; 83:23–29.

21. Dunaif A. Insulin resistance and the polycystic ovary syndrome: mechanism and implications for pathogenesis. Endocr Rev 1997; 18:774–800.

22. Book C-B, Dunaif A. Selective insulin resistance in the polycystic ovary syndrome. J Clin Endocrinol Metab 1999; 84:3110–3116.

23. Dunaif A, Xia J, Book C, Schenker E, Tang Z. Excessive insulin receptor serine phosphorylation in cultured fibroblasts and in skeletal muscle: a potential mechanism for insulin resistance in the polycystic ovary syndrome. J Clin Invest 1995; 96:801–810.

24. Kruszynska Y, Olefsky J. Cellular and molecular mechanisms of non-insulin dependent diabetes mellitus. J Invest Med 1996; 44:413–428.

25. O'Meara N, Blackman J, Ehrmann D, Barnes R, Jaspan J, Rosenfield R, Polonsky K. Defects in beta cell function and insulin action in functional ovarian hyperandrogenism. J Clin Endocrinol Metab 1993; 76:1241–1247.

26. Polonsky KS, Given BD, Hirsch L, Beebe C, Rue P, Pugh W, Frank BH, Galloway JA, Van Caute E. Abnormal patterns of insulin secretion in non-insulin dependent diabetes. N Engl J Med 1988; 318:1231–1239.

27. Polonsky KS, Sturis J, Bell BI. Non-insulin-dependent diabetes mellitus—a genetically programmed failure of the beta cell to compensate for insulin resistance. N Engl J Med 1996; 334:777–783.

28. Holte J, Bergh T, Berne C ea. Enhanced early insulin response to glucose in relation

to insulin resistance in women with polycystic ovary syndrome and normal glucose tolerance. J Clin Endocrinol Metab 1994; 78:1052–1058.

29. Kahn S, Prigeon R, McCulloch D, Boyko E, Bergman R, Schwartz M, Neifing J, Ward W, Beard J, Palmer J, Porte D. Quantification of the relationship between insulin sensitivity and β-cell function in human subjects. Evidence for a hyperbolic function. Diabetes 1993; 42:1663–1672.

30. Dunaif A, Finegood DT. β-cell dysfunction independent of obesity and glucose intolerance in the polycystic ovary syndrome. J Clin Endocrinol Metab 1996; 81:942–947.

31. Elbein SC, Hasstedt SJ, Wegner K, Kahn SE. Heritability of pancreatic beta-cell function among nondiabetic members of Caucasian familial type 2 diabetic kindreds. J Clin Endocrinol Metab 1999; 84:1398–1403.

32. Pimenta W, Korytkowski M, Mitrakou A, Jenssen T, Yki Jarvinen H, Evron W, Dailey G, Gerich J. Pancreatic beta-cell dysfunction as the primary genetic lesion in NIDDM. Evidence from studies in normal glucose-tolerant individuals with a first-degree NIDDM relative [see comments]. JAMA 1995; 273:1855–1861.

33. Zimmermann S, Phillips RA, Dunaif A, Finegood DT, Wilkenfeld C, Ardeljan M, Gorlin R, Krakoff LR. Polycystic ovary syndrome: lack of hypertension despite profound insulin resistance. J Clin Endocrinol Metab 1992; 75:508–513.

34. Dahlgren E, Janson P, Johansson S, Lapidus L, Oden A. Polycystic ovary syndrome and risk for myocardial infarction. Acta Obstet Gynecol Scand 1992; 71:599–604.

35. Baron AD. Vascular reactivity. Am J Cardiol 1999; 84:25J–27J.

36. Hsueh WA, Law RE. Insulin signaling in the arterial wall. Am J Cardiol 1999; 84: 21J–24J.

37. Schneider DJ, Nordt TK, Sobel BE. Attenuated fibrinolysis and accelerated atherogenesis in type 2 diabetic patients. Diabetes 1993; 42:1–7.

38. Colwell JA. Vascular thrombosis in type 2 diabetes mellitus [editorial]. Diabetes 1993; 42:8–11.

39. Ehrmann D, Schneider D, Sobel B, Cavaghan M, Imperial J, Rosenfield R, Polonsky K. Troglitazone improves defects in insulin action, insulin secretion, ovarian steroidogenesis, and fibrinolysis in women with polycystic ovary syndrome. J Clin Endocrinol Metab 1997; 82:2108–2116.

40. Keber I, Keber D. Increased plasminogen activator inhibitor activity in survivors of myocardial infarction is associated with metabolic risk factors of atherosclerosis. Haemostasis 1992; 22:187–194.

41. Juhan-Vague I, Valadier J, Alessi MC, Aillaud MF, Ansaldi J, Philip-Joet C, Holvoet P, Serradimigni A, Collen D. Deficient t-PA release and elevated PA inhibitor levels in patients with spontaneous or recurrent deep venous thrombosis. Thromb Haemost 1987; 57:67–72.

42. Nilsson IM, Ljungner H, Tengborn L. Two different mechanisms in patients with venous thrombosis and defective fibrinolysis: low concentration of plasminogen activator or increased concentration of plasminogen activator inhibitor. Br Med J (Clin Res Ed) 1985; 290:1453–1456.

43. Sampson M, Kong C, Patel A, Unwin R, Jacobs HS. Ambulatory blood pressure profiles and plasminogen activator inhibitor (PAI-1) activity in lean women with

and without the polycystic ovary syndrome. Clin Endocrinol (Oxf) 1996; 45:623–629.

44. Nordt TK, Schneider DJ, Sobel BE. Augmentation of the synthesis of plasminogen activator inhibitor type-1 by precursors of insulin. A potential risk factor for vascular disease. Circulation 1994; 89:321–330.

45. Vague P, Juhan-Vague I, Alessi M, Badier C, Valadier J. Metformin decreases the high plasminogen activator inhibition capacity, plasma insulin and triglyceride levels in non-diabetic obese subjects. Thromb Haemostas 1987; 57:326–328.

46. Velazquez EM, Mendoza SG, Wang P, Glueck CJ. Metformin therapy is associated with a decrease in plasma plasminogen activator inhibitor-1, lipoprotein(a), and immunoreactive insulin levels in patients with the polycystic ovary syndrome. Metabolism 1997; 46:454–457.

47. Wild RA, Painter PC, Coulson PB, Carruth KB, Ranney GB. Lipoprotein lipid concentrations and cardiovascular risk in women with polycystic ovary syndrome. J Clin Endocrinol Metab 1985; 61:946–951.

48. Talbott E, Guzick D, Clerici A, Berga S, Detre K, Weimer K, Kuller L. Coronary heart disease risk factors in women with polycystic ovary syndrome. Arterioscler Thromb Vasc Biol 1995; 15:821–826.

49. Rajkhowa M, Neary RH, Kumpatla P, Game FL, Jones PW, Obhrai MS, Clayton RN. Altered composition of high density lipoproteins in women with the polycystic ovary syndrome. J Clin Endocrinol Metab 1997; 82:3389–3394.

50. Wild RA, Alaupovic P, Givens JR, Parker IJ. Lipoprotein abnormalities in hirsute women. II. Compensatory responses of insulin resistance and dehydroepiandrosterone sulfate with obesity. Am J Obstet Gynecol 1992; 167:1813–1818.

51. Slowinska-Srzednicka J, Zgliczynski S, Wierzbicki M, Srzednicki M, Stopinska-Gluszak U, Zgliczynski W, Soszynski P, Chotkowska E, Bednarska M, Sadowski Z. The role of hyperinsulinemia in the development of lipid disturbances in nonobese and obese women with the polycystic ovary syndrome. J Endocrinol Invest 1991; 14:569–575.

52. Pierpoint T, McKeigue PM, Isaacs AJ, Wild SH, Jacobs HS. Mortality of women with polycystic ovary syndrome at long-term follow-up. J Clin Epidemiol 1998; 51:581–586.

53. Wild RA, Grubb B, Hartz A, Van Nort JJ, Bachman W, Bartholomew M. Clinical signs of androgen excess as risk factors for coronary artery disease. Fertil Steril 1990; 54:255–259.

54. Birdsall MA, Farquhar CM, White HD. Association between polycystic ovaries and extent of coronary artery disease in women having cardiac catheterization [see comments]. Ann Intern Med 1997; 126:32–35.

55. Guzick DS, Talbott EO, Sutton-Tyrrell K, Herzog HC, Kuller LH, Wolfson SK, Jr. Carotid atherosclerosis in women with polycystic ovary syndrome: initial results from a case-control study. Am J Obstet Gynecol 1996; 174:1224–1229; discussion 1229–1232.

56. Fogel RB, Malhotra A, Pillar G, Pittman SD, Dunaif A, White DP. Increased prevalence of obstructive sleep apnea syndrome in obese women with polycystic ovary syndrome. J Clin Endocrinol Metab 2001; 86:1175–1180.

57. Vgontzas AN, Legro RS, Bixler EO, Grayev A, Kales A, Chrousos GP. Polycystic ovary syndrome is associated with obstructive sleep apnea and daytime sleepiness: role of insulin resistance. J Clin Endocrinol Metab 2001; 86:517–520.
58. Hla KM, Young TB, Bidwell T, Palta M, Skatrud JB, Dempsey J. Sleep apnea and hypertension. A population-based study. Ann Intern Med 1994; 120:382–388.
59. Lavie P, Herer P, Hoffstein V. Obstructive sleep apnoea syndrome as a risk factor for hypertension: population study. BMJ 2000; 320:479–482.
60. Miller WP. Cardiac arrhythmias and conduction disturbances in the sleep apnea syndrome. Prevalence and significance. Am J Med 1982; 73:317–321.

10

Detection and Diagnosis of Heart Disease in Diabetic and Prediabetic Subjects

Srihari Thanigaraj and Julio E. Pérez
Washington University School of Medicine, and Barnes–Jewish Hospital, St. Louis, Missouri

I. INTRODUCTION

Cardiovascular diseases account for a major component of the morbidity and mortality afflicting patients with diabetes. Nearly 77% of all hospitalizations attributable to medical complications in patients with diabetes are cardiovascular in nature. Cardiovascular disease event rates and mortality among patients with diabetes are on the rise, although they are decreasing in individuals without diabetes (1,2). The effect of diabetes on the heart includes a wide spectrum of abnormalities that extends from subtle subclinical findings to overt clinical manifestations that may be considered under three broad categories: (1) coronary atherosclerosis; (2) diabetic cardiomyopathy; and (3) diabetic autonomic neuropathy. There is growing evidence that an early and tailored management strategy can limit or slow down the progression of diabetic heart disease and may also potentially reduce the cardiovascular event rate in this group of patients (3). This underscores the need for early and accurate detection of the manifestations of heart disease in patients with diabetes. This chapter summarizes the various diagnostic tools that are available to the clinician for the diagnosis of diabetic heart disease, and their value and utility in clinical practice. This chapter does not attempt to consider independently the important differences among patients with type 1 and type 2 diabetes, but rather addresses patients with diabetes in general, specifically referring to either type when issues unique to them are discussed.

II. CORONARY ATHEROSCLEROSIS

Several clinical observations, most notably those reported from the Framingham study, have shown that the incidence and prevalence of the major clinical manifestations of atherosclerotic coronary artery disease (CAD) are increased in patients with diabetes (4). This is independent of the other risk factors such as arterial hypertension, male gender, and dyslipidemia. CAD is the major cause of morbidity and mortality in patients with diabetes, with a mortality rate that is three times as high as in those without diabetes. The clinical indications for performing noninvasive and invasive tests for the purpose of detection or risk stratification of CAD in patients with diabetes largely parallel those of the nondiabetic population. However, certain aspects with regard to evaluation of CAD in patients with diabetes merit special consideration.

Although a standard exercise treadmill test is economical and widely available, in diabetic patients who are at an increased risk for CAD a treadmill test is less sensitive; hence a stress imaging test would be more valuable. The sensitivity and specificity for the detection of coronary artery disease among patients with diabetes was 75% and 77% for the exercise test and 80% and 87% for thallium myocardial scintigraphy (5). This supports the use of noninvasive imaging tests for the detection of coronary artery disease, especially in those patients who have multiple cardiac risk factors. The sensitivity and specificity of stress echocardiography is comparable to that of nuclear SPECT imaging study in the general population, and it is reasonable to assume that the same should also be true for diabetic patients, although comparative studies are not available. The decision to refer a patient for a nuclear or echocardiographic stress test should be based on the available resources and local expertise. Among diabetics with significant peripheral vascular disease, a pharmacological stress test may lend higher sensitivity and specificity for the detection of significant CAD. It should be noted that, in some studies, exercise electrocardiography as well as radionuclide imaging are somewhat less accurate in patients with hypertension, established diabetic or autonomic cardiomyopathy, renal insufficiency, or microvascular disease (3).

The clinical impression that patients with diabetes tend to have a higher incidence of silent myocardial infarctions was challenged with data emerging from the 30-year follow-up analysis of the Framingham study (6). Nevertheless, it has been clearly established that the prevalence of significant CAD in asymptomatic diabetic patients is substantially higher compared to nondiabetic control subjects. In diabetic patients with additional risk factors for coronary atherosclerosis, periodic thorough clinical examination and resting ECG may fail to detect significant CAD (7). Thus, it is reasonable to consider noninvasive imaging stress tests as part of the periodic care, especially in those with two or more cardiovascular risk factors like hypertension, dyslipidemia, family history of CAD, and smoking, as well as in sedentary patients beginning a vigorous exercise program. The yield of noninvasive testing of patients identified in this fashion is between 10 and 20% (3). Screening for CAD markers such as lipoprotein (a), fibrinogen levels, C-reactive protein, and homocysteine levels may add further to the identification of patients at increased risk. According to ACC–AHA guidelines, stress testing in an asymptomatic diabetic patient with multiple cardiac risk factors is considered to be a class IIb indication (usefulness is less well established by evidence/opinion) if performed in men over 40 years and women over 50 years of age (8). A functional study in an asymptomatic diabetic patient may be well justified based on the findings of the Asymptomatic Cardiac Ischemia Pilot (ACIP) study that concluded that revascularization may improve survival in these patient groups (9,10). It is important to remember that most of the coronary events occur due to plaque rupture from minor, non-flow-limiting stenoses rather than from critical coronary artery stenoses (11). With respect to diabetic patients who also have evidence of atherosclerosis in the peripheral or cerebral arterial circulation, there is a very high likelihood of concomitant CAD. Peripheral arterial disease, for example, is associated with a fourfold increase in CAD risk. Patients with macroalbuminuria have markedly increased CAD risk as well (3), and hence diagnostic testing in such patients to evaluate for significant CAD, even if asymptomatic, should be considered appropriate.

With respect to the performance of coronary angiography in patients with diabetes, the use of low osmolar and nonionic contrast agents are preferred, especially in those patients with compromised left ventricular systolic or diastolic function and impaired renal function. Both pathological as well as angiographic studies have demonstrated that patients with diabetes are more likely to have significant three-vessel CAD rather than single-vessel involvement by angiography. Although distal coronary vessel involvement has been noted to be more common in diabetics, studies have also shown that there is an increased frequency of left main coronary narrowing. Despite the common impression that coronary atherosclerosis in patients with diabetes is more a diffuse than a focal process, data pertaining to this fact are conflicting (12). Recent intravascular ultrasound (IVUS) studies suggest that the conventional angiogram may not be a good predictor of the degree of CAD. There is often eccentric arterial narrowing, which may not be well detected by angiography. Furthermore, the concentrically narrowed lumen may be of lesser risk than one with eccentric narrowing because of the likelihood that the latter contains a lipid-rich plaque more susceptible to rupture. In general, patients who have had a coronary angiogram and subsequently have sustained a myocardial infarction were frequently noted to have less than 50% narrowing of the infarct-related coronary artery (11).

Although the use of electron beam computerized tomography (EBCT) for screening of CAD is considered controversial, there is evidence that EBCT may be a useful approach for patients with diabetes since coronary calcification is common in this population, as is the case for asymptomatic or subclinical CAD (3,13). In a recent study (13), coronary calcification scores over 82 gave 68% sensitivity and 68% specificity for the detection of CAD, whereas a score exceeding 200 gave a 62% sensitivity and 98% specificity in patients with diabetes. Higher HbA1c, lower HDL cholesterol, and coronary calcium score, but not arterial blood pressure, age, or total cholesterol, were predictors of angiographic coronary disease in this group of patients.

III. DIABETIC CARDIOMYOPATHY

Patients with diabetes have a four- to fivefold increased risk for developing heart failure; thus, diabetes has a greater influence on the incidence of congestive heart failure than CAD. Using multivariate analysis, it has been shown that patients with diabetes have substantially higher incidence of congestive heart failure even after accounting for CAD, arterial blood pressure, cholesterol levels, and body weight. While it is common for many patients with diabetes to have various other contributing factors for heart failure, such as hypertension and ischemic heart disease, diabetic cardiomyopathy as a disease entity should be strictly limited by definition to the manifestation of myocardial dysfunction stemming primarily from diabetes. Studies have suggested that approximately one-third of diabetic patients have subclinical or asymptomatic myocardial dysfunction that is primarily attributable to the metabolic derangements of diabetes.

Possible mechanisms underlying cardiomyopathy in patients with diabetes include abnormalities of the microvasculature, interstitial fibrosis, extravascular deposition of collagen and triglyceride and cholesterol esters, and, at the molecular level, metabolic derangements that alter actomyosin and myosin adenosine triphosphatase activities. Based on experimental animal model data it is hypothesized that the structural manifestations of diabetic cardiomyopathy consist of two major components. The first involves changes in the intercalated disk and capillaries, including their basal laminae which are reversible, short-term, physiological adaptations to metabolic alterations. The other represents focal, yet progressive, degenerative changes such as loss of myofibrils, transverse tubules, and sarcoplasmic reticulum for which the myocardium has only a limited capacity for repair. Metabolic abnormality that is present since the prestage of type 2 diabetes has been suggested to be at the center of these structural alterations with resultant myocardial dysfunction. Studies in experimental animals and in patients with type 2 diabetes have shown that left ventricular function improves concomitantly with insulin therapy and improvement in metabolic control. Although type 1 diabetic patients studied thus far in the context of diabetic cardiomyopathy have longer duration of diabetes and higher HbA1c values, the prevalence of ventricular diastolic dysfunction are more commonly seen in those with type 2 diabetes.

Ever since its first description in the early 1970s, the evidence in support of a discrete and clinically definable diabetic cardiomyopathy has been steadily accumulating (14,15). Several M-mode and Doppler echocardiography studies, as well as radionuclide ventriculographic studies have shown evidence of systolic and diastolic left ventricular (LV) function abnormalities in asymptomatic diabetic patients in whom arterial hypertension, CAD, and valvular heart disease were excluded. It is suggested that diastolic and systolic dysfunction abnormalities represent intrinsic reduction in LV compliance and decreased myocardial contractility, respectively. Despite some of the differences that may be encountered in these studies, largely attributable to the methodological variations and disparity in patient selection, there is a broad consensus with respect to the general features of diabetic cardiomyopathy. In essence, these studies indicate that the earliest and predominant functional abnormality is primarily diastolic in nature. In general, the systolic function is normal at rest but fails to augment in response to exercise (16,17), which, as discussed later, may at least in part be related to autonomic dysfunction (18). The exercise-induced global LV dysfunction seen in patients with diabetes does not seem to follow the known clinical course of diabetic microvascular complications. Overall, diabetics tend to have a smaller LV end-diastolic cavity dimension, which does not change during exercise. The decreased LV performance during exercise in diabetic subjects is most likely secondary to reduced LV diastolic filling, as indicated by their generally smaller LV cavity size, rather than due to higher afterload, but impairment of contractile function may also play a role. A higher incidence of left ventricular hypertrophy has also been a consistent finding in patients with presumed diabetic cardiomyopathy as supported by pathologic, echocardiographic, and electrocardiographic studies. From the SOLVD trial, it is apparent that the all-cause patient mortality is higher in the presence of LV hypertrophy for the same degree of LV dysfunction. Recent studies have shown that treatment with angiotensin converting enzyme inhibitors results in regression of hypertrophy in patients with type 2 diabetes independent of the reduction achieved in arterial blood pressure (19).

At the risk of oversimplifying, it is reasonable to summarize diabetic cardiomyopathy as a primary myocardial disease, wherein the earliest functional cardiac manifestations, albeit subtle, are primarily diastolic in nature, but over an extended period of time may progress and result in clinically manifest heart failure, which then may be exclusively diastolic or a combination of systolic and diastolic dysfunction. At present, there are several diagnostic techniques that are readily available to the clinician for diagnosing diabetic cardiomyopathy, which can be of both diagnostic and prognostic value (20). These are predominantly echocardiography techniques, but radionuclide ventriculography can also be useful. Since echocardiography is comparatively simple and easy to perform and provides a wealth of physiological information, it has been the test most frequently utilized for assessing patients with possible diabetic cardiomyopathy. Because the evaluation of LV diastolic function is more germaine to the entity of diabetic cardiomyopathy, the following discussion encompasses the assessment of LV filling in general terms, not particularly different for patients with diabetes as compared to patients in general.

A. Assessment of Diastolic Function

Diastolic dysfunction is the hallmark of diabetic cardiomyopathy and echocardiography is invariably the most commonly employed test at the present time to reliably assess diastolic functional abnormalities. Left ventricular diastolic filling abnormalities in patients with diabetes do not correlate with the duration of diabetes nor with the presence of other complications such as retinopathy, nephropathy, or peripheral neuropathy. In diabetic cardiomyopathy, the initial abnormality of diastolic filling is characterized by a slowed or impaired myocardial relaxation as is the case for most other cardiac diseases. It should be noted that there is a gradual impairment of myocardial relaxation with normal aging, but in pathological states it is more pronounced than what is usually expected for the patient's age. With continued progression of the disease, LV compliance is reduced and elevation in left atrial pressure results in a restrictive LV filling pattern, which initially may be reversible, but eventually becomes fixed. Based on the pulsed-wave spectral Doppler flow patterns measured at the mitral valve tips, as well as at the entrance of the pulmonary veins into the left atrium, the spectrum of diastolic abnormality has been generally classified into four stages as discussed below.

1. Impaired Relaxation Pattern—Grade 1

In this stage of the disease, the mitral inflow Doppler pattern is characterized by prolonged isovolumic relaxation time (>90 ms), prolonged deceleration time (>240 ms), and reversal of the E and the A wave ratio (E/A <1) for patients in sinus rhythm. The systolic flow velocity at the pulmonary vein location is more prominent compared to the diastolic flow.

2. Pseudonormal Pattern—Grade 2

As the diastolic function continues to deteriorate, a transition phase ensues when the mitral inflow Doppler has an apparent normal pattern. But the pulmonary venous Doppler pattern now becomes abnormal and the diastolic flow is much more prominent than the systolic flow.

3. Restrictive Filling Pattern—Reversible Grade 3 and Irreversible Grade 4

This phase is characterized by shortened isovolumic relaxation time (<70 ms), markedly shortened deceleration time (<160 ms), and very prominent E wave resulting in a E- to A-wave ratio of greater than 2 on the mitral inflow Doppler spectra. On the pulmonary vein Doppler flow pattern, the diastolic flow is markedly prominent compared to the systolic flow component. With appropriate treatment, such as afterload reduction, the restrictive filling pattern may revert back to impaired relaxation pattern in the earlier stages (Grade 2) of the disease. But, with continued progression of the disease, the restrictive pattern becomes irreversible despite treatment (Grade 4). A restrictive filling pattern indicates poor prognosis and with medical management the return of an impaired relaxation pattern denotes an improvement in clinical outcome. Thus, in addition to its prognostic value, these parameters may also serve to assess the response to treatment.

As noted above, during the pseudonormal phase of the diastolic functional impairment, the mitral inflow Doppler pattern may erroneously appear normal to a simple visual assessment. However, a reduction in the preload by Valsalva maneuver usually unmasks the underlying impaired relaxation of the LV. Alternatively, administration of sublingual nitroglycerin achieves a comparable effect in those patients who cannot effectively perform a Valsalva maneuver. It should be noted that the pulmonary vein flow does continue to reflect the diastolic impairment even when the mitral flow pattern portrays a pseudonormal pattern. Employing this approach, recent studies have shown that diastolic abnormalities are much more common than previously reported in type 2 diabetic patients with otherwise good glycemic control who are free of clinically detectable heart disease (21). Thus, the value of a comprehensive Doppler assessment of the mitral tips and pulmonary veins flow patterns cannot be overemphasized.

B. Tissue Doppler Imaging

While the conventional Doppler evaluates the relatively higher blood flow velocity, low-amplitude profile, tissue Doppler imaging permits the selective evaluation of the low-velocity high-amplitude displacement of the LV myocardium movements at the mitral annulus. The mitral annulus velocity profile during diastole reflects the rate of changes in the longitudinal dimension and in LV volume and can be obtained by sampling at the septum or the LV lateral wall as visualized from an apical four-chamber view. Normally the early diastolic annular velocity (E' or Em) is greater than the late diastolic annular velocity (A' or Am). But, when LV diastolic function is impaired, the E' is equal to or smaller than the A', regardless of the stage of the diastolic functional impairment (22,23). Thus, in those patients who exhibit a pseudonormal mitral inflow Doppler pattern, tissue Doppler imaging can be very valuable to establish the presence of diastolic function impairment. Furthermore, the absolute values of the mitral annular velocities by tissue Doppler echocardiography have been shown to be relatively preload independent and hence can be employed not only to assess relaxation, but also, in the context of the mitral inflow velocity data, they permit an indirect assessment of the left atrial pressure (23).

C. Myocardial Ultrasound Tissue Characterization

Ultrasound tissue characterization with backscatter analysis is a reliable method for the direct and quantitative assessment of the physical state of the myocardium. With backscatter analysis, abnormal myocardial tissue acoustic properties can be detected even in the absence of overt contractile dysfunction or alterations in chamber dimensions. Two main indices are obtained from backscatter analysis: (1) absolute integrated backscatter (analogous to the tissue echodensity) values that are linked to the structural and histological component of the myocardial tissue such as the collagen content; and (2) cyclic (systolic to diastolic) variations in integrated backscatter values that reflect myocardial contractile properties. Studies in asymptomatic type 1 diabetic patients with normal resting systolic function have demonstrated that the absolute values of integrated backscatter are increased and that the cyclic variation of tissue-integrated backscatter is blunted (24,25). These alterations of myocardial acoustic properties may be considered an early preclinical phenomenon, potentially related to collagen deposition that signals the subsequent development of diabetic cardiomyopathy, although no correlative histological or biochemical tissue assessment was carried out in these studies. Nevertheless, based on the clinical and experimental animal data available thus far, it is reasonable to state that ultrasound tissue characterization that evaluates the myocardial tissue itself can be a useful tool in the preclinical detection of diabetic cardiomyopathy in otherwise healthy and asymptomatic diabetic patients.

IV. DIABETIC CARDIAC AUTONOMIC NEUROPATHY

The pathophysiological association of cardiac autonomic dysfunction with other manifestations of heart disease in diabetes has been well demonstrated in several studies. Cardiac autonomic neuropathy is suspected to be a major contributor to manifestations of myocardial dysfunction in patients with diabetes. Studies have demonstrated that approximately one-third of patients with diabetes have evidence for depressed LV function in the absence of significant coronary atherosclerosis (12). Furthermore, the extent of cardiac dysfunction has been shown to be related to the severity of cardiac autonomic neuropathy, rather than to age, sex, duration or control of diabetes, microvascular complications, or plasma norepinephrine levels (26).

Cardiac autonomic dysfunction in patients with diabetes has also been linked to the incidence of lethal arrhythmia and sudden cardiac death. In asymptomatic diabetic patients, the presence of cardiac autonomic dysfunction appears to be a better predictor of major cardiac events than myocardial ischemia itself. The risk of events due to cardiac autonomic dysfunction appears to be independent of documented myocardial ischemia, although it is higher when associated with myocardial ischemia (27).

Cardiac autonomic dysfunction is a common, albeit less well recognized, consequence of diabetes on the cardiovascular system. This type of neuropathy is clinically perceived to be far less ominous when compared to other deleterious effects of diabetes on the heart, but is very closely intertwined within the manifestations of diabetic heart disease. In this context, it is important to note that patients with diabetes afflicted with autonomic neuropathy exhibit decreased survival and an increased risk of sudden death. Clinically, cardiac autonomic neuropathy may be apparent by the relatively fixed and rapid heart rate that barely responds to physiological stimuli, such as the Valsalva maneuver, carotid sinus pressure, standing, and tilting, and to the administration of drugs such as atropine or beta-blockers. The most notable manifestation of cardiac autonomic dysfunction is the impaired hemodynamic response to exercise. During exercise, the physiological augmentation in heart rate and systolic blood pressure are blunted in patients with cardiac autonomic dysfunction related to diabetes. In these patients, it is the severity of cardiac autonomic neuropathy that correlates with the maximal increase in heart rate, as opposed to the patient's age, duration of diabetes, or the presence and severity of microvascular disease. The diagnosis of cardiac autonomic dysfunction can be made when two or more of the following criteria are present:

1. *Resting Heart Rate*: Defined as a resting heart rate of 100 beats per minute or more after 15 min of rest in a supine position (in the absence of other causes).
2. *Beat-to-Beat Variability*: Defined as a lack of beat-to-beat variability of less than 10 beats per minute, determined as the difference between minimum and maximum heart rate on a resting electrocardiogram, obtained during normal inspiration and expiration with the patient breathing at least at 16 times per minute.
3. *R-R Interval Ratio During a Valsalva Maneuver*: Defined as the ratio of the longest electrocardiographic R-R interval to the shortest R-R

interval after and during (respectively) the Valsalva maneuver, obtained with the patient blowing into a manometer at 40 mmHg for 15 s. A ratio of less than 1.10 is suggestive of autonomic neuropathy.

4. *Heart Rate Response to Standing*: Using continuous electrocardiographic tracing, the ratio of the R-R interval of the 30th beat after assuming the standing position to the R-R interval of the 15th beat is calculated. A ratio less than 1 indicates an abnormal response.

5. *Blood Pressure Response to Standing*: A decrease in the systolic blood pressure of more than 30 mmHg after 1 min of standing is considered to be consistent with the diagnosis of autonomic neuropathy.

Autonomic dysfunction may involve the sympathetic and/or the parasympathetic nervous system. The progress of cardiac parasympathetic dysfunction in patients with diabetes may parallel that of the involvement of the sympathetic system. Myocardial ^{123}I-Metaiodobenzylguanidine (MIBG) scan can evaluate cardiac sympathetic dysfunction, whereas analysis of the heart rate variability reflects the involvement in cardiac parasympathetic activity (28). Reduced myocardial MIBG accumulation is associated with autonomic dysfunction in diabetic patients, although it can also occur to a lesser extent in some patients with diabetes without apparent autonomic neuropathy. Indices of heart rate spontaneous beat-to-beat variability (such as Ewing's) are consistently related to the degree of cardiac autonomic dysfunction. The Z method and spectral analysis of heart rate also reliably detect cardiac baroreflex impairment in diabetic patients (29). These methods, although not routinely used in the clinical setting, may be clinically relevant in detecting early manifestations of cardiac autonomic neuropathy in individual patients at specialized testing laboratories. Because the early stage of puberty is a critical period for the development of diabetic cardiac autonomic dysfunction, some studies have suggested that all type 1 diabetic patients should be screened for this complication by heart rate variability analysis beginning at the first stage of puberty, regardless of illness duration, microalbuminuria, and level of metabolic control (30).

In patients with diabetes, despite normal resting LV systolic function, a blunted recruitment of myocardial contractility plays an important role in determining exercise-induced LV dysfunction. This abnormal response to exercise may be related in part to an impairment of cardiac sympathetic innervation. Clinical studies have also shown that the limited cardiac output response to exercise in patients with diabetes is related to a reduction in cardiac parasympathetic nervous system activity and can be manifested by an abnormal electrocardiographic RR variation. This index of parasympathetic nervous system activity can identify that subset of diabetic patients who may need special consideration when exercise training is prescribed.

Cardiac autonomic neuropathy is also believed to contribute to diastolic dysfunction (26). In patients with diabetes, alterations in sympathetic nervous system activity, as evidenced by decreased myocardial MIBG uptake, is associated with abnormalities of LV diastolic filling. Nocturnal elevations in arterial blood pressure have been suggested to be the link between autonomic neuropathy and diastolic ventricular dysfunction (18). Of the various tests of autonomic nervous system function, the one that correlates the best to impaired diastolic filling is an abnormal response to orthostasis, measured as the extent of reduction in systolic blood pressure upon standing.

V. HEART DISEASE AND PREDIABETIC STATES

The duration of diabetes influences the development of CAD in patients with type 1 diabetes, but such a relationship has not been demonstrated in those with type 2. Therefore, it is unclear whether the duration of asymptomatic hyperglycemia, or the state of impaired glucose tolerance, may have an important role on the development of CAD preceding the overt manifestations of type 2 diabetes (31,32). Several studies have shown that the mortality rate due to CAD was higher in patients with impaired glucose tolerance compared to normoglycemic men, although it was smaller when compared to that of patients with overt diabetes. At least one study has demonstrated that the risk of CAD increases linearly with fasting blood glucose levels in patients with impaired glucose tolerance, whereas the fasting insulin level has been implicated as a possible independent risk factor for CAD mortality in another study. Early impairment of LV diastolic function has been documented not only in patients with type 2 diabetes, but also in those with impaired glucose tolerance, independent of the confounding role of myocardial ischemia, body weight, and levels of arterial blood pressure (33). Similarly, early atherosclerotic changes, as well as borderline impairment of cardiac autonomic function, could be demonstrated in those subjects with impaired glucose tolerance. The various diagnostic tests previously reviewed that are useful in the diagnosis of heart disease in patients with previously diagnosed diabetes can also be applied to those with impaired glucose tolerance or prediabetic states, although the clinical benefits and cost effectiveness of a strategy directed to screen for early cardiac abnormalities in asymptomatic subjects with prediabetic states or impaired glucose tolerance remains to be established.

REFERENCES

1. Wingard D, Barrett-Conor E. Heart disease and diabetes. In: Harris MI, eds. Diabetes in America. Bethesda, MD: NIH publication No. 95–1468, 1995:429–448.
2. Kleinman JC, Donahue RP, Harris MI, Finucane FF, Madans JH, Brock DB.

Mortality among diabetics in a national sample. Am J Epidemiol 1988; 128:389–401.

3. Bloomgarden ZT. American Diabetes Association 60th Scientific Sessions, 2000 Cardiovascular disease in diabetes. Diabetes Care 2001; 24 399–404.

4. Garcia MJ, McNamara PM, Gordon T, Kannel WB. Morbidity and mortality in diabetics in the Framingham population. Sixteen year follow-up study. Diabetes 1974; 23:105–111.

5. Paillole C, Ruiz J, Juliard JM, Leblanc H, Gourgon R, Passa P. Detection of coronary artery disease in diabetic patients. Diabetologia 1995; 38:726–731.

6. Kannel WB. Silent myocardial ischemia and infarction: insights from the Framingham Study. Cardiol Clin 1986; 4:583–591.

7. Paillole C, Passa P, Paycha F, Juliard JM, Steg PG, Leblanc H, Philippe L, Gourgon R. Non-invasive identification of severe coronary artery disease in patients with long-standing diabetes mellitus. Eur J Med 1992; 1:464–468.

8. Gibbons RJ, Balady GJ, Beasley JW, Bricker JT, Duvernoy WF, Froelicher VF, Mark DB, Marwick TH, McCallister BD, Thompson PD, Jr., Winters WL, Yanowitz FG, Ritchie JL, Cheitlin MD, Eagle KA, Gardner TJ, Garson A, Jr., Lewis RP, O'Rourke RA, Ryan TJ. ACC/AHA Guidelines for Exercise Testing. A report of the American College of Cardiology/American Heart Association Task Force on Practice Guidelines (Committee on Exercise Testing). J Am Coll Cardiol 1997; 30: 260–311.

9. Stone PH, Chaitman BR, Forman S, Andrews TC, Bittner V, Bourassa MG, Davies RF, Deanfield JE, Frishman W, Goldberg AD, MacCallum G, Ouyang P, Pepine CJ, Pratt CM, Sharaf B, Steingart R, Knatterud GL, Sopko G, Conti CR. Prognostic significance of myocardial ischemia detected by ambulatory electrocardiography, exercise treadmill testing, and electrocardiogram at rest to predict cardiac events by one year (the Asymptomatic Cardiac Ischemia Pilot [ACIP] study). Am J Cardiol 1997; 80:1395–401.

10. Davies RF, Goldberg AD, Forman S, Pepine CJ, Knatterud GL, Geller N, Sopko G, Pratt C, Deanfield J, Conti CR. Asymptomatic Cardiac Ischemia Pilot (ACIP) study two-year follow-up: outcomes of patients randomized to initial strategies of medical therapy versus revascularization. Circulation 1997 95:2037–2043.

11. Topol EJ, Nissen SE. Our preoccupation with coronary luminology. The dissociation between clinical and angiographic findings in ischemic heart disease. Circulation 1995; 92:2333–2342.

12. Riff ER, Riff KM. Abnormalities of myocardial depolarization in overt, subclinical and prediabetes. A vectorcardiographic study. Diabetes 1974; 23:572–578.

13. Schurgin S, Rich S, Mazzone T. Increased prevalence of significant coronary artery calcification in patients with diabetes. Diabetes Care 2001 24:335–338.

14. LeWinter MM. Diabetic cardiomyopathy: an overview. Coron Artery Dis 1996; 7: 95–98.

15. Spector KS. Diabetic cardiomyopathy. Clin Cardiol 1998; 21:885–887.

16. Poirier P, Garneau C, Marois L, Jobin JF, Dumesnil JG. Impact of diastolic dysfunction on maximal treadmill performance in type 2 diabetic subjects without clinical heart disease. Med Sci Sports Exercise Med 1999; 31:S361.

17. Vered A, Battler A, Segal P, Liberman D, Yerushalmi Y, Berezin M, Neufeld HN.

Exercise-induced left ventricular dysfunction in young men with asymptomatic diabetes mellitus (diabetic cardiomyopathy). Am J Cardiol 1984; 54:633–637.

18. Monteagudo PT, Moises VA, Kohlmann O, Jr., Ribeiro AB, Lima VC, Zanella MT. Influence of autonomic neuropathy upon left ventricular dysfunction in insulin-dependent diabetic patients. Clin Cardiol 2000; 23:371–375.

19. Nielsen FS, Sato A, Ali S, Tarnow L, Smidt UM, Kastrup J, Parving HH. Beneficial impact of ramipril on left ventricular hypertrophy in normotensive nonalbuminuric NIDDM patients. Diabetes Care 1998; 21:804–809.

20. Tischler MD. Clinical abnormalities of cardiac function and echocardiographic tissue characterization in diabetes mellitus. Coron Artery Dis 1996; 7:139–142.

21. Poirer P, Bogaty P, Garneau C, Marois L, Dumesnil JG. Diastolic dysfunction in normotensive men with well-controlled type 2 diabetes—Importance of maneuvers in echocardiographic screening for preclinical diabetic cardiomyopathy. Diabetes Care 2001; 24:5–10.

22. Nagueh SF, Middleton KJ, Kopelen HA, Zoghbi WA, Quinones MA. Doppler tissue imaging: a noninvasive technique for evaluation of left ventricular relaxation and estimation of filling pressures. J Am Coll Cardiol 1997; 30:1527–1533.

23. Sohn DW, Chai IH, Lee DJ, Kim HC, Kim HS, Oh BH, Lee MM, Park YB, Choi YS, Seo JD, Lee YW. Assessment of mitral annulus velocity by Doppler tissue imaging in the evaluation of left ventricular diastolic function. J Am Coll Cardiol 1997; 30:474–480.

24. Di Bello V, Talarico L, Picano E, Di Muro C, Landini L, Paterni M, Matteucci E, Giusti C, Giampietro O. Increased echodensity of myocardial wall in the diabetic heart: an ultrasound tissue characterization study. J Am Coll Cardiol 1995; 25:1408–1415.

25. Perez JE, McGill JB, Santiago JV, Schechtman KB, Waggoner AD, Miller JG, Sobel BE. Abnormal myocardial acoustic properties in diabetic patients and their correlation with the severity of disease. J Am Coll Cardiol 1992; 19:1154–1162.

26. Zola B, Kahn JK, Juni JE, Vinik AI. Abnormal cardiac function in diabetic patients with autonomic neuropathy in the absence of ischemic heart disease. J Clin Endocrinol Metab 1986; 63:208–214.

27. Valensi P, Sachs RN, Harfouche B, Lormeau B, Paries J, Cosson E, Paycha F, Leutenegger M, Attali JR. Predictive value of cardiac autonomic neuropathy in diabetic patients with or without silent myocardial ischemia. Diabetes Care 2001; 24:339–343.

28. Mustonen J, Mantysaari M, Kuikka J, Vanninen E, Vainio P, Lansimies E, Uusitupa M. Decreased myocardial ^{123}I-Metaiodobenzylguanidine uptake is associated with disturbed left ventricular diastolic filling in diabetes. Am Heart J 1992; 123:804–805.

29. Ducher M, Cerutti C, Gustin MP, Abou-Amara S, Thivolet C, Laville M, Paultre CZ, Fauvel JP. Noninvasive exploration of cardiac autonomic neuropathy. Four reliable methods for diabetes? Diabetes Care 1999; 22:388–393.

30. Massin MM, Derkenne B, Tallsund M, Rocour-Brumioul D, Ernould C, Lebrethon MC, Bourguignon JP. Cardiac autonomic dysfunction in diabetic children. Diabetes Care 1999; 22:1845–1850.

31. Haffner SM. Cardiovascular risk factors and the prediabetic syndrome. Ann Med 1996; 28:363–370.
32. Haffner SM. The prediabetic problem: development of non-insulin-dependent diabetes mellitus and related abnormalities. J Diabetes Complic 1997; 11:69–76.
33. Celentano A, Vaccaro O, Tammaro P, Galderisi M, Crivaro M, Oliviero M, Imperatore G, Palmieri V, Iovino V, Riccardi G, et al. Early abnormalities of cardiac function in non-insulin-dependent diabetes mellitus and impaired glucose tolerance. Am J Cardiol 1995; 76:1173–1176.

11

Treatment of Diabetes: Implications for Heart Disease

Thomas A. Buchanan, Howard N. Hodis, and Wendy J. Mack
University of Southern California Keck School of Medicine,
Los Angeles, California

I. OVERVIEW

There are three general levels of glycemic control that can be set as goals in the management of patients with type 1 or type 2 diabetes: (1) keep patients out of ketoacidosis and hyperosmolar coma; (2) prevent symptoms of hyperglycemia (e.g., polyuria) and catabolism (fatigue, weight loss, and hyperphagia); and (3) prevent long-term complications associated with diabetes. In the absence of extenuating social or medical circumstances that make prevention of long-term complications irrelevant (e.g., terminal illness) or infeasible (e.g., inability of the patient to cooperate with a complex care program), the third level should be the standard of care for people with diabetes. The effectiveness of good glycemic control in slowing or preventing the development of diabetic retinopathy, nephropathy, and neuropathy has been demonstrated in several well-controlled clinical trials and is beyond question. Whether good glycemic control has a beneficial effect on the risk of atherosclerosis and its clinical manifestations remains controversial. In this chapter, we will illustrate that improved glycemic control is beneficial for reducing the risk of clinical atherosclerotic events, but that methods of achieving good control may differ in their impact on such events.

II. APPROACHES TO GLYCEMIC CONTROL

There is normally a curvilinear relationship between the degree of tissue sensitivity to insulin and the amount of insulin required to maintain normal glycemia

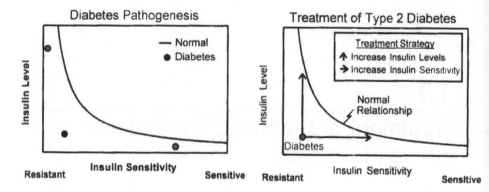

Figure 1 *Left panel*: Schematic diagram of relationship between insulin sensitivity and insulin levels in pathogenesis of diabetes. Curved line represents relationship in cross-section of normal people with a wide range of insulin sensitivity. Closed circles represent the different relationships that can lead to diabetes because insulin levels are below insulin requirements. *Right panel*: Schematic diagram of approaches to the treatment of insulin-resistant people with type 2 diabetes. A normal relationship between insulin levels and requirements can be achieved by increasing insulin levels (vertical arrow), increasing insulin sensitivity (horizontal arrow), or both (not shown).

(Fig. 1, left). People who have less insulin in their blood than required by their tissues have hyperglycemia. In patients with type 1 diabetes, the insulin deficiency is generally absolute, occurring as a result of autoimmune destruction of pancreatic B cells in the absence of tissue resistance to insulin. Type 2 diabetes is a more heterogeneous group of disorders in which there is generally tissue insensitivity to insulin that is associated with inadequate pancreatic B-cell compensation for the insulin resistance. The B-cell inadequacy tends to be progressive over time, leading to marked insulin deficiency in patients who have had type 2 diabetes for many years.

Successful treatment of hyperglycemia requires reestablishment of the normal relationship between insulin levels and insulin needs. For patients with type 1 diabetes, the therapeutic choices are relatively simple. Insulin deficiency can be treated with exogenous insulin or transplantation of new insulin-secreting tissue. The end result of a successful treatment program for type 1 diabetes is normal blood sugars with mild hyperinsulinemia owing to the fact that endogenous insulin is secreted directly into the portal vein and substantially cleared during the first pass through the liver, while exogenous insulin is administered into the peripheral circulation. Whole pancreas transplantation also results in insulin delivery to the peripheral circulation and modest hyperinsulinemia, while recently successful transplantation of pancreatic islets into the liver holds the promise of direct hepatic delivery and less hyperinsulinemia.

Treatment options for type 2 diabetes are more varied. For many years the only pharmacological therapies available in the United States were sulfonylurea drugs and insulin. Both therapies are capable of attaining good blood glucose control by increasing circulating insulin levels (vertical arrow in Fig. 1, right panel). More recently, drugs that alter hepatic glucose metabolism (metformin) or peripheral insulin resistance (thiazolidinedione drugs like pioglitazone and rosiglitazone) have become available for clinical use. These drugs offer the potential for improving glycemia without increasing (and in many cases decreasing) circulating insulin levels (horizontal arrow in Fig. 1, right panel). Combinations of two or more approaches (e.g., a peripheral or hepatic insulin-sensitizing agent and either an insulin secretogogue or exogenous insulin) appear to be additive in their effects on glycemia; the insulin sensitizers reduce the need for endogenous or exogenous insulin when such combination therapy is employed. Thus, clinicians now have an extensive armamentarium of medications that can be used to achieve hemoglobin A_{1C} concentrations in the low-risk range of 7% or less in people with type 2 diabetes. Treatment to this target can greatly reduce the risk of diabetic eye, kidney, and nerve disease. Indeed, any lowering of average glycemia and hemoglobin A_{1C} concentrations can lower the risk of all three of these complications.

III. IMPACT ON CARDIOVASCULAR DISEASE: THE DCCT AND UKPDS STUDIES

Clinical atherosclerosis results largely from acute embolic or thrombotic events that arise from long-term changes in the arterial wall. The pathogenesis of the arterial wall changes in relation to the metabolic abnormalities that attend poorly controlled diabetes are not well known in humans. Epidemiological studies indicate that both hyperglycemia and hyperinsulinemia increase the risk of atherosclerosis and of the acute clinical complications of that condition. The high triglyceride and low HDL cholesterol concentrations that frequently attend hyperglycemia may contribute as well. Animal studies suggest that good blood glucose control can mitigate the effects of diabetes on the arterial wall. Cross-sectionally, worsening glycemia is associated with thickening of the intima and media layers of the common carotid arteries. Intervention studies to test the impact of improved glycemic control on this or other measures of atherosclerosis are lacking. However, there is mounting evidence that the risk of acute clinical complications of atherosclerosis can be reduced by good glycemic control.

The Diabetes Control and Complications Trial (DCCT) was the first large study that examined the impact of lowering glycemia on the risk of long-term diabetic complications. Patients had type 1 diabetes, so they were mostly children or young adults. They were randomized to an intensive care arm (management by a multidisciplinary diabetes care team, intensive glucose self-monitoring, diabetes self-management with multiple daily insulin injections or an insulin infusion pump) or to standard care (less intensive management, one or two shots of insulin per day, no multidisciplinary care team). During a median follow-up of 6.5 years, median hemoglobin A_{1C} levels were 8.9% and 7.0% in standard and intensive management arms, respectively. The lower HbA_{1c} concentrations in the intensive arm were associated with 40 to 60% reductions in the development or progression of retinopathy, nephropathy, and neuropathy. Clinical cardiovascular events were uncommon in the DCCT, presumably owing to the relatively young age of the patients. Nonetheless, there clearly was no increase in such events in the intensively managed patients. Rates for all cardiovascular and peripheral events combined were 0.8 and 0.5 events per 100 patient-years in standard and intensive management groups. Intensive management reduced by 34% the number of patients who developed a serum cholesterol concentration >160 mg/dL during the trial. Thus, intensive treatment with insulin did not increase the risk of vascular events, as had been feared prior to the DCCT. Indeed, the actual frequency of events was slightly, but not significantly, lower in the intensive treatment group. Lipid profiles were better in the intensive management arm.

An analogous study to examine the effects of improved glycemic control on the risk of long-term complications was conducted in patients with type 2 diabetes—the United Kingdom Prospective Diabetes Study (UKPDS). The study design was quite complex. In essence, newly diagnosed type 2 diabetic patients were given 3 months of intensive dietary treatment, then randomized to receive one of two stepped-care management strategies. With the first strategy, patients were maintained on diet therapy alone unless fasting plasma glucose exceeded 270 mg/dL (15 mmol/L), at which time they were randomized to insulin, sulfonylurea, or metformin. Medication doses were adjusted or another medication was added to keep patients free of symptoms of hyperglycemia and to keep fasting plasma glucose <270 mg/dL. With the second strategy, patients were initially assigned to insulin, sulfonylurea, or metformin therapy. Medication doses were adjusted to achieve a fasting plasma glucose of <90 mg/dL (6 mmol/L). Additional medications were added if fasting glucose concentrations exceeded 270 mg/dL on maximum dose of sulfonylurea or metformin. The overall study contained more than 4000 patients and lasted for 12 years. Patients assigned to the second strategy (more intensive glucose management) had a mean HbA_{1C} that was ~1% lower than the HbA_{1C} of the less intensive management group. HbA_{1C} levels increased in both groups over time. The development of eye, kidney, and nerve complications of diabetes was reduced by 12 to 34% in the intensive therapy arm. The reductions were of similar magnitude regardless of whether the initial treatment was with insulin, a sulfonylurea, or metformin. Myocardial infarction was reduced by 16% when intensive management was initiated with insulin or sulfonylurea and by 39% when intensive management was initiated with metformin. The results of metformin-first treatment are not directly comparable to the results of insulin- or sulfonylurea-first treatments, since randomizations for those two parts of the UKPDS were performed several years apart. Nonetheless, the results of the UKPDS suggest very strongly that (1) the risk of acute cardiovascular events such as myocardial infarction is reduced by lowering circulating glucose concentrations in patients with type 2 diabetes; and (2) the risk reduction may be greater with regimens that lower (i.e., metformin), rather than raise (e.g., sulfonylureas or exogenous insulin), circulating insulin concentrations. It is also important to note that lowering blood pressure was effective in reducing cardiovascular events in the UKPDS. The effects of improved glycemia and improved blood pressure were independent of one another.

IV. FEWER CARDIOVASCULAR EVENTS WHEN GLUCOSE CONTROL IMPROVES

Improved blood glucose control is associated with a number of effects that could contribute to a reduction in the risk of clinical cardiovascular events such as myocardial infarction and stroke. Improved glycemia lowers PAI-1 concentrations and reduces platelet adhesiveness and aggregability. Chronic amelioration of hyperglycemia reduces glycation of proteins in the arterial wall and in circulating lipoproteins. Improved glycemia is associated with an amelioration of the circulating lipid abnormalities, especially the elevated triglycerides and low HDL cholesterol that are typical of poorly controlled type 1 or type 2 diabetes. No clinical trial has been conducted exclusively in patients with diabetes to determine the effects of lipid lowering per se on cardiovascular events. However, several lipid-lowering trials have included patients with type 2 diabetes. Post hoc analysis of those trials is informative about the potential role of hyperlipidemia in the genesis of atherosclerosis in patients with diabetes. The topic has also been reviewed recently by Goldberg (see Suggested Reading).

In the Scandinavian Simvastatin Survival Study (4S), simvastatin significantly reduced coronary mortality (42%) in the 2221 subjects randomized to lipid-lowering therapy relative to the 2223 placebo-treated subjects. Total mortality was also significantly reduced (30%) in the simvastatin-treated group. In the subgroup of 202 diabetic subjects, coronary events were significantly reduced (55%) with lipid-lowering therapy. Coronary and total mortality were nonsignificantly reduced (28% and 21%, respectively). All subjects in 4S had established cardiovascular disease prior to randomization and the average LDL-C level prior to treatment was 186 mg/dL in the subgroup of diabetic subjects. In the Cholesterol and Recurrent Events (CARE) study, coronary mortality was reduced 24% in the

2081 subjects randomized to pravastatin therapy relative o the 2078 subjects randomized to placebo treatment. Lipid-lowering therapy in CARE significantly reduced coronary events (25%) in the subgroup of 586 diabetic subjects. CARE was a secondary prevention trial and all subjects randomized to this trial had a previous myocardial infarction. The baseline LDL-C level was 136 mg/dL in the subgroup of diabetic subjects. In the Long-Term Intervention with Pravastatin in Ischemic Disease (LIPID) trial, coronary death was significantly reduced (24%) in the 4512 subjects randomized to pravastatin therapy relative to the 4502 subjects randomized to placebo treatment. Total mortality was also significantly reduced (22%) in the pravastatin-treated group. Lipid-lowering therapy in LIPID reduced fatal and nonfatal myocardial events 19% in the subgroup of 782 diabetic subjects. LIPID was a secondary prevention trial and the baseline LDL-C level was 150 mg/dL in the subgroup of diabetic subjects. The Air Force/Texas Coronary Atherosclerosis Prevention Study (AFCAPS) was a primary prevention trial in which the primary endpoint of fatal or nonfatal myocardial infarction, unstable angina, or sudden death was reduced 37% in the 3304 subjects treated with lovastatin relative to the 3301 subjects randomized to placebo. Lipid-lowering therapy reduced the primary endpoint 42% in the subgroup of 155 diabetic subjects. Baseline LDL-C in this trial was 150 mg/dL.

In summary, aggressive LDL-lowering therapy that resulted in LDL-C reductions of 25 to 35% reduced recurrent and first cardiovascular events by 19 to 55% in subjects with diabetes mellitus. Although these trials were not specifically designed to determine the effects of lipid lowering in diabetic subjects, they clearly indicate benefit in this subgroup of individuals equal to or greater than nondiabetic subjects. The optimum goal for LDL-C levels in diabetic subjects is less than 100 mg/dL and for total triglyceride levels, less than 150 mg/dL. Every effort to raise HDL-C to the highest level possible should be attempted. Optimum control of hyperglycemia usually results in optimization of triglyceride and HDL-C levels.

V. THIAZOLIDINEDIONES

Drugs of the thiazolidinedione (TZD) class have recently been introduced for treatment of type 2 diabetes. The first drug in the class, troglitazone, caused liver failure on rare occasions and has been removed from clinical use. Two other TZDs, pioglitazone and rosiglitazone, appear to be safer and are currently marketed in the United States. As a class, the drugs bind to the nuclear receptor PPAR-γ and alter the transcription of a number of genes. Their effects on carbohydrate metabolism are manifested as an increase in the sensitivity of skeletal muscle and adipose tissue to insulin in vivo. The available thiazolidinediones are approximately equally potent to sulfonylureas and metformin in lowering glucose concentrations in patients with type 2 diabetes. Their glucose-lowering effects rely on the presence of insulin in the bloodstream, so they are not effective by themselves in patients with type 1 diabetes. Since TZDs have their primary effect on muscle and adipose tissue, their glucose-lowering effects are additive to the effects of metformin, sulfonylurea drugs, and exogenous insulin.

In addition to their effects on glycemia, TZDs have several actions that make them particularly attractive for use in people who have atherosclerosis or are at increased risk for that disease. They ameliorate hyperinsulinemia, which has been associated with an increased risk of atherosclerosis in epidemiological and animal studies. They also have potentially beneficial effects on circulating lipids, although these effects differ between the available TZDs. Pioglitazone lowers triglycerides and raises HDL and LDL cholesterol levels. Rosiglitazone raises LDL and HDL cholesterol but has no consistent impact on triglyceride levels. TZDs have also been reported to shift the pattern of LDL particle size from small and dense to larger and less atherogenic. Finally, TZDs inhibit the growth-promoting effects of some endogenous growth factors on vascular smooth muscle and endothelial cells. In animal models and in one human study, TZDs reduced the endothelial hypertrophy that follows experimental endothelial injury or coronary angioplasty, respectively. These extraglycemic effects suggest that TZDs may have specific antiatherogenic properties. However, they have not yet been rigorously tested for their effects on atherosclerosis or related clinical events in patients with type 2 diabetes. It is of note that our group has observed a 30% reduction in the rate of thickening of carotid intima and media layers in insulin-resistant, nondiabetic women treated with troglitazone. Whether the effect was due to reversal of insulin resistance, which did occur, or to direct vascular effects of the drug is unknown. Nonetheless, this finding raises the possibility that insulin resistance may become a target for clinical intervention in nondiabetic but insulin-resistant individuals in the future.

VI. SUMMARY

Worries that aggressive treatment of hyperglycemia with insulin or insulin secretogogues would increase the risk of clinical cardiovascular disease are not supported by existing data from clinical trials. In fact, aggressive management of glycemia has been associated with a decrease, rather than an increase, in events such as myocardial infarction and stroke. Results from the UKPDS and from studies with thiazolidinediones suggest that approaches to glycemic management focused on amelioration of hepatic or peripheral tissue insulin resistance may be preferable to approaches that raise circulating insulin concentrations. However, both approaches have some beneficial impact on the risk of cardiovascular events compared to allowing patients to maintain chronic hyperglycemia. Much work is needed to understand the impact of improved glycemia, changes in circulating lipids, and alterations in insulin resistance and insulin levels in the pathogenesis of the arterial wall changes of atherosclerosis and in the precipitation of clinical cardiovascular events. Based on current information regarding events, clinical care of patients with type 1 or type 2 diabetes who remain at risk for long-term diabetic complications should include a stepped-care approach to achieve low-risk glycemia (HbA$_{1C}$ <7%) in addition to low-risk lipid and blood pressure levels.

SUGGESTED READING

1. The Diabetes Control and Complications Research Group. The effect or intensive treatment of diabetes on the development and progression of long-term complications in insulin-dependent diabetes mellitus. N Engl J Med 1993 329:977–986.
2. UKPDS Study Group. Effect of intensive blood glucose control with sulphonylureas or insulin compared with conventional treatment and risk of complications in patients with type 2 diabetes (UKPDS 33). Lancet 1998; 352:837–853.
3. UKPDS Study Group. Effect of intensive blood glucose control with metformin on complications in overweight patients with type 2 diabetes (UKPDS 34). Lancet 1998; 352:854–865.
4. UKPDS Study Group. Tight blood pressure control and risk of macrovascular and microvascular complications in type 2 diabetes: UKPDS 38. Br Med J 1998; 317: 703–713.
5. Goldberg IJ. Diabetic dyslipidemia: causes and consequences. J Clin Endocrinol Metab 2001; 86:965–971.

12

Management of Patients with Diabetes and Coronary Artery Disease

William E. Boden
Hartford Hospital, Hartford, and University of Connecticut School of Medicine, Farmington, Connecticut

I. INTRODUCTION

Diabetes mellitus (DM) is a major risk factor for accelerated atherosclerosis, is associated with a markedly increased prevalence of coronary artery disease (CAD), myocardial infarction (MI), and cardiac death, and is rapidly becoming a major public health concern in Western countries. The overall prevalence of CAD, as assessed by various invasive and noninvasive measures, is as high as 55% among adult patients with DM, compared with 2 to 4% for the general population. Diabetes mellitus also represents an independent risk factor for morbidity and mortality. The cardiovascular mortality rate has more than *doubled* in men and more than *quadrupled* in women with DM, compared to their counterparts without DM, and post-MI prognosis is also significantly worse in these patients.

Because diabetes is becoming such a common disease, diabetic patients account for a significant percentage of patients undergoing coronary revascularization procedures; indeed, diabetics represent 15 to 25% of patients referred for percutaneous or surgical treatment of CAD. Importantly, DM is a recognized risk factor for adverse outcomes after either percutaneous coronary intervention (PCI) or coronary artery bypass graft (CABG) surgery.

In particular, after coronary revascularization, short- and long-term outcomes in diabetic subjects are less favorable than in nondiabetic patients. In patients undergoing CABG surgery, DM is an independent predictor of lesion progression, occlusion, and reduced long-term survival. PCI has gained acceptance as an alternative to CABG surgery in selected patients. By contrast, several studies have demonstrated that diabetic subjects have worse clinical outcomes after angioplasty (primarily balloon angioplasty) compared with surgical coronary revascularization. These observations have led some to suggest that multivessel balloon angioplasty should be abandoned in diabetic patients. Despite similar initial procedural success, diabetic patients have a higher incidence of subsequent MI, restenosis, repeat revascularization, and long-term mortality. Recent advances in technique and adjunctive therapy for PCI have not clarified the optimal therapeutic approach in managing diabetic patients. Accordingly, patients with diabetes represent a unique challenge for clinical and interventional cardiologists and cardiac surgeons.

II. ROLE OF DIABETES IN THE GENESIS OF CAD

There are several clinical, angiographic, and biological features particular to DM that increase the propensity for developing CAD in diabetic patients. In the aggregate, these risk factors increase the likelihood for sustaining a clinical event and have important prognostic implications. Endothelial dysfunction, platelet and coagulation abnormalities, and metabolic disorders associated with DM play a major role in accelerating the process of atherosclerosis and generating coronary thrombosis. The interplay of these factors and processes affects healing after arterial wall injury. The diffuse and distal nature of coronary atherosclerosis may contribute to incomplete revascularization and may increase the risk of surgical or percutaneous revascularization in diabetic patients.

A. Metabolic Syndrome

The metabolic abnormalities associated with DM are well recognized and include insulin resistance (or, more appropriately, dysinsulinemia), hyperglycemia, hypertension, and dyslipidemia. These factors are associated with a panoply of biological perturbations that result in endothelial dysfunction with impaired coronary flow reserve, increased platelet activity, increased thromboxane A_2 secretion, higher fibrinogen and factor VII levels, lower antithrombin III and plasma fibrinolytic activity, and higher concentrations of plasminogen activator inhibitor (PAI-1). It is thus axiomatic that the dysinsulinemia of type 2 DM as well as other traditional risk factors be treated aggressively to delay or impede the genesis of cardiovascular and cerebrovascular events. What remains uncertain, at present, is whether treating aggressively the insulin resistance (or metabolic) syndrome in the years leading up to frank type 2 DM will decrease the likelihood of subsequent clinical events. The metabolic syndrome, first described by Reaven, has been proposed as a "disease" that includes many of the clinical, biological, and vascular abnormalities observed in non-insulin-requiring DM patients.

The metabolic syndrome includes hyperinsulinemia (impaired glucose tolerance) an abnormal lipid profile characterized by elevated triglycerides, low levels of high-density-lipoprotein (HDL) cholesterol, and increased low-density-lipoprotein (LDL) cholesterol, hypertension, and central obesity with an increased waist-to-hip ratio. Many cross-sectional studies have indicated that insulin resistance is associated with ultrasonographically or angiographically demonstrable atherosclerosis, even in the absence of other risk factors for CAD. However, controversy still exists about the mechanisms by which the metabolic syndrome induces or accelerates atherogenesis. Some have proposed that "traditional" cardiac risk factors are enhanced by hyperinsulinemia and may account for accelerated atherogenesis. Reaven hypothesized that insulin resistance and compensatory hyperinsulinemia might be the primary, or inciting, event causing hypertension and leading in turn to an increased risk of CAD. The exact role of insulin remains to be defined.

B. Hyperglycemia

The so-called traditional cardiovascular risk factors account for only about 25 to 50% of the increase in risk for developing CAD among diabetic patients. Thus, the pivotal role of glycemic control in the management of diabetic patients with CAD cannot be overemphasized. Further, hyperglycemia and dyslipidemia associated with DM are central to the pathogenesis of CAD development in these patients. Several prospective studies have emphasized that poor glycemic control predicts CAD risk among diabetic subjects. Lehto et al. demonstrated that the concomitant presence of fasting hyperglycemia and abnormal blood lipids were associated with a threefold higher risk of CAD morbidity and mortality in over 1000 diabetic patients who were followed for up to 7 years.

Hyperglycemia induces several abnormalities that may accelerate atherosclerosis. It decreases endothelium-dependent vasodilatation in humans and produces adverse changes in lipid and coagulation factors. Chronic hyperglycemia leads to glycosylation of proteins that can induce renal injury and lead to vascular damage and secondary hypertension. These changes exert direct toxic effects on the vasculature and accelerate the development of atherosclerosis. Recent results suggest that the deleterious effects of insulin or proinsulin on native vessel walls and on vessels subjected to PCI may account for a higher incidence of adverse outcomes after PCI in diabetic patients who are treated with insulin or oral hypoglycemic agents compared with those who were treated with dietary management and exercise alone.

C. Dyslipidemia

Hypertriglyceridemia associated with increased concentrations of the atherogenic small, dense LDL cholesterol and low levels of HDL cholesterol are the most frequently observed lipid and lipoprotein abnormalities associated with type 2 diabetes. Baseline triglyceride levels change with the development of DM and correlate well with levels of fasting hyperglycemia. Control of hyperglycemia ameliorates but does not normalize these abnormalities. There is no consensus on the best method to assess CAD in diabetics or whether diabetics with CAD should have a more aggressive target for LDL cholesterol reduction (and HDL cholesterol augmentation) than nondiabetics. Nevertheless strategies based essentially on LDL reduction in these patients do provide a basis for treatment of the elevated LDL in facilitating diabetic vasculopathy and, hence, indirectly support a more aggressive approach to dyslipidemia management in diabetic subjects with CAD.

In summary, metabolic abnormalities associated with DM play a vital role in both the genesis and progression of atherosclerosis. It is imperative that control of these metabolic abnormalities, either through diet and exercise or the aggressive use of combination pharmacotherapy, can elicit a positive benefit in reducing cardiovascular and cerebrovascular events in diabetic patients with established CAD.

III. MEDICAL MANAGEMENT OF CAD IN DIABETIC SUBJECTS

A. General Principles

It is well recognized that diabetics—even those without overt manifestations of CAD—are at significantly increased risk for developing MI Finnish investigators reported that the risk of developing a MI was similar in diabetic patients without prior infarction compared with the risk in nondiabetic patients with a history of prior MI. Such a propensity for developing MI among diabetics without a history of MI argues persuasively for an aggressive strategy of primary prevention in diabetics that would parallel secondary prevention efforts in patients with established CAD. Regrettably, there is evidence that the majority of diabetic patients do not receive optimal medical therapy; there is suboptimal implementation of angiotensin converting enzyme (ACE) inhibitors and lipid-altering agents.

Vigorous control of hyperglycemia, hyperlipidemia, hypertension, and other risk factors is crucial to optimize risk reduction. Behavioral modifications are similarly important. Weight loss and increased physical activity are indicated because of their beneficial effects in improving control of insulin resistance, hyperglycemia, obesity, abnormal lipid profiles, as well as platelet and coagulation abnormalities. Cigarette smoking is recognized as an independent predictor of mortality in diabetic patients, especially diabetic women with insulin-requiring DM in whom the risk of cardiac mortality more than doubles compared to diabetic women who are nonsmokers. Thus, smoking cessation is imperative among diabetics.

B. Control of Hyperglycemia

Several studies demonstrate the importance of intensive glycemic control in preventing or reducing microvascular complications of DM. The effect of intensive glycemic control on macrovascular complications in type 1 and type 2 DM is not as convincing. The Diabetes Control and Complications Trial (DCCT) demonstrated compelling evidence in support of a major reduction in chronic microvascular complications among type 1 diabetics under tight glycemic control. In the same study, tight glycemic control was associated with a reduction in major macrovascular events by approximately 50% compared with that in those in whom glycemic control was conventional or less stringent. This difference did not achieve statistical significance. Similarly, the United Kingdom Prospective Diabetes Study (UKPDS) has shown that during 10 years of follow-up intensive glycemic control with either insulin or sulfonylureas decreased the risk of microvascular complications by 25% in non–insulin-requiring diabetics. The incidence of MI and diabetes-related mortality was reduced by 20% and 10%, respectively. Again, these differences did not achieve statistical significance. A similar reduction was observed in obese non–insulin-requiring diabetics who received metformin. In addition, a recent small-scale study showed that tight glycemic control in diabetic subjects reduced major cardiac adverse events (MACE) following balloon PCI. In the aggregate, these results support aggressive management of hyperglycemia in diabetics, especially in those who are candidates for coronary revascularization.

C. Use of Lipid-Altering Therapy

While there have been no prospective, randomized, clinical trials to evaluate the effects of lipid-altering therapy in the subsequent development of CAD among diabetic patients, there is a consistent body of scientific evidence derived from subset analyses. These results indicate that lipid-altering therapy is beneficial in both primary and secondary prevention. A subset analysis of the Scandinavian Simvastatin Survival Study (4S) showed that, in diabetic patients with elevated total cholesterol and LDL cholesterol, normal triglycerides, and established CAD, there was a significant reduction in major CAD and related atherosclerotic events.

Overall, 5-year cause-specific (cardiovascular) mortality was reduced by 43% in diabetic patients and by 29% in nondiabetic patients. Similar findings were observed in the Cholesterol And Recurrent Events (CARE) trial, where patients with documented CAD were randomized to pravastatin or placebo in the settings of "normal," or desirable, levels of LDL cholesterol following an index MI. The overall trial results showed a statistically significant benefit for all patients who received pravastatin. An even greater event rate reduction was seen in diabetic patients compared with the nondiabetic subjects. In particular, the relative risk reduction among the pravastatin-treated diabetics was significantly greater than among nondiabetics for major adverse cardiac events and the subsequent need for myocardial revascularization during a 5-year follow-up. The Long-term Intervention with Pravastatin in Ischemic Disease (LIPID) trial showed a similar approximate 20% reduction in the primary composite endpoint of coronary heart disease, death, or MI during a 6.1-year follow-up among diabetic patients compared with nondiabetic patients treated with pravastatin. These differences did not achieve statistical significance.

The Veterans Affairs–HDL Intervention Trial (VA–HIT) showed that gemfibrozil, administered to male veterans with established CAD and whose only lipid abnormality was "isolated low-HDL cholesterol" (mean baseline LDL cholesterol = 111 mg/dL), resulted in a 22% reduction in the trial primary endpoint of coronary heart disease death or nonfatal MI during a mean 5.1-year follow-up. The beneficial effects were observed equally among diabetic and nondiabetic subjects.

The role of niacin and its safety for use in diabetics has long been questioned. Certainly, short-acting (or immediate-release) niacin preparations are associated with disturbing side effects, notably cutaneous flushing. Sustained-released preparations (particularly those agents sold "over the counter" and in health food outlets) can be associated with dangerous hepatotoxicity, which may be even more problematic in the diabetic. Earlier studies with various niacin preparations in diabetics have revealed concerns about worsening glucose metabolism (by increasing fasting hyperglycemia and increasing insulin requirements) and increases in uric acid.

More recently, a once-daily, extended-release formulation of niacin (Niaspan) has been approved by the U.S. Food and Drug Administration. This agent has been tested extensively in unselected patients with dyslipidemia as well as in diabetic patients with dyslipidemia and/or features of the metabolic syndrome. Niaspan was shown to be efficacious in lowering elevated triglycerides and raising HDL cholesterol levels. Further, Niaspan was safe in diabetics and did not worsen glycemic control. Statin monotherapy is frequently suboptimal in diabetic patients because their atherogenic lipid profile may not be amenable to this form of treatment. Accordingly, Niaspan holds great promise as an important therapeutic agent in the management of diabetic dyslipidemia.

D. Antihypertensive Therapy

Among diabetics, achievement of blood pressure control is of paramount importance to reducing cardiovascular events that occur as a consequence of macrovascular complications. The previously cited UKPDS Trial showed that control of blood pressure with either a beta-blocker or ACE inhibitor was associated with an important salutary effect on microvascular complications. Uncertainty continues to exist concerning the "optimal" blood pressure target for diabetics—especially those with overt manifestations of CAD. In addition, there continues to be controversy regarding which classes of antihypertensive agents are most efficacious in diabetics. The most recent report from the Joint National Committee on Prevention, Detection, Evaluation and Treatment of Hypertension (JNC-6) recommended a blood pressure target of 130/85 mmHg for diabetic patients. First-line therapy should include ACE inhibitors, cardioselective beta-blockers, and diuretics. Each has been demonstrated to reduce morbidity and mortality in patients with diabetic nephropathy and in non-insulin-requiring patients with diabetes. Calcium antagonists can be used as second-line therapy or as part of combination therapy.

Approximately 80% of diabetic subjects will die of cardiovascular disease and more than half of those with type 2 diabetes, particularly women, are hypertensive by age 50 when the recently recommended target of 130/85 mmHg is used for the diagnosis of hypertension. The prevalence of hypertension in diabetic subjects is considerably higher than in the general population. Among diabetics, 40–50% are hypertensive compared with 20% of patients without DM. Among diabetic patients greater than age 75, 60% are hypertensive. The prevalence of essential hypertension in patients with type 2 DM is two to three times greater than it is among nondiabetics.

E. Use of Pharmacotherapy for CAD and MI in Diabetics

1. Fibrinolytic Agents

Numerous studies have demonstrated that DM is a major independent predictor of acute and long-term post-MI morbidity and mortality. This is particularly true in women and in non-insulin-requiring diabetics. Many factors, including a greater extent and magnitude of angiographically severe CAD, associated comorbidity, metabolic disturbances, silent myocardial ischemia, and late or atypical clinical presentation (often without chest discomfort) may contribute to a lower utilization of fibrinolytic agents and may be causally implicated in a worse post-MI prognosis among diabetic patients.

An overview by the Fibrinolytic Therapy Trialists' Collaborative Group evaluated results from 4529 diabetic patients from a total sample of 43,073 patients who presented with acute ST-segment-elevation MI. These results confirmed the important benefit of thrombolysis in diabetic patients. The absolute reduction in mortality was greater in diabetic patients than in nondiabetics (3.7% vs. 2.1%), despite a greater 35-day mortality rate in diabetics (13.6% vs. 8.7%). Diabetics also had a modestly higher absolute risk of developing hemorrhagic stroke than nondiabetics (0.6% vs. 0.4%). This difference was not statistically significant.

2. Insulin-Glucose Infusion

Long-term mortality in diabetic patients who are hospitalized for acute MI may be reduced by an insulin-glucose infusion followed by multidose insulin treatment. In the Diabetes and Insulin-Glucose Infusion in Acute Myocardial Infarction (DIGAMI) study, an infusion of insulin and glucose followed by daily subcutaneous injections of insulin resulted in a 52% reduction in mortality within 1 year after myocardial infarction among patients with DM. This beneficial effect was attributed to improved metabolic control in the presence of an extreme increase in the level of catecholamines in blood and ischemic myocardium that is associated with sudden ischemic episodes. Insulin therapy appeared to beneficially influence acute cardiovascular mortality. A striking reduction in the incidence of fatal reinfarction and left ventricular failure was seen. These results are consistent with favorable effects in reducing mortality among diverse groups of patients treated with a glucose–insulin–potassium infusion in the setting of acute MI.

3. Antiplatelet Agents (Aspirin, Thienopyridines, Platelet Glycoprotein IIb/IIIa Agents) and Antithrombin Agents

Platelet and coagulation abnormalities contribute to the development of CAD in diabetic patients. Results from diverse randomized clinical trials support the use of antiplatelet therapy in all diabetic patients. A meta-analysis of the Antiplatelet Trialists' Collaborative Group included over 47,000 patients (of whom approximately 10% were diabetics) and demonstrated an important benefit of aspirin therapy in diabetics with, or at increased risk for, vascular disease. The combined endpoint of vascular death, MI, or stroke was 22.3% in the control group and 18.5% in the aspirin group. The magnitude of benefit was similar in both diabetic and nondiabetic patients, and there was no evidence of excess bleeding in the former group. A preliminary report from the CURE trial investigators showed a significant 25% relative risk reduction in the composite endpoint of death and MI in 12,562 patients with acute coronary syndromes who were randomized to aspirin plus clopidogrel and compared with aspirin alone for up to 9 months of blinded therapy. The favorable treatment effects were seen across all subgroups of patients studied, including patients with diabetes.

Clinical trials with low-molecular-weight heparins (LMWH) indicate that these agents are more effective than placebo and as beneficial as, if not superior to, standard unfractionated heparin (UFH) in the management of patients with non-ST-segment elevation acute coronary syndromes (unstable angina or non-Q-wave MI). For the most part, these studies demonstrate a consistent treatment benefit among patient subgroups. The ESSENCE trial demonstrated comparable benefits among diabetics and nondiabetics. In the TIMI-11B trial, enoxaparin was found to be superior to UFH in preventing cardiac death and nonfatal cardiac events (MI and unstable angina). Beneficial effects of enoxaparin were greatest in high-risk patients. In the GUSTO IIB trial, hirudin, a direct thrombin inhibitor, was more effective than UFH in the treatment of diabetic patients who presented with an acute coronary syndrome (ACS) and was not associated with increased risk of bleeding.

Results from randomized trials provide strong evidence that platelet glyco-protein (GP) IIb/IIIa inhibitors reduce the early and short-term incidence of death, MI, and recurrent angina in patients who present with non-ST-segment elevation acute coronary syndromes. In the PRISM-PLUS study, the benefit associated with tirofiban plus heparin in reducing cardiac events compared to heparin alone was comparable for both diabetic and nondiabetic subjects. Importantly, combination therapy of tirofiban plus heparin compared with heparin alone reduced significantly the secondary endpoint of death and MI much more profoundly in the diabetic subjects compared with that in the overall study population (88% vs. 43%; $p = 0.005$). In the PURSUIT trial, death and nonfatal MI were also significantly reduced by eptifibatide compared to placebo in both diabetic and nondiabetic subgroups of non-ST-segment elevation ACS. However, compared to nondiabetic patients, 30-day mortality was reduced to a greater extent in insulin-requiring diabetic patients. A meta-analysis that pooled diabetic patients from 10 recent trials of GP IIb/IIIa inhibitors revealed that diabetics had *twice* the absolute reduction in cardiac event rates compared to nondiabetics. There was a strong trend favoring an interaction between DM and the use of GP IIb/IIIa agents, but this did not reach statistical significance. The role of this class of agents when used adjunctively during PCI will be discussed in the section that details outcomes among diabetics who undergo myocardial revascularization.

4. Beta-Blockers

Pooled data from several trials of beta-blockers administered as secondary prevention post-MI demonstrate an overall 25% mortality reduction and a 29% reduction in reinfarction. Diabetic subjects exhibit an almost threefold greater reduction in mortality compared to nondiabetics (37% vs. 13%). A similar reduction in the incidence of reinfarction was apparent in those with and without diabetes. The results unquestionably underscore the important role of beta-blocker therapy after MI in diabetic patients. Unless there is an overt contraindication, all diabetic patients with prior MI or established CAD should receive a betablocker as part of a standard secondary prevention regimen.

5. Angiotensin-Converting-Enzyme (ACE) Inhibitors

Post hoc analyses of many prospective, randomized studies indicate that the use of ACE inhibitors in diabetics with acute MI is associated with significant reductions in short-term mortality and occurrence rates of congestive heart failure. In addition, similar data support an important long-term benefit of these drugs in diabetic patients who have had an MI complicated by systolic left ventricular dysfunction. Recent results of the Danish TRACE trial revealed that the ACE inhibitor trandolapril after MI in diabetic patients with left ventricular dysfunction decreased mortality and reduced the risk of progression to severe heart failure. In addition, in studies of high-risk diabetic patients with CAD but no prior MI, ACE inhibitors have been shown to decrease cardiac events in those subjects with congestive heart failure. ACE inhibitors reduce morbidity and mortality to a greater extent in diabetic patients.

The Heart Outcomes Prevention Evaluation (HOPE) trial demonstrated the beneficial role of ACE inhibitors in high-risk diabetics with CAD. In this trial, a predefined group of 3651 middle-aged diabetic patients at risk for cardiovascular and renal disease were randomized to receive the ACE inhibitor ramipril or placebo for 4 years. The primary endpoint of cardiovascular death, MI, and stroke was reduced by 24% and mortality alone was reduced by 38% in the ramipril-treated patients. Moreover, diabetic complications and microvascular disease were reduced by 17%. An additional important finding of the HOPE trial was that the decrease in composite clinical events was similar among diabetic patients with or without systolic left ventricular dysfunction.

In summary, the data from numerous randomized, clinical trials assessing the impact of various pharmacotherapies on outcomes in diabetic patients provide abundant scientific evidence in support of a multifaceted, aggressive approach to medical treatment. All diabetic patients should receive intensive glycemic control. All diabetic patients should take 325 mg aspirin daily. Further analysis of the results of the CURE trial may lead to an additional recommendation for treatment with 75 mg clopidogrel daily. Hypertension should be managed aggressively with (preferably) an ACE inhibitor such as ramipril and, for diabetic patients who have sustained an MI, ACE inhibitor therapy should be administered as secondary prevention, along with a beta-blocker—ideally a cardioselective beta-blocker such as atenolol or metoprolol. These cardioselective beta-blockers should limit the masking of promonitory symptoms of hypoglycemia. Additionally, if diabetic patients with CAD or MI exhibit evidence of systolic left ventricular dysfunction, an ACE inhibitor will have important salutary effects on ventricular remodeling and decreased progression to advanced heart failure. In addition, several evidence-based pharmacological treatment strategies have shown convincing benefits in diabetic patients with CAD. Specifically, diabetic patients who present with non-ST-segment-elevation ACS should be treated with GP IIb/IIIa inhibitors such as tirofiban in combination with UFH or LMWH to decrease thrombotic complications and reduce clinical events. Additional randomized studies should evaluate the role of tight glycemic control on the reduction of major cardiovascular events with or without coronary revascularization. The Bypass Angioplasty Revascularization Investigation (BARI) 2D trial has been initiated recently, and will be discussed in greater detail in the section on myocardial revascularization of the diabetic patient.

IV. SURGICAL AND INTERVENTIONAL MANAGEMENT OF CAD IN DIABETICS

Several clinical trials have demonstrated that outcomes after myocardial revascularization are different in diabetic patients compared to nondiabetic patients. These differences should influence treatment decisions.

Over the last decade, percutaneous coronary intervention (PCI) has gained increasing acceptance as an alternative to CABG surgery in selected patients. However, several reports demonstrating reduced long-term survival in diabetic patients treated with standard coronary balloon angioplasty have led to concerns regarding the use of PCI in this group of patients. A complete understanding of the mechanisms responsible for the reduced survival is of critical importance in the management of diabetic patients.

The operative and procedural management of diabetics with symptomatic CAD will be discussed based on the type of intervention employed. This section will detail the short- and long-term clinical outcomes associated with standard balloon PCI, PCI with stents, and CABG surgery in diabetic subjects. Where it is germane, there will be a discussion of the role of adjunctive therapies—notably the GP IIb/IIIa inhibitors—in the management of the diabetic patient who is undergoing catheter-based revascularization.

A. Catheter-Based Revascularization

1. Role of "Standard" Balloon Angioplasty: In-Hospital Outcomes

Angiographic success rates (85 to 95%) following conventional balloon PCI in diabetics are similar to nondiabetics. The composite endpoint of mortality, nonfatal MI, and urgent target vessel revascularization (TVR) was 11.0% in diabetics compared with 6.7% in nondiabetics, respectively ($p < 0.0$) based on registry data derived from the National Heart, Lung and Blood Institute. Higher mortality rates were seen in diabetics (3.2%) compared with nondiabetics (0.5%; $p < 0.05$). However, lower mortality rates (<0.5%)—comparable to rates in nondiabetics— have also been reported.

2. Short- and Long-Term Follow-Up

High restenosis rates (up to 63% in some series) have been reported after balloon PCI in diabetic patients. Late clinical outcomes after balloon angioplasty in diabetics are also frequently unfavorable. Stein and coworkers reported that the 5-year MI-free survival rate was lower and that the subsequent revascularization was more frequent among 1333 diabetics compared with 9300 nondiabetics undergoing balloon PCI. Likewise, Kip et al. showed that the 9-year mortality was twice as high in diabetic patients treated with balloon angioplasty compared to nondiabetics (35.9 vs. 17.9%), respectively, with significantly higher rates of MI and repeat revascularization.

In the Bypass Angioplasty Revascularization Investigation (BARI) trial, post-balloon angioplasty 5-year survival was 73.3% in diabetics compared with 91.3% in nondiabetics ($p < 0.0001$). The benefit of CABG surgery was most evident in the non-insulin-requiring DM patients. More recently, the BARI investigators have reported 7-year outcomes. These results show that, for the entire study group of 1873 patients, the composite trial primary endpoint favors improved clinical outcomes in the patients who were randomized to CABG surgery, compared to balloon PCI; Kaplan-Meier estimates of 7-year survival for the total population were 84.4% for CABG and 80.9% for balloon PCI ($p = 0.043$). Further post hoc analyses of these findings indicate that all of the benefit associated with CABG surgery occurs in the diabetic subgroup; among the 353 patients with treated DM, the 7-year survival rate was 76.4% for CABG surgery versus 55.7% for balloon PCI ($p = 0.0011$). Among the remaining 1476 patients without treated DM, survival was virtually identical by assigned treatment (86.4% for CABG vs. 86.8% for balloon angioplasty; $p = 0.72$). Despite similar survival, the balloon PCI group had substantially higher subsequent revascularization rates than the CABG group (59.7% vs. 13.1%; $p < 0.001$).

Similar results were observed in the Coronary Angioplasty versus Bypass Revascularization Investigation (CABRI) trial. A trend toward superiority of CABG was observed in the BARI registry, even though CAD was less extensive in balloon PCI than in surgical patients.

On the other hand, better results after CABG were not observed in the small subgroup of diabetics enrolled in the first Randomized Intervention Treatment of Angina One (RITA-1) study and in the Emory Angioplasty Surgery Trial (EAST).

Five- and 10-year survival rates were similar in diabetic patients undergoing balloon angioplasty compared with CABG surgery in the large nonrandomized series (n = 2639) reported by Weintraub and coworkers. Comparable 6-year results were also reported by Gum et al. in 525 diabetics.

In summary, in the majority of published series, balloon PCI in diabetic patients is feasible technically with high rates of initial angiographic success. However, DM appears to be predictive of higher risk of in-hospital complications, substantially increased early and late restenosis rates, and relatively poor long-term clinical outcomes.

2. Role of Coronary Stenting: In-Hospital Outcomes

Angiographic success rates (92 to 100%) of stenting in diabetics rival rates observed in nondiabetics. The composite endpoint of mortality, nonfatal MI, and urgent CABG, ranging from 0.7% to 6.8%, is similar among diabetics and nondiabetics in most series. The in-hospital complications after stent implantation compare favorably to the 3% to 11% rates reported after balloon PCI in diabetes. In one study, there was a trend toward higher rates of subacute stent thrombosis in diabetics (3.2%) compared with nondiabetics (2.0%; p = 0.06).

3. Short- and Long-Term Follow-Up

Angiographic restenosis rates among diabetics range from 24 to 40% after stenting compared to rates of 20 to 25% in nondiabetics. However, some reports have found more favorable results in diabetics. In a series reported by Van Belle, restenosis rates were similar (25 vs. 27%) after stenting, but different (63 vs. 32%) after balloon PCI in diabetics compared to nondiabetics, respectively.

Major adverse cardiac events are lower in diabetics. Elezi and coworkers reported a 1-year event-free survival in diabetics of 73.1% compared with 78.8% in nondiabetics (p < 0.001). In contrast, other studies have shown that long-term outcome after stenting is not influenced by the presence of diabetes.

Some reports (generally post hoc analyses) suggest that multivessel coronary stenting is safe and feasible with a high initial angiographic success rate, low in-hospital major complication rate, and favorable long-term outcomes. Prospectively acquired data concerning the role of this therapeutic strategy in a specifically targeted group of patients with type 2 diabetes is lacking. The recently initiated BARI-2D trial will test an important hypothesis by randomizing diabetic subjects who have undergone diagnostic coronary angiography to one of two different glycemic control strategies. One, an insulin-sensitizing regimen, will entail reliance on the use of insulin sensitizers such as thiazolidinediones and metformin. The other strategy, an insulin-providing regimen, will target the same efficacy of glycemic control but will use agents such as sulfonlyureas and insulin.

BARI-2D will utilize a 2 × 2 factorial design whereby type 2 diabetics with objective evidence of ischemia will be randomized to one of these two glycemic treatment regimens and randomized also to an early invasive approach ("revascularization of choice," including PCI/stenting or CABG) or an initial medical treatment of angina. The primary endpoint is a cardiac death during 5 years of follow-up. A total of 2800 patients will be recruited from both U.S. and Canadian sites.

A similar study is underway in the United States and Canada. This study is known as the Clinical Outcomes Utilizing Revascularization and Aggressive druG Evaluation (COURAGE) trial and will enroll up to 3000 patients (diabetic and nondiabetic) with symptomatic CAD and objective evidence of myocardial ischemia and single- or multivessel CAD. Two treatment strategies will be employed: PCI/stenting plus multifaceted, aggressive medical therapy or intensive medical therapy alone. Patients will be followed for 3 to 5 years and the primary endpoint is a composite of death, MI, or a biomarker-positive acute coronary syndrome. Medical therapy in both groups will consist of aspirin, clopidogrel, simvastatin, metoprolol, lisinopril, long-acting nitrates, and tirofiban, if needed. The hypothesis of COURAGE is that the combination of PCI plus multifaceted, aggressive medical therapy will be superior to medical therapy alone. To date, 1400 patients have been randomized, of whom 28% are diabetic. Both BARI-2D and COURAGE will provide important answers to questions regarding aggressive medical therapy in the context of state-of-the-art coronary revascularization.

In summary, stenting is feasible in diabetics with favorable procedural and in-hospital success rates. However, angiographic restenosis rates and long-term outcome after stenting in this population require careful prospective evaluation in large-scale randomized, controlled studies of diabetic patients with symptomatic CAD.

4. Mechanisms of Restenosis After Balloon PCI and Stenting

The basic mechanisms responsible for restenosis after catheter-based revascularization in diabetics have not been fully elucidated. The metabolic, hematological, and biological abnormalities observed in these patients all participate in the complex restenotic reaction following vessel injury. These patients' coronary lesions are more often associated with thrombus formation as detected by coronary angioscopy. Intravascular ultrasound demonstrates that intimal hyperplasia is the main reason for increased restenosis in both stented and nonstented lesions in diabetics. By contrast, other studies have reported favorably lower rates of restenosis after stenting in diabetics, results that do not appear to support the "excessive intimal hyperplasia" hypothesis.

An inability to completely revascularize all ischemic territories, high restenosis rates, and rapid progression of atherosclerosis requiring repeat revascularization procedures are the most frequently cited reasons for the long-term unfavorable results in diabetics. Although several hypotheses have been advanced, no conclusive explanation for this so-called "diabetes–balloon angioplasty" interaction has been found.

Van Belle and coworkers recently characterized restenosis in 603 diabetic patients treated with balloon angioplasty and scheduled for repeat coronary angiography 6 months later. During an average of 6.5 years, the incidence of both nonocclusive and occlusive restenosis was higher in diabetic subjects compared to historical controls. Further, the finding of occlusive restenosis was "a strong, independent correlate of long-term mortality." These provocative observational findings implicate accelerated restenosis as both a *consequence* of diabetes and a *cause* for mortality after balloon PCI in diabetic patients. As Sobel cites in an accompanying editorial, there are distinct pathogenetic implications that diabetes accelerates restenosis following angioplasty in patients with dysinsulinemia. The deleterious effects of insulin, proinsulin, or both, which lead to accelerated macroangiopathy in type 2 DM alone or in association with elevated concentrations of free fatty acids and very-low-density lipoprotein (VLDL) cholesterol in blood, may result from abnormalities in platelet activation, the coagulation system, the fibrinolytic system in blood, and the proteo(fibrino)lytic system in vessel walls. Derangements in these systems can accelerate the evolution of macroangiopathy by exposing luminal surfaces of vessel walls to clot-associated mitogens and atherogenic stimuli. Whether increased long-term mortality in type 2 diabetics who undergo balloon PCI results from occlusive restenosis per se, or is a consequence of the nature of the restenotic lesion, remains unclear. Thus, the nature of the restenotic lesion in DM may be dominated by inhibition of proteolysis by PAI-1 during the evolution of lesion progression and associated with the accumulation of extracellular matrix and lipid, and the paucity of vascular smooth muscle cell migration. By contrast, proliferation typical of vascular smooth muscle cell–rich atherosclerotic lesions and restenosis may occur under other conditions.

In summary, intimal hyperplasia and late vessel occlusion (total or subtotal) contribute to the complex process of restenosis following angioplasty in diabetics with CAD. The potential role of hyperinsulinemia in the pathogenesis of restenosis and whether there is a putative role for insulin or proinsulin in the acceleration of restenosis in diabetes warrants further study.

5. Role of GP IIb/IIIa Inhibitors as Adjuncts to Catheter-Based Revascularization

The emerging role of GP IIb/IIIa agents as adjuncts to catheter-based revascularization in diabetics is predicated largely on post hoc analyses of existing clinical trials of unselected patients with CAD. Six prospective clinical trials have assessed the effects of glycoprotein IIb/IIIa inhibitors in CAD patients undergoing PCI. In the EPIC trial, abciximab therapy led to a 35% reduction in the primary endpoint of death, MI, and urgent revascularization at 1 month—with a similar risk reduction in both diabetic and nondiabetic subgroups. At 3 years of follow-up, however, the overall clinical benefit was sustained in the total population, but in diabetics there was a progressive deterioration with more clinical events than nondiabetics. In the EPILOG trial, abciximab therapy in diabetics under-going elective balloon PCI was associated with a significant reduction in death and MI at 30 days and 6 months, but target vessel revascularization was reduced only in the nondiabetic subgroup. Pooled data from the EPIC, EPILOG, and EPISTENT trials revealed that abciximab decreased 1-year mortality of diabetic patients compared to the placebo-treated diabetics. In the IMPACT-II trial, treat-ment with eptifibatide during coronary intervention reduced rates of early abrupt vessel closure and ischemic events at 30 days, and this benefit was observed equally in both diabetic and nondiabetic patients. In the RESTORE trial, tirofiban reduced early cardiac events in patients undergoing principally balloon PCI for acute coronary syndromes. Twenty-percent of all patients were diabetic, but no formal subgroup analysis was performed.

The EPISTENT trial evaluated the benefit of abciximab in patients with both stable and unstable CAD who were undergoing coronary stenting. Overall, this study showed a significant reduction in major adverse cardiac events at 30 days and 6 months in the abciximab-treated subjects compared with the stent-plus-placebo group. Importantly, the combination of stenting plus abciximab among diabetic patients resulted in a significant reduction in 6-month rates of death, MI, and target vessel revascularization compared with stent-plus-placebo or balloon angioplasty-plus-abciximab therapy. The significant reduction in target vessel revascularization associated with a significant increase in angiographic net gain and a trend toward a reduced late loss index in stented diabetic patients with CAD treated with abciximab compared to placebo suggests, for the very first time, a potential additive benefit of abciximab in reducing restenosis in diabetic patients treated with stents. The ERASER trial has shown that abciximab de-creases neointimal proliferation when stents were used in diabetic subjects com-pared with placebo. This proliferation was assessed with intracoronary vascular ultrasound and was not reduced in the study group as a whole.

In summary, the EPISTENT trial demonstrates a significant reduction of major ischemic cardiac events and target vessel revascularization when stents are used in diabetic patients with CAD. This study confirms the important role of adjunctive GP IIb/IIIa inhibitors in this population. Clearly, additional invest-igations are needed to clarify the interaction between abciximab and diabetes and whether these salutary effects can be replicated with other GP IIb/IIIa agents.

B. CABG Surgery in Patients with Symptomatic CAD and Diabetes Mellitus

It is well recognized that DM is a powerful risk factor for poor early and late outcome after CABG surgery. Further, DM is an important predictor of subsequent saphenous vein graft occlusion as well as progression of atherosclerosis in both bypassed and nonbypassed vessels.

As described previously, the BARI trial has shown that patients with DM and angiographic multivessel CAD randomized to an initial strategy of CABG surgery have a striking reduction in mortality compared to diabetic patients randomized to balloon PCI. Further, post hoc analyses of three smaller trials comparing CABG with balloon PCI in patients with stable CAD demonstrated potentially conflicting results in diabetic subjects. In the CABRI trial, diabetic patients fared worse in a manner similar to that seen in BARI. By contrast, the RITA-1 and EAST trials demonstrated similar outcomes in diabetic patients treated with CABG or balloon PCI.

Results from retrospective studies and registries bear on the role of CABG in diabetic subjects. A caveat in the interpretation of these results is that such databases of diabetic patients who have undergone coronary intervention may not be generalizable to more unselected groups. Further, the prognosis in such nonrandomized cohorts can be influenced by physician practice patterns and potential bias regarding the selection and choice of intervention. These limitations aside, however, there are two sizeable databases that have evaluated clinical outcomes among diabetic and nondiabetic patients treated with PCI or CABG surgery. In the Emory University study, only insulin-requiring diabetic patients treated with balloon PCI demonstrated lower 5- and 10-year survival compared with the CABG-treated patients. In the large Duke University registry, DM was associated with a significantly worse 5-year survival, but the effect of DM on prognosis was similar in both revascularization strategies.

In patients undergoing CABG surgery, the long-term patency of internal mammary artery (IMA) conduits to the left anterior descending coronary artery compared to autologous saphenous vein grafts (SVGs) has been shown to be unquestionably superior. It is thus not surprising that the results of the BARI trial, which showed the benefit of CABG over balloon PCI in diabetics, was confined to those patients who had at least one IMA graft. Whether bilateral IMA grafts afford additional benefit in diabetic patients is unknown, especially since this technique may be associated with a greater risk of sternal wound complications in diabetic patients.

In summary, the superiority of CABG surgery over angioplasty in diabetics with symptomatic CAD, as was observed in the BARI trial, has not been definitively established. These findings represent a post hoc analysis, and neither stents nor GP IIb/IIIa agents were available for use in the BARI trial diabetic patients. Thus, we must await the results of ongoing, prospective, randomized trials in diabetic patients, such as the BARI-2D and COURAGE trial.

V. SUMMARY

The management of the diabetic patient with symptomatic CAD is both complex and challenging for the clinician. Advances in our understanding of the pathogenesis of vascular injury in diabetic patients, and the role of metabolic, biological, and hematological abnormalities in the genesis of accelerated atherosclerosis in both native vessels and following angioplasty, should continue to drive improvements in the care of diabetic patients. The evolution of catheter-based technologies including heparin-coated and drug-eluting stents coupled with the increasing use of adjunctive antiplatelet and antithrombin therapies offer promise that we will be able to alter the natural history and clinical course of diabetic patients who are at such high risk for death and MI.

Newer technologies, such as locally delivered ionizing radiation (brachytherapy) to prevent or reduce in-stent restenosis and the use of gene-based therapy to promote neovascularization in high-risk diabetics with CAD are being explored actively. Nevertheless, we must not lose sight of the more "traditional" lifestyle modification interventions (weight loss, regular aerobic exercise, smoking cessation) and aggressive, multifaceted medical therapy directed toward optimized glycemic control, management of hypertension and dyslipidemia, and other secondary prevention strategies—all of which, in the aggregate, are critical to enhancing improved event-free survival. This is especially important in the diabetic patient with established CAD; however, the influence of aggressive primary prevention in the "at-risk" diabetic is equally compelling.

The role and timing of myocardial revascularization requires further study. The evolution of catheter-based technology and of adjuvant therapy is likely to benefit both diabetic and nondiabetic patients. Results from ongoing, randomized clinical trials will improve our understanding of the pathogenesis and management of vascular disease in diabetic patients as we focus on ways to improve survival, functional status, and quality of life in a notoriously high-risk group of patients with a high prevalence of CAD.

SUGGESTED READING

1. Abbott RD, Donahue RP, Kannel WB, et al. The impact of diabetes on survival following myocardial infarction in men vs. women: the Framingham Study. JAMA 1988; 260:3456–3460.

2. Agewall S, Fagerberg B, Attwall S, et al. Carotid artery wall intima-media thickness is associated with insulin-mediated glucose disposal in men at high and low coronary risk. Stroke 1995; 26:956–960.

3. Alderman EL, Corley SD, Fisher LD, et al. The CASS Participating Investigators and Staff. Five-year angiographic follow-up of factors associated with progression of coronary artery disease in the Coronary Artery Surgery Study (CASS). J Am Coll Cardiol 1993; 22:1141–1154.

4. Al-Rashdan JR, Rankin JM, Elliott TG, et al. Glycemic control and major adverse cardiac events after PTCA in patients with diabetes mellitus. J Am Coll Cardiol 1999; 33:97 (abstr).

5. Ambrosioni E, Borghi C, Magnani B, for the Survival of Myocardial Infarction Long-term Evaluation (SMILE) Study Investigators. The effect of the angiotensin-converting-enzyme inhibitor zofenopril on mortality and morbidity after anterior myocardial infarction. N Engl J Med 1995; 332:80–85.

6. American Diabetes Association. Diabetes mellitus and exercise. Diabetes Care 1998; 21(suppl 1):S40–54.

7. American Diabetes Association. Standards of medical care for patients with diabetes mellitus. Diabetes Care 1997; 20(suppl 1):S5–S13.

8. Antiplatelet Trialists' Collaboration. Collaborative overview of randomized trials of antiplatelet therapy-I: prevention of death, myocardial infarction, and stroke by prolonged antiplatelet therapy in various categories of patients. Br Med J 1994; 308:81–106.

9. Aronson D, Bloomgarden Z, Rayfield EJ. Potential mechanisms promoting restenosis in diabetic patients. J Am Coll Cardiol 1996; 27:528–535.

10. BARI Investigators. Influences of diabetes on 5-year mortality and morbidity in randomized trial comparing CABG and PTCA in patients with multivessel disease. Circulation 1997; 96:1761–1769.

11. Barsness GW, Peterson ED, Ohman EM, et al. Relationship between diabetes mellitus and long-term survival after coronary bypass and angioplasty. Circulation 1997; 96:2551–2556.

12. Bernink PJLM, Antman EM, McCabe CH, et al. Treatment benefit with enoxaparin in unstable angina is greatest in patients at highest risk: a multivariate analysis from TIMI 11B. J Am Coll Cardiol 1999; 33(suppl A):352 (abstr).

13. Bhatt D. Marso S, Lincoff M, et al. Abciximab reduces mortality in diabetics following percutaneous coronary intervention. J Am Coll Cardiol 2000; 35:922–928.

14. Bierman EL. Atherogenesis in diabetes. Atheroscler Thromb 1992; 12:647–656.

15. Bressler P, Bailey SR, Marsuda M, DeFronzo RA. Insulin resistance and coronary disease. Diabetologia 1996; 39:1345–1350.

16. CABRI. Long-term follow-up of European revascularization trials. Presented at the 68th Scientific Plenary Session XII, of the American Heart Association, Nov. 16, 1995, Anaheim, California.

17. Ceriello A. Coagulation activation in diabetes mellitus: a role of hyperglycemia and therapeutic prospects. Diabetologia 1993; 1119–1125.

18. Chowdhury TA, Lasker SS, Dyer PH. Comparison of secondary prevention measures after myocardial infarction in subjects with and without diabetes mellitus. J Intern Med 1999; 245:565–570.

19. Cohen M, Demers C, Gurfinkel EP, et al, for the ESSENCE Study Group. Low molecular weight heparins in non-ST-segment elevation eschemia: the ESSENCE trial. Am J Cardiol 1998; 82:19L–24L.

20. Cohen M, Demers C, Gurfinkel EP, et al. for the Efficacy and Safety of Subcutaneous Enoxaparin in Non-Q-Wave Coronary Events Study Group. A comparison of low-molecular-weight heparin with unfractionated for unstable coronary artery disease. N Engl J Med 1997; 337:447–452.

21. Cohen RA, Dysfunction of vascular endothelium in diabetes mellitus. Circulation 1993; 87(suppl 5):67–76.

22. Davi G, Catalano I, Averna M, et al. Thromboxane biosynthesis and platelet function in type II diabetes mellitus. N Engl J Med 1990; 322:1769–1774.

23. Detre KM, Guo P, Holubkov R, et al. Coronary revascularization in diabetic patients. A comparison of the randomized and observational components of the Bypass Angioplasty Revascularization Investigation (BARI). Circulation 1999; 99: 633–640.

24. Dias R, Paolasso E, Piegas L, et al. for the ECLA (Estudios Cardiologicos Latinoamerica) Collaborative Group. Metabolic modulation of acute myocardial infarction: the ECLA Glucose-Insulin-Potassium Pilot Trial in Acute Myocardial Infarction. Circulation 1998; 98:2227–2234.

25. Estacio RO, Jeffers BW, Hiatt WR, et al. The effect of nisoldipine as compared with non-insulin-dependent diabetes and hypertension. N Engl J Med 1998; 338: 645–652.

26. Fein F, Scheur J. Heart disease in diabetes mellitus: theory and practice. In: Rifkin H, Porte D Jr., eds. New York: Elsevier, 1990:812–823.

27. Fibrinolytic Therapy Trialists' Collaborative Group. Indications for fibrinolytic therapy in suspected acute myocardial infarction: collaborative overview of early mortality and major morbidity results from all randomized trials of more than 1000 patients. Lancet 1994; 343:311–322.

28. Fragmin during Instability in Coronary Artery Disease study group. Low-molecular weight heparin during instability in coronary artery disease. Lancet 1996; 347:561–568.

29. Gerstein HC, Bosch J, Pogue J, et al. Rationale and design of a large study to evaluate the renal and cardiovascular effects of an ACE inhibitor and vitamin E in high-risk patients with diabetes. The MICRO-HOPE study. Diabetes Care 1996; 19:1225–1228.

30. Godsland JK, Stevenson JC. Insulin resistance: syndrome or tendency? Lancet 1995; 346:100–103.

31. Goldberg RB, Mellies MJ, Sacks FM, et al. Cardiovascular events and their reduction with pravastatin in diabetic and glucose-intolerant myocardial infarction survivors with average cholesterol levels. Circulation 1998; 98 2513–2519.

32. Gustafsson, J, Torp-Pedersen C, Kober L, et al. Effect of the angiotensin-converting enzyme inhibitor trandolapril on mortality and morbidity in diabetic patients with left ventricular dysfunction after acute myocardial infarct on. J Am Coll Cardiol 1999; 34:83–89.

33. Haffin M, Lehto S, Ronnemax T, Pyorala L, Laakso M. Mortality from coronary

heart disease in subjects with type 2 diabetes and non-diabetic subjects with and without prior myocardial infarction. N Engl J Med 1998; 339:229–234.

34. Haffner SM. The Scandinavian Simvastatin Survival Study (4S) subgroup analysis of diabetic subjects: implications for the prevention of coronary heart disease. Diabetes Care 1997; 20:469–471.

35. Haffner SM, Lehto S, Ronnemaa T, et al. Mortality from coronary heart disease in subjects with type 2 diabetes and in non-diabetic subjects with and without prior myocardial infarction. N Engl J Med 1998; 339:229–234.

36. Hammoud T, Tanguay J, Bourassa M. Management of coronary artery disease: therapeutic options in patients with diabetes. J Am Coll Cardiol 2000; 36:355–361.

37. Herlitz J, Karlson BW, Wogensen GB, et al. Mortality and morbidity in diabetic and non-diabetic patients during a 2-year period after coronary artery bypass grafting. Diabetes Care 1996; 19:698–703.

38. Hermann HC, Tirofiban—an overview of the phase III trials. J Invas Cardio 1999; 11(suppl C):7C–13C.

39. Higgs ER, Parfitt VI, Harney BA, Harlog M. Use of thrombolysis for acute myocardial infarction in the presence of diabetic retinopathy in the UK, and associated ocular haemorrhagic complications. Diabetic Med 1995; 12:426–428.

40. Howard G, O'Leary DH, Zaccaro D, et al. for the IRAS Investigators. Insulin sensitivity and atherosclerosis. Circulation 1996; 93:1809–1817.

41. Jacoby RM, Nesto RW. Acute myocardial infarction in the diabetic patient: pathophysiology, clinical course and prognosis. J Am Coll Cardiol 1992; 20:736–744.

42. Jilma B, Fasching P, Ruthner C, et al. Elevated circulating P-selectins in insulin dependent diabetes mellitus. Thromb Haemost 1996; 328–332.

43. Jonas M, Reicher-Reiss H, Royko V, et al. Usefulness of beta-blocker therapy in patients with non-insulin-dependent diabetes mellitus and coronary artery disease. Am J Cardiol 1996; 77:1273–1277.

44. Kannel W. Lipids, diabetes, and coronary heart disease: insights from the Framingham Study. Am Heart J 1985; 110:1100–1107.

45. Kendall MJ, Lynch KP, Hjalmarson A, Kjekshus J. Beta-blockers and sudden cardiac death. Ann Intern Med 1995; 123:358–367.

46. Kip KE, Faxon DP, Detre KM, et al, for the investigators of the NHLBI PTCA registry. Coronary angioplasty in diabetic patients: the National Heart, Lung, and Blood Institute Percutaneous Transluminal Coronary Angioplasty Registry. Circulation 1996; 94:1818–1825.

47. Kip KE, Faxon DP, Detre KM, Yeh W, Kelsley SF, Currier JW, for the Investigators of the NHLBI PTCA Registry. Coronary angioplasty in diabetic patients. The National Heart, Lung, and Blood Institute Percutaneous Transluminal Coronary Angioplasty Registry. Circulation 1996; 94:1818–1825.

48. Klein W, Buchwald A, Hillis SE, et al, for the FRISC Investigators. Comparison of low-molecular-weight heparin with unfractionated heparin acutely and with placebo for 6 weeks in the management of unstable coronary artery disease. Fragmin in Unstable Coronary Artery Disease Study (RIC). Circulation 1997; 96:61–68.

49. Koskinen P, Manttari M, Manninen V, Huttunen JK, Heinonen OP, Frick MH.

Coronary heart disease incidence in NIDDM patients in the Helsinki Heart Study.
Diabetes Care 1992; 15:820–825.

50. Kreisberg RA. Diabetic dyslipidemia. Am J Cardiol 1998; 82:67U–73U.

51. Kuntz RE. Importance of considering atherosclerosis progression when choosing
a coronary revascularization strategy. The diabetes-percutaneous transluminal coronary angioplasty dilemma. Circulation 1999; 99:847–851.

52. Laakso M, Sarlund H, Salonen R, et al. Asymptomatic atherosclerosis and insulin
resistance. Arterioscler Thromb 1991; 11:1068–1076.

53. Lorenzi, Cagliero E, Toledo S. Glucose toxicity for human endothelial cells in
culture. Delayed replication, disturbed cell cycle with accelerated death. Diabetes
1985; 34:621–627.

54. Mak KH, Moliterno DJ, Granger CB, et al., for the GUSTO-1 Investigators. Influence of diabetes mellitus on clinical outcome in the thrombolytic era of acute myocardial infarction. J Am Coll Cardiol 1997; 30:171–179.

55. Malmberg K, Norhammar A, Wedel II, Ryden L. Glucometabolic state at admission: important risk market of mortality in conventionally treated patients with diabetes mellitus and acute myocardial infarction. Long-term results from the Diabetes
and Insulin-Glucose Infusion in Acute Myocardial Infarction Study. Circulation
1999; 99:2626–2632.

56. Malmberg K, Ryden L., Hamsten A, Herlitz J, Waldenstrom A, Wedel H, on behalf
of the DIGAMI Study Group. Effects of insulin treatment on cause-specific one-
year mortality and morbidity in diabaetic patients with acute myocardial infraction.
Eur Heart J 1996; 17:1337–1344.

57. McGuire, DK, Emanuelsson H, Granger CB, White HD. Diabetes mellitus is associated with worse clinical outcomes across the spectrum of acute coronary syndromes
results from GUSTO-IIb. Circulation 1999; 100(suppl 1):432 (abstr).

58. Miettenen H, Lehto S, Salomaa V, et al. Impact of diabetes on mortality after the
first myocardial infarction: The FINMONICA Myocardial Infarction Register
Study Group. Diabetes Care 1998; 21:69–75.

59. Morris JJ. Smith LR Jones RH, et al. Influence of diabetes and mammary artery
grafting on survival after coronary bypass. Circulation 1991; 84(suppl 3):275–284.

60. Moye LA, Pfeffer MA, Wun CC, et al. for the SAVE Investigators. Uniformity of
captopril benefit in the SAVE study; subgroup analysis. Eur Heart J 1994; 15(suppl
B):2–8.

61. Nahser PJ, Brown RE, Oakarsson H, Winniford MD, Rossen JD. Maximal coronary
flow reserve and metabolic coronary vasodilation in patients with diabetes mellitus.
Circulation 1995; 91:635.

62. Nishimoto Y, Miyazaki Y, Toki Y, et al. Enhanced secretion of insulin plays a role
in the development of atherosclerosis and restenosis of coronary arteries: elective
percutaneous transluminal coronary angioplasty in patients with effort angina. J
Am Coll Cardiol 1998; 32:1624–1629.

63. Niskanen L, Tarpeinen A, Penttila I, Uusitupa MIJ. Hyperglycemia and compositional lipoprotein abnormalities as predictors of cardiovascular mortality in type 2
diabetes: a 15-year follow-up from the time of diagnosis. Diabetes Care 1998; 21:
1861–1869.

64. Nitenberg A, Paycha F, Ledoux S, Sachs R, Attali JR, Valensi P. Coronary artery

responses to physiological stimuli are improved by deferoxamine but not by L-arginine in non-insulin-dependent diabetic patients with angiographically normal coronary arteries and no other risk factors. Circulation 1998; 97:736–743.

65. Nordescgaard BG, Agerholm-Larsen B, Stender S. Effect of exogenous hyperinsulinemia on atherogenesis in cholesterol-fed rabbits. Diabetologia 1997; 40:512–520.

66. Nordt TK, Sawa H, Sobel BE. Induction of plasminogen activator inhibitor type-1 (PAC-1) by proinsulin and insulin in vivo. Circulation 1995; 91:764–770.

67. O'Neill WW. Multivessel balloon angioplasty should be abandoned in diabetic patients. J Am Coll Cardiol 1998; 31:20–22.

68. Pyorala M, Miettinen H, Laakso M, Pyorala K. Hyperinsulinemia predicts coronary heart disease risk in healthy middle-aged men. The 22-year follow-up results of the Helsinki Policemen Study. Circulation 1998; 98:398–404.

69. Ramanathan AV, Miller DP, Kleimar, NS. Effect of GP IIb/IIIa antagonists in patients with diabetes mellitus; a meta-analysis. Circulation 1999; 100(suppl I):640 (abstr).

70. Reaven GM. Hypertension and associated metabolic abnormalities—the role of insulin resistance and the sympathoadrenal system. N Engl J Med 1996; 334:374–381.

71. Reaven GM. Role of insulin resistance in human disease. Diabetes 1998; 37:1595–1607.

72. Ruige JB, Assendelft WJJ, Dekker JM, Kostense PJ, Bouter LM. Insulin and risk of cardiovascular disease. Circulation 1998; 97:996–1001.

73. Sawicki PT, Berber M. Pharmacological treatment of diabetic patients with cardiovascular complications. J Intern Med 1998; 243:181–189.

74. Scala, Laporte R, Dorman J, et al. Insulin dependent diabetes mellitus mortality: the risk of cigarette smoking. Circulation 1990; 82:37–43.

75. Serne EH, Stehouwer CDA, Maaten JC, et al. Microvascular function relates to insulin sensitivity and blood pressure in normal subjects. Circulation 1999; 99:896–902.

76. Smith LR, Harrell FE, Rankin JS et al. Determinants of early versus late cardiac death in patients undergoing coronary artery bypass graft surgery. Circulation 1991; 84(suppl 3):245–253.

77. Sobel BE. Acceleration of restenosis by diabetes. Pathogenetic implications. Circulation 2001; 103:1185–1187.

78. Solang L, Malmberg K, Ryden L. Diabetes mellitus and congestive heart failure. Eur Heart J 1999; 20:789–795.

79. Stamler J, Vaccaro O, Neaton JD, et al. Diabetes, other risk factors, and 12-year cardiovascular mortality for men screened in the Multiple Risk Factor Intervention Trial. Diabetes Care 1993; 16:434–444.

80. Stein B, Weintraub WS, Gebhart SSP, et al. Influence of diabetes mellitus on early and late outcome after percutaneous transluminal coronary angioplasty. Circulation 1995; 91:979–989.

81. Stern MP. Do non-insulin-dependent diabetes mellitus and cardiovascular disease share common antecedents? Ann Intern Med 1996; 93:1780–1783.

82. Stern, MP, Mitchell, BD, Haffner SM, Hazuda HP. Does glycemic control of type 2 diabetes suffice to control diabetic dyslipidemia? Diabetes Care 1992; 15:638–644.

83. Stout RW. Insulin and atheroma: 20-year perspective. Diabetes Care 1990; 13:631–654.
84. Strano A, Davi G, Patrono C. In vivo platelet activation in diabetes mellitus (review). Semin Thromb Haemost 1991; 17:422–425.
85. The BARI Investigators. Influence of diabetes on 5-year mortality and morbidity in a randomized trial comparing CABG and PTCA in patients with multivessel disease. The Bypass Angioplasty Revascularization Investigation (BARI). Circulation 1997; 96:1761–1769.
86. The Bypass Angioplasty Revascularization Investigation (BARI) Investigators. Comparison of coronary bypass surgery with angioplasty in patients with multivessel disease. N Engl J Med 1996; 335:217–225.
87. The Diabetes Control and Complications Trial (DCCT) Research Group. Effect of intensive diabetes management on macrovascular events and risk factors in the Diabetes Control and Complications Trial. Am J Cardiol 1995; 75:894–903.
88. The Diabetes Control and Complications Trial Research Group. The effect of intensive treatment of diabetes on the development and progression of long-term complications in insulin-dependent diabetes mellitus. N Engl J Med 1993; 329:977–986.
89. The HOPE study. Results in diabetic patients. Presented at the XXIst Congress of the European Society of Cardiology, August 31, 1999; Barcelona, Spain.
90. The Long-Term Intervention with Pravastatin in Ischaemic Disease (LIPID) Study Group. Prevention of cardiovascular events and death with pravastatin in patients with coronary heart disease and a broad range of initial cholesterol levels. N Engl J Med 1998; 339:1349–1357.
91. The Platelet Receptor Inhibition for Ischemic Syndrome Management in Patients Limited by Unstable Signs and Symptoms (PRISM-PLUS) Study Investigators. Inhibition of the platelet glycoprotein IIb/IIIa receptor w th tirofiban in unstable angina and non-Q-wave myocardial infarction. N Engl J Med 1998; 338:1488–1497.
92. The Platelet Receptor Inhibition in Ischemic Syndrome Management (PRISM) Study Investigators. A comparison of aspirin plus tirofiban with aspirin plus heparin for unstable angina. N Engl J Med 1998; 338:1498–1505.
93. The PURSUIT Trial Investigators. Inhibition of platelet glycoprotein IIB/IIIa with eptifibatide in patients with acute coronary syndromes. N Engl J Med 1998; 339:436–443.
94. Tschoepe D. Roesen P, Esser J, et al. Large platelets circu ate in an activated state in diabetes mellitus. Semin Thromb Haemost 1991; 17:433–438.
95. UK Prospective Diabetes Study (UKPDS) Group. Effect of intensive blood-glucose control with metformin on complications in over-weight patients with type 2 diabetes (UKPDS 34). Lancet 1998; 352:854–865.
96. UK Prospective Diabetes Study (UKPDS) Group. Intensive blood glucose control with sulphonylureas or insulin compared with conventional treatment and risk of complications in patients with type 2 diabetes (UKPDS 33). Lancet 1998; 352:837–853.
97. UK Prospective Diabetes Study Group. Tight blood pressure control and risk of macrovascular and microvascular complications in type 2 diabetes (UKPDS 38). Br Med J 1998; 317:703–713.

98. Van Belle E, Abolmaali K, Bauters C, et al. Restenosis, late vessel occlusion and left ventricular function six months after balloon angioplasty in diabetic patients. J Am Coll Cardiol 1999; 34:476–485.

99. Weintraub WS, Stein B, Kosinski A, et al. Outcome of coronary bypass surgery versus coronary angioplasty in diabetic patients with multivessel coronary artery disease. J Am Coll Cardiol 1998; 31:10–19.

100. Williams SB, Goldfine AB, Timimi FK et al. Acute hyperglycemia attenuates endothelium-dependent vasodilation in humans in vivo. Circulation 1998; 97:1695–1701.

101. Windgard DL, Barrett-Connor E. Heart disease and diabetes. In: National Diabetes Data Group. Diabetes in America, 2nd ed. Washington, DC: Government Printing Office, 1995:429–448. (NIH publication number 95-1468).

102. Wingard DL, Barrett-Connor EL, Ferrara A. Is insulin really a heart disease risk factor? Diabetes Care 1995; 18:1299–1304.

103. Winocour, PD, Platelet abnormalities in diabetes mellitus. Diabetes 1992; 41(suppl 2):26–31.

104. Winocour PD, Richardson M, Kinlough-Rathbone RI. Continued platelet interaction with de-endothelialized aorta associated with slower re-endothelization and more extensive intimal hyperplasia in spontaneously diabetic BB Wistar rats. Int J Exp Pathol 1993; 74:603–613.

105. Woodfield SL, Lundergan CF, Reiner JS, et al. Angiographic findings and outcome in diabetic patients treated with thrombolytic therapy for acute myocardial infarction: the GUSTO-1 experience. J Am Coll Cardiol 1996; 28:1661–1669.

106. Wright RS, Kopecky SL, Barsness GW, Tuttle RH. Impact of diabetes mellitus on outcome in non-ST elevation myocardial infarction and unstable angina: is there a benefit from treatment with eptifibatide? Circulation 1999; 100(suppl I):640 (abstr).

107. Yokoyama I, Momomura SI, Ohtake T, et al. Reduced myocardial flow reserve in non-insulin-dependent diabetes mellitus. J Am Coll Cardiol 1997; 30:1472–1477.

108. Young, MH, Jeng CY, Sheu WHH, et al. Insulin resistance, glucose intolerance, hyperinsulinemia and dyslipidemia in patients with angiographically demonstrated coronary disease. Am J Cardiol 1993; 72:458–460.

109. Zuanerti G, Latini R, Maggioni AP, et al. Effect of the ACE inhibitor lisinopril on mortality in diabetic patients with acute myocardial infarction: data from the GISI1-3 study. Circulation 1997; 96:4239–4245.

110. Zunnetti G, Latini R, Maggioni AP, Santoro L, Franzosi PG, for the GISSI-2 Investigators. Influence of diabetes on mortality in acute myocardial infarction: data from the GISSI-2 study. J Am Coll Cardiol 1993; 22:1788–1794.

13

Pathophysiology and Management of Congestive Heart Failure in Patients with Diabetes Mellitus

Martin M. LeWinter
*University of Vermont College of Medicine,
Burlington, Vermont*

I. BACKGROUND

Diabetes mellitus is a major risk factor for development of congestive heart failure (CHF). Data from the Framingham Study and other epidemiological databases indicate that diabetic patients have on the order of a two to threefold increase in the risk of developing CHF. Conversely, there is an overrepresentation of diabetic subjects in the population of patients with chronic CHF, including patients with dilated cardiomyopathy who do not have coronary artery disease or hypertension. (The term coronary artery disease is used here to denote the presence of what are considered to be hemodynamically significant stenoses in vessels large enough to be assessed by contrast angiography.) The common presence of coexistent hypertension markedly potentiates the risk of CHF, suggesting specific, deleterious interactions of the two disease processes. Diabetes, in addition to being a major risk factor *for* coronary artery disease, also has a potent and deleterious interaction *with* coronary disease with respect to the development of CHF. This is most striking in the setting of acute myocardial infarction, where diabetic patients have about a twofold greater risk of CHF and death compared to nondiabetic patients. This difference is not accounted for by the occurrence of large infarcts in diabetics. Not surprisingly, the "triple threat" combination of diabetes, hypertension, and coronary disease is especially lethal.

These powerful epidemiological associations suggest the possibility that diabetes has deleterious effects on the myocardium independent of those mediated by coexistent hypertension and/or coronary disease and have spurred investigations into whether a specific diabetic cardiomyopathy exists. If such an entity does exist, it would obviously strongly influence our thinking about the pathophysiology of CHF in diabetic patients and, potentially, its treatment.

II. DIABETIC CARDIOMYOPATHY: DOES IT EXIST?

In addition to the epidemiological data mentioned above, there are a host of other observations, both clinical and experimental, that point toward cardiomyopathic manifestations specifically related to the presence of diabetes. (In reviewing clinical data for this purpose, it is important to search for evidence of cardiomyopathy in the absence of the confounding presence of coronary artery disease and hypertension, both of which can cause CHF by themselves.)

The occurrence of dilated cardiomyopathy in patients with diabetes who do not have coronary disease or hypertension is well documented. In an individual patient, it is impossible to know whether this represents a specific diabetic cardiomyopathy or simply the chance occurrence of two common diseases. Stronger evidence of a specific, underlying cardiomyopathic process comes from studies of patients with diabetes, typically younger, who do not have clinical signs or symptoms of heart disease. These subjects have normal contraction patterns but a high incidence (on the order of one-third to one-half) of abnormal mitral inflow patterns detected by Doppler echocardiography (e.g., increased E to A ratios) consistent with slowed myocardial relaxation and/or decreased compliance. In addition, they have on average a larger myocardial mass than age-matched controls and frequently have increased myocardial ultrasonic backscatter. The latter is a nonspecific finding that can be caused by abnormalities of the myocardial tissue (e.g., increased collagen content and possibly other alterations of matrix proteins). Several studies demonstrate abnormal left ventricular contractile responses during dynamic exercise in asymptomatic diabetic patients, although this finding has not been uniform. It is noteworthy that the cardiomyopathic abnormalities described above have been reported in a broad spectrum of diabetic patients, including juvenile and adult onset, and insulin and non-insulin-requiring subjects. In general, clinical signs of cardiomyopathy are positively correlated with the prevalence and severity of other complications of diabetes such as retinal vasculopathy, nephropathy, and neuropathy.

Recently, we have obtained preliminary evidence of a depressed force-frequency relationship (FFR) in strips dissected from left ventricular epicardial biopsies obtained from diabetic patients undergoing coronary bypass surgery compared with nondiabetic controls (Fig. 1). Although the presence of coronary

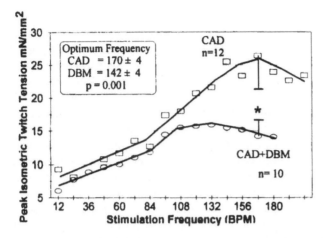

Figure 1 Relation between isometric twitch force and frequency of stimulation in isolated myocardial strips obtained from patients with diabetes (DBM) and coronary artery disease (CAD) and nondiabetic CAD controls at time of coronary bypass surgery. Note reduced augmentation of force in diabetic patients as well as lower optimum frequency (see text).

artery disease is a potential confounding feature, we restricted our studies to patients with a normal left ventricular contraction pattern who did not have either hypertension or a clinical history of myocardial infarction. Thus, we excluded patients with conventional markers of ischemic myocardial dysfunction. As shown in Figure 1, normal humans have a markedly positive FFR (i.e., an increase in contractility as a function of stimulation frequency until an optimal frequency is reached, at which point contractility decreases as rate increases further). The positive FFR is thought to result from frequency-dependent increases in calcium pumping by the sarcoplasmic reticulum, with resultant increased calcium delivery to the myofilaments. Phosphorylation of phospholamban by calcium activated calmodulin kinase may be an important mechanism. The positive FFR is of great physiological importance because it is the most important mechanism whereby myocardial function is augmented during dynamic exercise. In contrast, patients with dilated cardiomyopathy have repeatedly been shown to have marked depression of the FFR as well as a decrease in optimal frequency; indeed, many have an inverted FFR, with decreasing contractility as frequency increases. These abnormalities have been correlated with alterations in calcium cycling protein expression.

As shown in Figure 1, diabetic patients are indistinguishable from nondiabetics at typical basal frequencies of around 60/min, but have a smaller augmentation in contractile performance as frequency is increased and a lower optimal frequency. This extent of FFR depression is less marked than that observed in patients with dilated cardiomyopathy patients, but could account for abnormal functional responses during exercise. It is tempting to speculate that it could also contribute to impaired contractile responses during myocardial infarction with resultant heart failure.

Various experimental animal preparations have been used to delineate the effects of diabetes on the myocardium. The most common utilize destruction of pancreatic islet cells by streptozotocin, but a number of others have also been employed, including obese, insulin-resistant rat strains and genetically engineered mice lacking insulin receptors. Some animal models display evidence of impaired coronary tone consistent with endothelial dysfunction, but they do not exhibit the type of coronary artery disease present in diabetic patients that confounds efforts to distinguish the effects of diabetes on the myocardium from those of coronary stenoses. However, great caution must be exercised in extrapolating results from experimental animal models to patients, in whom diabetes is obviously much more chronic. Nonetheless, although the details differ, it is remarkable that cardiac functional abnormalities can be detected in almost any experimental model of diabetes. These abnormalities include depressed contractile performance, slowed relaxation, and, in some instances, decreased diastolic compliance. Defects in both excitation–contraction coupling due to abnormal calcium cycling and in the contractile machinery have been documented as factors underlying the abnormalities of contraction and relaxation.

Thus, in patients selected to exclude other diseases that could alter myocardial function, as well as in a number of experimental diabetes models, there is considerable evidence supporting the concept of a diabetic cardiomyopathy. The manifestations are diverse, and it is not yet clear how or if they relate to each other mechanistically.

III. MECHANISMS CONTRIBUTING TO DIABETIC CARDIOMYOPATHY

There is virtually no definitive evidence delineating the mechanism(s) of diabetic cardiomyopathy in patients. This applies to both proximate mechanisms (e.g., defects in excitation–contraction coupling) and "upstream" mechanisms (e.g., possible alterations in gene expression that result in changes in the proteins responsible for excitation–contraction coupling). Even in experimental animal preparations, it is at present impossible to understand fully all of the potentially causative factors activated as a result of the presence of diabetes. Despite the paucity of hard evidence, there are a number of putative candidates as well as approaches that can be taken to at least ask the right questions about mechanism(s) and begin to make correlations in patients. This section will address some of the proposed mechanisms. What follows, however, is an incomplete list.

Microvascular disease related to diabetes has often been considered to be a mechanism underlying diabetic cardiomyopathy. Myocardial abnormalities in diabetic patients without clinically manifest heart disease are correlated with microvasculopathy in other organs. As judged from endomyocardial biopsy studies, there is no question that myocardial microvessels are affected in patients with diabetes even in the absence of confounding features such as hypertension or large-vessel coronary disease. Thus, microvessels (small arteries, arterioles, capillaries) display "diabetic" histological abnormalities such as thickening of the medial layer and basement membrane and capillary microaneurysms. As in other organs, myocardial capillaries are "leaky" in animal models with diabetes. In vivo coronary flow velocity studies in patients reveal evidence of endothelial dysfunction. What is unclear is how these microvascular abnormalities could actually cause cardiomyopathy. Animal models are of little use in clarifying this issue because they do not manifest microvascular disease comparable to that of human patients.

In the absence of angiographically detectable coronary artery disease and/ or hypertension, there is little to suggest ischemic dysfunction at the microvascular level (e.g., areas of microinfarction with replacement fibrosis or dysfunction consistent with stunned and/or hibernating myocardium). As an alternative to microvascular ischemia, local elaboration by the endothelium of various growth factors and cytokines that influence myocardial signaling pathways and can also impair contractile function is a possible mechanism. High levels of circulating insulin and PAI-1, present in many diabetic patients, could be involved in causing and/or reflecting abnormal signaling.

The heart has usually been considered to be an organ in which the metabolic substrate is primarily fatty acids. However, normal myocardium does take up glucose to a limited extent at rest, and glucose uptake and use of the glycolytic pathway are substantially increased with stress. Moreover, certain key ion pumps, for example, the myocardial sarcoplasmic reticulum calcium ATPase (SERCA-2), may be particularly dependent on glycolytic energy supply. Human myocardium is insulin sensitive. Thus, the metabolic consequences of impaired glucose entry should be considered as a possible mechanism contributing to diabetic cardiomyopathy. In animal preparations, impaired glucose entry with associated increased fatty acid oxidation results in accumulation of toxic intermediates, especially long-chain acyl carnitines, that can result in free-radical-mediated damage to both the sarcolemma and intracellular membranes. This in turn could result in impaired ion pumping and exchange mechanisms. The latter are well described in the myocardium in experimental diabetes and in nonmyocardial tissue in diabetic patients, and include abnormalities of calcium pumping and exchange as well as the sarcolemmal Na-K ATPase. Although there is no information with regard to free-radical-mediated damage in human myocardium, in view of the results in experimental diabetes this could contribute to the depressed FFR discussed earlier.

Hyperglycemia per se may cause myocardial damage by glycation of myocardial matrix proteins with formation of advanced glycosylation end-products (AGEs) and associated free-radical-mediated damage that, in the case of collagen, causes increased cross-linking. This may be the mechanism underlying the common histological finding of increased PAS positive material in myocardium from diabetic patients and is an attractive possibility as an explanation for echocardiographic Doppler findings consistent with decreased compliance. However, very limited immunohistopathological studies directed specifically at detection of AGEs in myocardium of autopsied patients with diabetes have not shown extensive deposition. In very small studies examining the histological appearance of myocardium obtained by endomyocardial biopsy in diabetic patients with evidence of cardiomyopathy who do not have coronary artery disease or hypertension, only very modest increases in connective tissue have been reported, and most of it has been perivascular. Increased cross-linking, however, may be at least as important functionally as changes in collagen content or type. When diabetes is combined with hypertension, however, the result seems to be much more pronounced increases in connective tissue. It is also possible for cytosolic proteins, including contractile proteins, to be glycated. Although abnormalities of myofilament calcium sensitivity have been reported in experimental diabetes, it is unknown whether this is due to glycation. This question has not been studied in patients.

Three other putative abnormalities that could cause a cardiomyopathy in patients with diabetes merit consideration. First, a defect in pyruvate kinase activity has been observed in some diabetic patients. If present in human myocardium, it could contribute to abnormal carbohydrate metabolism. Second, mitochondrial damage in diabetic myocardium could limit energy reserves derived from oxidative metabolism during stress. However, there is at present no objective evidence to support this. In our studies on the FFR, diastolic tension does not rise at high stimulation frequencies, as would be expected if energy reserves were exceeded because of increased demand. Third, protein kinase C (PKC) has been found to be activated in some forms of experimental diabetes. PKC activation is thought to occur in dilated cardiomyopathy and is known to depress crossbridge cycling and may also have deleterious effects on excitation–contraction coupling. Moreover, transgenic mice with selective overexpression of a specific PKC isoform develop a dilated cardiomyopathy. However, it is unknown whether PKC is activated in human diabetes.

From the above, it is apparent that there are a number of different manifestations as well as potential mechanisms underlying diabetic cardiomyopathy. It is not known which manifestations and mechanisms are actually operative in patients. Indeed, it may well be that they can be multiple in a given patient and perhaps vary with age, gender, ethnicity, and duration and severity of diabetes. As noted above, there have not been obvious differences in the clinical manifestations of diabetic cardiomyopathy with respect to the type of diabetes or insulin use, although such differences may emerge.

IV. MECHANISMS UNDERLYING HEART FAILURE IN PATIENTS WITH DIABETES

Most diabetic patients with CHF have it in conjunction with some other known cause(s) of CHF, usually coronary artery disease and/or hypertension. Thus, there are relatively few patients with CHF in whom the only predisposing factor is diabetes. Stated another way, although there is strong evidence that cardiomyopathy is caused by diabetes, it is unusual for it to account for overt CHF by itself. Moreover, in an individual patient, it is usually impossible to delineate the qualitative and quantitative contributions of diabetic cardiomyopathy as opposed to hypertension or ischemia caused by coronary artery disease. As noted above, diabetes in combination with hypertension and coronary artery disease is not merely additive, but interacts with either or both in a way that seems to potentiate myocardial failure.

Accordingly, when diabetic patients have CHF in association with coronary artery disease, they typically have conventional manifestations of myocardial ischemia (i.e., acute and chronic infarction, stunned and/or hibernating myocardium) that result in both systolic failure, characterized by a reduced ejection fraction and ventricular chamber dilatation (when the process is chronic), and diastolic failure, characterized by upward displacement of the diastolic pressure–volume relationship due to slowed or incomplete relaxation and/or decreased passive compliance (with or without a decrease in ejection fraction). In addition, remodeling of noninfarcted myocardium in patients with chronic infarction may also contribute to systolic failure. A depressed and even inverted FFR is a common manifestation of ischemic as well as nonischemic dilated cardiomyopathy.

The cellular and molecular mechanisms of systolic failure specifically related to ischemia are multiple, and include necrosis, apoptosis, reversible proteolytic damage to calcium cycling, and contractile proteins and perhaps phenotypic changes in these same proteins. In addition, a variety of mechanisms are generic to dilated cardiomyopathy, both ischemic and nonischemic, such as downregulation of calcium cycling proteins, alterations in protein kinase A and C activity, and neurohumoral and cytokine-mediated adverse effects on the myocardium. Ischemia causes diastolic failure mediated by some of the same phenomena (e.g., impaired function or damage to calcium cycling proteins), and also by virtue of scar formation following infarction. In addition, because they often do not have typical chest discomfort in conjunction with ischemia, diabetic patients with "demand ischemia" may present with exertional dyspnea as the main symptom. Dyspnea caused by demand ischemia is a form of reversible heart failure primarily ascribable to diastolic dysfunction.

Hypertension, when present in diabetic patients, can also cause CHF through multiple mechanisms. When hypertension is "compensated" (i.e., ejection fraction is normal), it causes concentric left ventricular hypertrophy, which in turn can cause symptoms of CHF (mainly dyspnea). This form of diastolic dysfunction may result from depressed calcium pumping by the sarcoplasmic reticulum and reduced chamber compliance related to decreased volume:mass ratio and increased connective tissue content. Concentric hypertrophy can cause subendocardial ischemia when energy demands increase even in the absence of coronary artery disease. When concentric hypertrophy becomes decompensated, the ejection fraction decreases and systolic failure ensues.

In view of the manifestations of and mechanisms underlying diabetic cardiomyopathy discussed above, it is not difficult to envision how the presence of diabetes might interact with both the ischemic consequences of coronary artery disease and hypertension to increase the incidence and worsen the manifestations of CHF. A few examples make this clear. Diabetes-related damage to ion exchange and pumping functions would obviously be expected to compound abnormalities of calcium cycling and further compromise systolic function and relaxation. A depressed FFR limits an important adaptation to acute stress and may help explain the high incidence of heart failure in diabetic subjects who sustain an acute myocardial infarction. Diabetes-related alterations in connective tissue would compound the effects of increased collagen due to myocardial ischemia and/or hypertension. In fact, the combination of hypertension and diabetes seems to result in much more exuberant fibrosis than that seen with either alone. Although little is known about the contribution of microvasculopathy to diabetic cardiomyopathy, interactions may exist related to the endothelial dysfunction that is common to coronary atherosclerosis, hypertension, and diabetes.

V. MANAGEMENT OF HEART FAILURE IN DIABETIC SUBJECTS

A. Acute Heart Failure

Treatment of acute CHF is for all intents and purposes identical in diabetic and nondiabetic patients and will not be discussed here. However, control of diabetes is impaired in the setting of poorly controlled CHF (both acute and chronic); conversely, the stress of hyperglycemia and associated metabolic imbalances complicate treatment of CHF. Thus, careful attention to management of blood glucose with insulin treatment, if necessary, is needed in diabetic patients with acute CHF.

B. Chronic Heart Failure

Most principles of the management of chronic, low-ejection-fraction CHF in patients with diabetes are similar to those in patients without diabetes, and have been published in the form of guidelines (for this purpose, a low ejection fraction is usually considered to be less than .40). After review of some general measures, these principles will be discussed, with special consideration and emphasis pertinent to diabetic patients. Patients with primarily diastolic heart failure (i.e., those with normal ejection fraction) will be considered subsequently.

1. General Measures

A low-salt diet (usually 2 g) with carbohydrate content tailored to the severity of diabetes is appropriate. It is rarely necessary to restrict salt to such a degree that the patient's diet is unpalatable nor is it ordinarily necessary to restrict water intake. Unless there is active and potentially dangerous demand ischemia or exercise-induced arrhythmias, physical activity need not be curtailed other than as dictated by symptoms. Indeed, regular aerobic exercise should be encouraged, and organized exercise conditioning programs may be beneficial. Such programs have not been convincingly shown to enhance cardiac function, but they increase exercise tolerance and have been reported to improve endothelial function. In diabetic patients, they offer the additional benefits of weight loss and enhanced control of blood glucose. Of course, smoking cessation is imperative. Smoking has specific, deleterious effects in heart failure because of vasoconstriction and reduced oxygen-carrying capacity caused by carbon monoxide. Treatment of hyperlipidemia, with its clearly demonstrated long-term benefits in patients with coronary artery disease, may improve endothelial function in the short term. It is important to be alert to and address concurrent problems that can induce and/ or make management of CHF more difficult (e.g., fever, occult infection, altered thyroid function, anemia, and, of course, poorly controlled diabetes).

2. Pharmacological Therapy of Low-Ejection-Fraction Heart Failure

Diuretics.   All patients should receive diuretic therapy with the exception of those who do not actually develop volume overload (strictly speaking, these patients do not have congestive heart failure). The latter include asymptomatic patients with depressed ejection fraction and patients with symptoms that occur exclusively with stress, provided they do not have evidence of systemic or pulmonary venous congestion under basal conditions. "Loop" diuretics, usually furosemide, are most effective in patients with CHF. Furosemide has several attractive features for CHF patients: potency, including the fact that increasing doses usually cause incremental diuretic effects, low toxicity, and low cost. As with all diuretics, especially in diabetic patients who may have nephropathy, care must be taken to avoid prerenal azotemia. Thiazide diuretics should generally be avoided in diabetic patients with CHF because of adverse effects on blood glucose. In patients with severe or refractory volume overload, especially when the systemic venous pressure is particularly high, it may be useful to add a second diuretic agent. Metalozone and spironolactone are often effective. As discussed below, spironolactone improves survival and clinical class in patients with CHF and a low ejection fraction in doses that are thought to be too low to have a significant diuretic effect. When used for the specific purpose of stimulating diuresis, however, spironolactone should be used in "diuretic" doses, typically 25 mg p.o. three times daily. Supplemental potassium should ordinarily be discontinued when initiating spironolactone therapy and serum potassium should be monitored. Many diabetic patients manifest modest hyporeninemia and hypokalemia. Thus, use of diuretics and potassium supplementation requires careful attention to potential changes in electrolytes over time.

   Digitalis.   After many years of controversy, the role of digitalis glycosides as a component of the modern therapy of CHF has been resolved with the recent publication of a large, randomized trial. These data show that routine administration of digitalis reduces long-term morbidity, reflected in a reduced hospital readmission rate, but does not alter long-term survival. Thus, there is objective justification for administration of digitalis. When administered with careful attention to dose selection in relation to age and renal function, digoxin can be used with very low toxicity. The higher incidence of renal insufficiency in diabetic subjects should of course engender extra caution in regard to dose selection as well as judicious monitoring of serum digoxin levels.

   It is likely that digitalis is effective in CHF because of resensitization of blunted baroreceptor responses with attendant deactivation of the sympathetic nervous system rather than because of its effects on cardiac contractility, which are actually very modest. It is not known whether this effect is altered in diabetic subjects with autonomic neuropathy.

   Angiotensin-Converting-Enzyme Inhibitors.   In chronic CHF neurohumoral activation, including the renin-angiotensin-aldosterone and sympathetic nervous systems, has long-term adverse effects. Several large, controlled clinical trials have firmly established angiotensin-converting-enzyme (ACE) inhibitors as one of the cornerstones of the modern pharmacological therapy of low-ejection-fraction myocardial failure, both ischemic and nonischemic in etiology. The tissue-specific myocardial renin-angiotensin system is markedly activated in failing myocardium, with resultant adverse effects on a number of cellular responses that occur in the evolution of cardiac hypertrophy, including promotion of calcium overload and matrix remodeling with increased fibrosis. Moreover, ACE inhibitors are nonspecific kininases. As a consequence, they potentiate the effects of bradykinin, a property that may have clinical significance and benefit.

ACE inhibitors improve long-term survival as well as clinical class in patients with low-ejection-fraction CHF. The SOLVD trials demonstrated that ACE inhibitors also have positive effects on postinfarction remodeling, resulting in reduced development of heart failure after an index myocardial infarction. ACE inhibitors may be especially important in diabetic patients because of their salutary influence on the progression of diabetic nephropathy and apparently favorable effects on carbohydrate metabolism with possible delay of onset of overt diabetes. Moreover, the HOPE trial documented reduced coronary event rates in diabetic patients receiving ACE inhibitors. This effect may be related to the observation that ACE inhibitors decrease PAI-1 levels in diabetic patients. Accordingly, in the absence of a specific contraindication and/or unacceptable side effects, virtually all patients with a low ejection fraction, including those with diabetes, should receive an ACE inhibitor. Relatively high doses are currently recommended, although what constitutes a truly optimal dose is uncertain. In patients who may be volume depleted there is a risk of induction of renal insufficiency and hyperkalemia when ACE inhibitors are employed, especially early after initiation of therapy. However, the presence of preexisting renal insufficiency per se is not a contraindication to the use of ACE inhibitors, but rather a signal to use them with extra caution. Many patients should have diuretics held or doses reduced as ACE inhibitor therapy is begun. BUN, creatinine, and electrolytes should be carefully monitored. Induction of renal insufficiency should alert the physician to the possibility of renal artery stenosis.

ACE inhibitors are well-tolerated in the vast majority of patients, with cough being the most common side effect responsible for discontinuation of therapy. Because diabetes is associated with a high incidence of coexisting renal insufficiency, extra vigilance to detect induction of renal toxicity is appropriate.

Beta-Adrenergic Blockers. Beta-adrenergic blocking drugs very significantly reduce mortality in CHF patients with low ejection fraction, once again consistent with the adverse effects of neurohumoral activation. Although these drugs have impressive effects on survival, their effects on clinical class are more subtle. Carvedilol is the beta-adrenergic blocker that has been used most extensively in published studies. This drug is unique in that it is also an alpha-adrenergic blocker and has antioxidant properties, both of which have theoretical benefit. There is also considerable experience with metoprolol and bucindolol. Presently,

published data do not support the use of one particular beta-blocker in low-ejection-fraction CHF, although it is prudent to use agents with which there is published experience. Beta-adrenergic blockers are currently recommended for all
but Class IV patients with CHF and low ejection fraction. The recently completed
but not yet published (as of this date) COPERNICUS study suggests that beta-
blockers are indicated in Class IV patients as well. Until COPERNICUS has been
peer reviewed, it is prudent to wait until Class IV patients have improved in
clinical class before starting beta-blockers. This does not preclude starting beta-
blockers in Class IV patients who are doing poorly on conventional management.

Beta-blocker therapy is initiated at very low doses, with progressive increases approximately every 2 weeks until a target dose is achieved over a period
of 2 to 3 months. Symptoms, weight, and physical findings should be carefully
monitored during this period. This approach is well tolerated in the vast majority
of patients. A small number develop worsening symptoms, usually mild, during
initiation of therapy. In most instances, this can be managed by slowing the dose
progression and/or increasing diuretics. Beta-blockers should not be considered
a form of therapy that will improve clinical class and circulatory congestion on a
short-term basis. Indeed, many patients with low ejection fractions will seriously
decompensate if these drugs are administered in full beta-blocking doses without
gradual dose progression.

There is no evidence that beta-blockers are more or less effective in diabetic
patients with low-ejection-fraction CHF than in nondiabetic patients. As with the
use of beta-blockers in general, in patients with diabetes the possibility of inducing and/or potentiating hypoglycemia should be kept in mind, but this is mainly
an issue in patients who require insulin therapy and have a history of hypoglycemia. Other cautions in the use of beta-blockers are identical to those for nondiabetic patients and include adverse conduction system effects, induction of bron-
chospasm, and central nervous system side effects.

Spironolactone.   The recently published RALES study, a large, controlled
clinical trial of spironolactone 25 mg daily in Class III–IV patients with low-
ejection-fraction CHF, demonstrated improved survival. The patients recruited
for the RALES trial received concomitant conventional therapy with diuretics,
digitalis, and ACE inhibitors, but very few received beta-blockers. Accordingly,
the potential use of spironolactone in conjunction with beta-blockers was not
clarified. *Current* recommendations are that spironolactone should be administered in addition to conventional therapy to sicker (Class III–IV) patients,
whereas beta-blockers should be withheld in Class IV patients. (The COPERNI-
CUS results may modify these recommendations.) This obviously leaves some
uncertainty for treatment of Class III patients. Our current practice is to prescribe
beta-blockers first in Class III patients and add spironolactone in patients who
have had a suboptimal clinical response.

The dose of spironolactone employed in the RALES study was smaller than that ordinarily employed when the drug is used primarily for its diuretic effect. This suggests that some nondiuretic effect is responsible for the favorable effect on survival, for example, inhibition of aldosterone-induced fibrosis. It is well-established that ACE inhibitors do not effectively block synthesis of aldosterone or its effects; indeed, this was a main rationale for undertaking the RALES study.

There is no evidence that spironolactone is more or less effective in diabetic compared with nondiabetic patients with low-ejection-fraction CHF. Patients with creatinine greater than 2.5 were excluded from RALES; certainly, caution should be exercised in diabetic patients with renal insufficiency. Serum potassium should be checked before starting spironolactone and monitored during therapy. Even though the recommended dose is low, it is wise to discontinue supplemental potassium when spironolactone is administered. With the above precautions, spironolactone was very well tolerated by patients enrolled in the RALES study.

Anticoagulation. All patients with CHF (regardless of ejection fraction) and atrial fibrillation and/or a history of thromboembolism should be treated with warfarin unless there is a contraindication. There is at present no objective information available with regard to prophylactic anticoagulation in patients with CHF who are in sinus rhythm.

Other Drugs. A significant number of patients do not tolerate ACE inhibitors. These patients should ordinarily be treated with some other form of vasodilator therapy. The most logical alternatives are combined hydralazine and isosorbide dinitrate or angiotensin receptor blockers (ARBs). As demonstrated in the VHEFT-I trial, the combination of hydralazine and isosorbide is the only other vasodilator treatment besides ACE inhibitors that has been shown to improve survival. ARBs are a logical choice. However, ACE inhibitors have effects other than inhibition of the conversion of angiotensin I to angiotensin II. Because large-scale trials of ARBs in patients with low-ejection-fraction CHF are nearing completion and publication, clarification of their effects on survival should be forthcoming. Some difficult patients with low-ejection-fraction CHF respond symptomatically to long-acting nitrates, especially those with inducible myocardial ischemia. Some Class IV patients have a favorable symptomatic response to periods of intensive therapy with intravenous dobutamine or phosphodiesterase inhibitors.

Myocardial Revascularization. A significant number of patients with low ejection fraction and coronary artery disease, including those with diabetes, have regions of hibernating myocardium, that is, regions supplied by stenotic vessels with depression of contractile function that is reversible by revascularization.

The mechanisms underlying hibernating myocardium are poorly understood, but appear to involve both acute and chronic feedback whereby reduced energy supply induces decreased contractile function and attendant reduced energy consumption. By maintaining the balance between supply and demand, ischemia is avoided and tissue survival is possible. Although often difficult to distinguish from hibernating myocardium with routine testing, stunned myocardium connotes a reversible ischemic injury in contrast to hibernating myocardium in which no injury is thought to occur. Clinically applicable measures of metabolism (e.g., with PET scanning) are depressed in hibernating myocardium but normal in stunned myocardium. Thus, PET scanning is an excellent way to identify poorly contracting but viable myocardium. Other useful approaches include dobutamine echocardiography, thallium redistribution studies, and "scar imaging" with nuclear magnetic resonance. Revascularization in patients with depressed but viable myocardium has been shown to improve function, and is therefore appropriate therapy for CHF. With the following exception, there are no special considerations in the identification and management of hibernating myocardium in diabetic compared with nondiabetic patients. The BARI study showed that diabetic patients with multivessel coronary disease with indications for revascularization fared much better in terms of survival when revascularization was accomplished surgically rather than percutaneously by balloon angioplasty. Coronary stenting combined with new approaches to prevention of restenosis (especially brachytherapy) may modify this conclusion, but for the time being diabetic patients with low-ejection-fraction CHF, significant areas of viable myocardium, and multivessel coronary disease should generally be treated with surgical rather than percutaneous revascularization.

Transplantation and Mechanical Assist Devices. Cardiac transplantation is appropriate treatment for the relatively small number of severely compromised CHF patients for whom suitable donor organs can be identified. In the past, diabetic patients had been considered to be suboptimal candidates for transplantation. However, with improvements in immunosuppressive regimens, the outlook for diabetic patients undergoing transplantation, providing they do not have extensive end organ damage, has become quite acceptable. As transplantation has come of age, great strides have been made in the development of ventricular assist devices. These devices now have portable power supplies and are being used increasingly for prolonged periods of time with acceptably low complication rates, although their role remains primarily that of a bridge to transplantation. As further advances in this technology occur, including continued development of a totally implantable mechanical heart, mechanical assist devices are likely to emerge as viable treatment approaches independent of transplantation for both diabetic and nondiabetic patients.

3. Heart Failure with Normal Ejection Fraction

Epidemiology, Clinical Features, and Pathophysiology.   Approximately 30 to 40% of patients with CHF have a normal or well-preserved ejection fraction (the latter usually defined as $>.45$). The differential diagnosis includes entities such as constrictive pericarditis, restrictive cardiomyopathy, and hypertrophic cardiomyopathy. However, the most common etiologic substrate is concentric left ventricular hypertrophy caused by systolic hypertension in elderly patients, most often women with noncompliant systemic arteries. Many of these patients have concomitant coronary artery disease that undoubtedly contributes to the pathophysiology of CHF, especially since demand ischemia causes increased left ventricular filling pressure with relatively little effect on ejection fraction. Thus, demand ischemia is itself a cause of transient CHF with well-preserved ejection fraction.

The presumption is that patients with CHF and normal ejection fraction have elevated cardiac filling pressures reflecting diastolic dysfunction that is in turn caused by slowed or incomplete myocardial relaxation and/or decreased passive compliance. This is obvious in patients with constrictive pericarditis and restrictive cardiomyopathy, who have major structural impediments to ventricular filling. However, the more commonly encountered patients with underlying concentric hypertrophy also have abnormalities of relaxation and filling, including possible depression of sarcoplasmic reticulum calcium pumping, increased ratio of wall thickness to chamber volume, and very likely increased myocardial connective tissue. In addition, concentric hypertrophy is a substrate for subendocardial ischemia when energy demands increase even in the absence of coronary artery disease. Patients with underlying concentric hypertrophy and CHF with normal ejection fraction present typically with acute pulmonary edema in conjunction with markedly elevated blood pressure and often tachycardia. This suggests an important role for increased myocardial energy demands and subendocardial ischemia superimposed on resting abnormalities of relaxation and filling.

Echocardiographic-Doppler abnormalities consistent with abnormal diastolic function are common in patients with diabetes, and left ventricular mass is increased compared with that in otherwise matched nondiabetic subjects. Moreover, diabetic patients are over-represented in the population of patients with CHF and normal ejection fraction. Thus, although not generally considered an independent etiology of CHF with normal ejection fraction, diabetic cardiomyopathy may contribute to the pathophysiology of this syndrome.

Management.   The general measures described above also apply to patients with CHF and normal ejection fraction. For the vast majority of patients with this syndrome and underlying concentric hypertrophy caused by systolic hypertension, therapy is otherwise exclusively pharmacological. The same special considerations pertinent to diabetic patients with low ejection fractions are applicable to these patients. In contrast to low-ejection-fraction heart failure, there are no large clinical trials available to date to help guide therapy. Accordingly, current recommendations are empirical.

Control of hypertension should be a major goal, with regression of left ventricular hypertrophy a hoped-for outcome. For this purpose, ACE inhibitors appear to be especially useful. They are usually well tolerated and may have advantages over other agents with respect to regression of hypertrophy and minimizing associated matrix remodeling. ARBs are a reasonable alternative. Careful attention should be paid to the presence of tachycardia. Either beta-adrenergic blockers or calcium channel antagonists that slow heart rate (usually diltiazem) should be considered in any patient with a tendency to tachycardia at rest or with CHF exacerbations. Long-term treatment with diuretic therapy is often useful, although particular attention should be paid to avoidance of excess intravascular volume depletion. Long-acting nitrates are also useful in some of these patients. There is no role for digitalis glycosides.

4. Management of Diabetes in Patients with Heart Failure

Poorly controlled diabetes should be managed aggressively in any patient with CHF because the attendant metabolic stress can certainly have adverse effects on myocardial function. Stringent control of blood glucose reduces the incidence of several complications of diabetes, specifically retinopathy, neuropathy, and nephropathy, but no data are available pertaining to the long-term effects of stringent control on diabetic cardiomyopathy or CHF in general in patients with diabetes. To the extent that diabetic cardiomyopathy is caused by hyperglycemia per se (e.g., matrix glycosylation) or the intracellular metabolic effects of reduced glucose transport (e.g., free radical damage to membranes), normalization of carbohydrate metabolism makes intuitive sense. Moreover, stringent control has been shown to modestly reduce event rates after an index myocardial infarction. On the other hand, prolonged hyperinsulinemia may be atherogenic and prothrombotic in type II diabetic patients. Thus, it is appropriate to achieve stringent control with the lowest possible doses of insulin or secretagogues, including sulfonylureas. The use of insulin sensitizers (thiazoladinediones) and biguanides may facilitate achieving this objective.

The use of insulin-sensitizing agents in CHF patients (especially the PPAR ligand thiazolidinedione class) has considerable potential attractiveness. Such agents should in theory improve the defects in carbohydrate metabolism that are likely significant causes of diabetic cardiomyopathy. In contrast to insulin, their salutary effects on various determinants of and risk factors for atherosclerosis and vasculopathy have obvious potential benefit. Recent preliminary reports also indicate that these agents can inhibit ventricular hypertrophy caused by mechanical stimuli. It is interesting to speculate that they might reverse the elevations in left ventricular mass observed in diabetic patients. Despite their promise, troglitazone, the first thiazolidinedione to be released (and subsequently withdrawn) was relatively contraindicated in symptomatic CHF because it can worsen volume overload and edema. Hopefully, newer thiazolidinediones will be better tolerated. Metformin, which also has insulin-sensitizing properties, is relatively contraindicated in CHF because of potential exacerbation of volume overload, induction of prerenal azotemia, and risk of lactic acidosis.

To reiterate, management of diabetes in patients with CHF should focus on stringent control with minimization of hyperinsulinemia. If insulin therapy cannot be avoided, the overall advantages of stringent control outweigh its potential disadvantages.

VI. SUMMARY

Diabetes is a powerful risk factor for the development of CHF, a major cause of morbidity and mortality in diabetic patients. A multifactorial cardiomyopathy occurs in patients with diabetes that is usually asymptomatic by itself. However, the cardiomyopathy seems to interact with and potentiate coexistent causes of hypertrophy and CHF, especially hypertension and ischemia resulting from coronary artery disease. Management of CHF in diabetic patients is quite similar to management in nondiabetic patients, with a few important differences. ACE inhibitors are very likely even more valuable in diabetic than in nondiabetic patients. Insulin-sensitizing drugs are promising but must be used very cautiously in the presence of heart failure.

SUGGESTED READING

1. Borow KM, Jaspan JB, Williams KA, Neumann A, Wolinski-Wally P, Lag R. Myocardial mechanics in young adult patients with diabetes mellitus: effects of altered load, inotropic state and dynamic exercise. J Am Coll Cardiol 1990;15:1508–1517.
2. Brownlee M. Glycation and diabetic complications. Diabetes 1994;43:836–841.
3. The Bypass Angioplasty Revascularization Investigation (BARI) Investigators. Comparison of coronary artery bypass surgery with angioplasty in patients with multivessel disease. N Engl J Med 1996;335:217–225.
4. Cohn JN, Johnson G, Zeische S, Cobb F, Francis G, Tristani F, Smith R, Dunkman WB, Loeb H, Wong M. A comparison of enalapril with hydralazine-isosorbide dinitrate in the treatment of congestive heart failure. N Engl J Med 1991;325:303–310.
5. Detre KM, Lombardero MS, Brooks MM, Hardison RM, Holubkov R, Sopko G, Frye RL, Chaitman BR, for the Bypass Angioplasty Revascularization Investigation Investigators. N Engl J Med 2000;342:989–997.

6. Dhalla NS, Elimban V, Rupp H. Paradoxical role of lipid metabolism in heart function and dysfunction. Mol Cell Biochem 1992;116:3–9.

7. DiBello V, Talerico L, Picano E, Di Muro C, Landini L, Paterni M, Matteucci E, Giusti C, Giampietro O. Increased echodensity of myocardial wall in the diabetic heart: an ultrasound tissue characterization study. J Am Coll Cardiol 1995;25:1408–1413.

8. The Digitalis Investigation Group. The effect of digoxin on mortality and morbidity in patients with heart failure and normal sinus rhythm. N Engl J Med 1997;336:525–533.

9. Galderisi M, Anderson KM, Wilson PWF, Levey D. Echocardiographic evidence for the existence of a distinct diabetic cardiomyopathy. Am J Cardiol 1991;68:85–89.

10. Geffner ME, Golde DW. Selective insulin action on skin, ovary, and heart in insulin-resistant states. Diabetes Care 1988;11:500–505.

11. Gu K, Cowie CC, Harris MI. Diabetes and decline in heart disease mortality in US adults. JAMA 1999;281:291–297.

12. Haffner SM, Lehto S, Ronnemaa T, Pyorala K, Lsaakso M. Mortality from coronary heart disease in subjects with type 2 diabetes and in nondiabetic subjects with and without prior myocardial infarction. N Engl J Med 1998;339:229–234.

13. Jaffe AS, Spadaro JJ, Schechtman K, Roberts R, Geltman EM, Sobel BE. Increased congestive heart failure after myocardial infarction of modest extent in patients with diabetes mellitus. Am Heart J 1984;108:31–37.

14. Kannel WB, Hijortland M, Castelli WP. Role of diabetes in congestive heart failure: the Framingham Study. Am J Cardiol 1974;34:29–34.

15. LeWinter MM, ed. Review in depth: Diabetic cardiomyopathy. Coronary Artery Dis 1996;7:94–142.

16. Libby P. Molecular bases of the acute coronary syndromes Circulation 1995;91:2844–2855.

17. Lind L, Anderson PE, Andren B. Left ventricular hypertrophy in hypertension is associated with the insulin resistance metabolic syndrome. J Hypertens 1992;19(suppl I):116–118.

18. Malhotra A, Reich D, Nakouzi A, Sanghi V, Geenen DL, Buttrick PM. Experimental diabetes is associated with functional activation of protein kinase C epsilon and phosphorylation of troponin I in the heart, which are prevented by angiotensin II receptor blockade. Circ Res 1997;81:1027–1033.

19. Malmberg K. Prospective randomised study of intensive insulin treatment on long term survival after acute myocardial infarction in patients with diabetes mellitus. Br Med J 1997;314:1512–1515.

20. Mulieri L, LeWinter MM. Depressed force-frequency relationship in diabetic patients undergoing coronary bypass grafting. In preparation.

21. Nahser PJ Jr, Brown RE, Oskarsson H, Winniford MD, Rossen JD. Maximal coronary flow reserve and metabolic coronary vasodilatation in patients with diabetes mellitus. Circulation 1995;91:635–640.

22. Olefsky JM. Treatment of insulin resistance with peroxisome proliferator-activated receptor γ agonists. J Clin Invest 2000;106:467–472.

23. Orlander PR, Goff DC, Morrissey M, Ramsey DJ, Wear ML, Labarthe DR, Nicha-

man MZ. The relation of diabetes to the severity of acute myocardial infarction and post-myocardial infarction survival in Mexican-Americans and non-Hispanic whites. The Corpus Christi Heart Project. Diabetes 1994;43:897–902.

24. Packer M, Bristow MR, Cohn JN, Colucci WS, Fowler MB, Gilbert EM, Shusterman NH, for the U.S. Carvedilol Heart Failure Study Group. The effect of carvedilol on morbidity and mortality in patients with chronic heart failure. N Engl J Med 1996; 334:1349–1355.

25. Pailolle C, Dahan M, Paycha F, Cohen A, Passa P, Gourgon R. Prevalence and significance of left ventricular filling abnormalities determined by Doppler echocardiography in young type I (insulin-dependent) diabetic patients. Am J Cardiol 1990; 64:1100–1106.

26. Pitt B, Zannad F, Remme WJ, Cody R, Castaigne A, Perez A, Palensky J, Wittes J. The effect of spironolactone on morbidity and mortality in patients with severe heart failure. Randomized Aldactone Evaluation Study Investigators. N Engl J Med 1999;341:709–717.

27. Plutzky J. Peroxisome proliferator-activated receptors in vascular biology and atherosclerosis: Emerging insights for evolving paradigms. Curr Atherosclerosis Rep 2000;2:327–335.

28. Regan TJ, Weisse AB. Diabetic cardiomyopathy. J Am Coll Cardiol 1992;19:1165–1166.

29. Rodrigues B, McNeill JH. The diabetic heart: metabolic causes for the development of a cardiomyopathy. Cardiovasc Res 1992;26:913–922.

30. The SOLVD Investigators. Effect of enalapril on survival in patients with reduced left ventricular ejection fractions and congestive heart failure. N Engl J Med 1991; 325:293–302.

31. The SOLVD Investigators. Effect of enalapril on mortality and the development of heart failure in asymptomatic patients with reduced left ventricular ejection fractions. N Engl J Med 1992;327:685–691.

32. Stanley WC, Lopaschuk GD, McCormack JG. Regulation of energy metabolism in the diabetic heart. Cardiovasc Res 1997;34:25–33.

33. Uehara M, Kishikawa H, Isami S. Effect on insulin sensitivity of angiotensin converting enzyme inhibitors with and without a sulfhydryl group: bradykinin may improve insulin resistance in dogs and humans. Diabetologia 1994;37:300–307.

34. UK Prospective Diabetes Study Group. Intensive blood-glucose control with sulphonylureas or insulin compared with conventional treatment and risk of complications in patients with type 2 diabetes. Lancet 1998;352:837–853.

35. Vered A, Battler A, Segal P, Liberman D, yerushalmi Y, Berezin M, Nuefeld HN. Exercise-induced left ventricular dysfunction in young men with asymptomatic diabetes mellitus (diabetic cardiomyopathy). Am J Cardiol 1984;54:633–637.

14

Special Therapeutic Considerations: Coronary Interventions and Coronary Surgery

John S. Douglas, Jr.
Emory University School of Medicine,
Atlanta, Georgia

Diabetes mellitus is a commonly encountered condition that affects more than 16 million Americans who consume one of every four Medicare dollars and strongly increases their risk of coronary artery disease, myocardial infarction, and cardiac death. It has been estimated that over 50% of adult diabetics have significant coronary atherosclerotic disease (CAD), approximately 10 times the prevalence in the general population, and it is clear that in those afflicted, coronary disease progression is more rapid than in nondiabetics (1). About 80% of diabetics die of atherosclerotic causes, and although cardiac mortality has been decreasing in the general population in recent years, diabetic men and women have not enjoyed this decrease in cardiac mortality (1–3).

Coronary revascularization procedures performed in over a million Americans annually constitute one of the most commonly applied and effective strategies to palliate patients with severe coronary disease. Although about 25% of patients undergoing coronary artery revascularization are diabetic, attempts to intervene with revascularization therapy in diabetic patients with symptomatic and/or advanced coronary atherosclerosis have been frustrated by multiple problems, including difficulty in recognizing those patients most likely to benefit, increased initial morbidity and mortality associated with revascularization in diabetics, and disappointing long-term results in diabetics compared to nondiabetic patients. In addition, there are limited trials comparing percutaneous and surgical revascularization therapy, and those that have been completed utilized balloon angioplasty techniques, which are now outdated, without the benefit of stents, IIb/IIIa platelet receptor inhibitors, thienopyridines, or the aggressive therapy of diabetes and hyperlipidemia that has been recently shown to enhance outcomes of revascularization therapy. In addition, only now are patients who participated in percutaneous coronary intervention (PCI) versus coronary artery bypass graft surgery (CABG) trials reaching the time after surgery when deterioration of saphenous vein grafts becomes a major factor limiting long-term outcomes of surgically treated patients. Cardiologists, internists, and general practitioners who care for adult diabetics with and without known coronary atherosclerosis therefore face a plethora of issues beginning with questions regarding which patients should be screened for possible revascularization, how they should be screened, and which revascularization techniques are most appropriate for a given patient. After revascularization, how should patients be treated in light of the potential benefits of glycemic control and lipid-lowering, ACE inhibitors, long-term antiplatelet and beta-blocker therapy in this population? This chapter addresses these issues.

I. REVASCULARIZATION BENEFITS INCLUDE PROLONGATION OF LIFE

Coronary artery revascularization with PCI and CABG provides symptomatic palliation superior to that achieved with medical therapy. The degree of ischemia relief and symptomatic benefit obtained by diabetics, however, may be difficult to determine because of a blunted appreciation of ischemia and absence of typical anginal symptoms. The strongest case for benefit from coronary revascularization comes from the randomized trials of CABG and medical therapy, where CABG was life prolonging in patients with left main coronary artery stenosis, three-vessel coronary disease with abnormal LV function, and two- or three-vessel disease and >75% stenosis of the left anterior descending coronary artery. A meta-analysis of three major randomized trials comparing CABG with medical therapy also confirmed a survival benefit was achieved by surgery for patients with one-vessel disease involving the left anterior descending coronary artery (Table 1) (4). Although these trials did not specifically test outcomes in diabetics, there is reason to believe that diabetics do benefit especially in the more severely diseased subsets. This position is strongly supported by the Bypass Angioplasty Revascularization Investigation (BARI), which compared CABG with PCI in multivessel disease and reported that CABG prolonged life at 5 years in treated diabetics, a benefit that persisted at 7-year follow-up (survival of 84.4% with CABG vs. 80.9% with PCI; $p = 0.043$) (see Fig. 1) (5). It is important to note, however, that this survival benefit was confined to patients receiving an internal mammary artery graft, a strategy that is already firmly in place in most centers.

Table 1 Medical Therapy vs
Revascularization with CABG

CABG prolongs life in the following subgroups

Left main coronary stenosis
Three-vessel disease with LV dysfunction[a]
Two- or three-vessel disease and >75% LAD
One-vessel disease involving LAD[b]

---

[a] Benefit increases with increasing left ventricular (LV)
dysfunction.
[b] From meta-analysis by Yusuf et al. (4).
CABG = coronary bypass surgery; LAD = left anterior
descending coronary artery.

To restate, coronary bypass surgery has a potential for prolonging life in diabetics with severe coronary disease. Consequently, aggressive screening for this problem is justified in the diabetic population where severe coronary disease is common and underdiagnosed.

II. IDENTIFYING DIABETIC CANDIDATES FOR REVASCULARIZATION

A. Asymptomatic Patients

Diabetic patients frequently do not sense myocardial ischemia and this factor contributes to a significant increase in unrecognized myocardial infarction and sudden cardiac death (6) and greatly enhances the difficulty of recognizing the figurative iceberg of coronary disease that is present in the adult diabetic population. The prevalence of significant coronary artery disease in the adult diabetic population estimated by a variety of diagnostic methods is over 50% (1–7). Diabetes negates the cardioprotective effect of being female, a fact that mandates screening of adult women with diabetes in a manner comparable to that used in men. In reported series of patients undergoing revascularization, diabetic women are disproportionally represented compared to their nondiabetic counterparts. Diabetes alone accounts for about one-half of the increased mortality experienced by diabetics. The remainder is contributed by the presence of additional risk factors. Stamler et al. reported diabetes alone produced an absolute risk of cardiac death of 25 per 10,000 patient-years, which was increased to 47 by one additional risk factor (hypertension, hyperlipidemia, or smoking) and to 78 by all three (8). These observations emphasize the importance of the presence of multiple risk factors in identifying high-risk patients, and this is reflected in the consensus conference recommendations for cardiac testing in diabetics reproduced in

A. Survival–All Patients

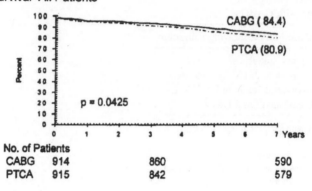

No. of Patients
CABG   914   860   590
PTCA   915   842   579

B. Survival–Patients with Treated Diabetes

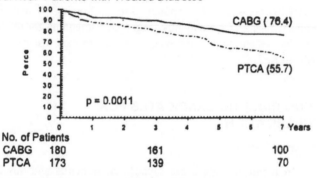

No. of Patients
CABG   180   161   100
PTCA   173   139   70

C. Survival–Patients without Treated Diabetes

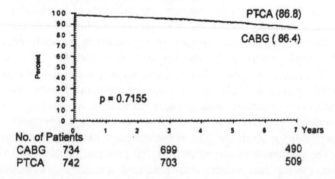

No. of Patients
CABG   734   699   490
PTCA   742   703   509

Figure 1 Survival curves of patients randomized to PTCA and CABG in BARI. (A) All patients included. (B) Survival of diabetic patients treated with PTCA and CABG. (C) Survival of patients without treated diabetes. (From Ref. 5.)

Table 2 Indications for Cardiac Testing in Diabetic Patients

1. Typical or atypical cardiac symptoms.
2. Resting ECG suggestive of ischemia or infarction.
3. Peripheral or carotid occlusive arterial disease.
4. Sedentary lifestyle, age ≥35 years, and plans to begin a vigorous exercise program.
5. Two or more of the following risk factors in addition to diabetes:
   a. Total cholesterol ≥240, LDL ≥160, or HDL <35 mg/dL.
   b. Blood pressure >140/90.
   c. Smoking.
   d. Family history of premature CAD.
   e. Positive micro/macroalbuminuria test.

Source: From Ref. 9.
ECG = electrocardiogram; LDL = low-density lipoprotein cholesterol; HDL = high-density lipoprotein cholesterol; CAD = coronary artery disease.

Table 2 (9). This report recommends that, in addition to patients with anginal symptoms, certain ECG abnormalities or evidence of noncardiac atherosclerotic disease, asymptomatic individuals with multiple risk factors should undergo cardiac testing. The primary reason for such testing is to identify candidates for life-prolonging revascularization, but major secondary gains from identifying diabetics with CAD include the opportunity to institute anti-ischemic therapy, angiotensin-converting-enzyme (ACE) inhibitors, and to aggressively pursue glycemic control and lipid lowering, strategies also capable of prolonging life. Beta-blockers alone reduced mortality as much as 50% in some subgroups (10), and of course there was a marked reduction of CAD event rates for diabetics treated with simvastatin in the 4S trial (11) and a reduced mortality demonstrated by ACE inhibitor therapy (12). Although cardiac screening is clearly beneficial, the best method of accomplishing this and the exact population that should be screened is less certain. Although routine treadmill testing and stress echocardiography have been used for this purpose, myocardial perfusion SPECT has recently been shown to be very effective in risk stratification in diabetics (13,14), and this method is selected in many centers. Cerisier and colleagues performed SPECT imaging in 383 totally asymptomatic patients with diabetes of 10 years' duration plus at least one additional risk factor. They found ischemia in 124 (32%) and, on the basis of higher subsequent cardiac events in those managed conservatively, recommended coronary angiography in similar patients with perfusion defects on screening SPECT studies (15). At Emory University, asymptomatic or mildly symptomatic diabetic patients with multiple risk factors and suggestive symptoms or ECG findings are commonly referred directly for coronary angiography without noninvasive screening. This is a Class I indication for coronary angiography when the patient has "clinical characteristics that indicate a high likelihood of severe CAD," a condition that applies in diabetics so defined (16). Coronary angiography has the marked advantage of defining revascularization options, risk stratification, and providing some guidance for the frequency and type of subsequent testing to monitor disease progression.

B. Chronic Stable Angina

The general population of patients with nondisabling chronic angina have a significant prevalence of advanced coronary disease. Douglas and Hurst reported that 11% of male patients with mild chronic angina evaluated angiographically had left main coronary disease, 28% had three-vessel disease, and 22% had two-vessel disease (17). The severity of symptoms does not correlate well with the severity of disease in nondiabetics, and this discrepancy is even more marked in diabetics. Diabetics not only have more advanced disease than nondiabetics, but, also are at higher risk for progression of disease and subsequent cardiac events. For these reasons, aggressive risk stratification is indicated with noninvasive testing (stress ECG, stress echocardiography, or perfusion SPECT) (13–15) or coronary angiography in patients who have angina, even if it is not disabling. Patients preferentially selected for coronary angiography include those with multiple coronary risk factors (Table 2), prior infarction, evidence of left ventricular dysfunction, symptoms of congestive heart failure, noninvasive testing results indicating high risk, and symptoms that are inadequately controlled with medical therapy. These recommendations comply with ACC/AHA/ACP–ASIM guidelines (16). In addition, diabetic patients with any evidence of ischemia on myocardial scans, shown by Kang et al. to have increased subsequent occurrence of hard cardiac endpoint events, should be offered angiographic evaluation (13).

C. Acute Coronary Syndromes

Management of diabetic patients presenting with acute coronary syndromes is detailed in Chapters 12 and 13. Current guidelines offer the option of conservative or invasive methods to risk stratify patients with unstable angina and non-ST-elevation infarction (18). However, recently presented data analyzing contemporary treatment with low-molecular-weight heparin, early catheterization, and stent-supported percutaneous or surgical revascularization when appropriate, support an early invasive approach in these patients (19,20). Given the marked increase in acute and subsequent mortality in diabetics with acute coronary syndromes, an invasive approach is generally favored in diabetics if there is no contraindication. Knowledge of coronary anatomy permits identification of those patients likely to benefit from life-prolonging CABG as well as other revasculari-

zation options, and allows for orderly planning for subsequent pharmacotherapy
and follow-up.

III. REVASCULARIZATION IN THE DIABETIC PATIENT

A. Balloon Angioplasty

Although patients with diabetes typically have more diffuse coronary atherosclerosis than nondiabetics, the initial angiographic success rates in diabetic patients
selected for balloon angioplasty have been comparable to those of nondiabetics.
In the National Heart, Lung, and Blood Institute (NHLBI) PTCA Registry, outcomes of 281 diabetic and 1833 nondiabetic balloon angioplasty patients were
analyzed. Diabetic patients were older, more likely to be female, and had more
comorbidity at baseline, triple-vessel disease, and atherosclerotic lesions (21).
Angiographic success and revascularization completeness were comparable, but
diabetics experienced more death and nonfatal myocardial infarction. A composite endpoint of death, myocardial infarction, or urgent revascularization occurred
in 11.0% of diabetics, but in only 6.7% of nondiabetics ($p < 0.01$). Female
diabetics were particularly at risk, with a striking in-hospital mortality of 8.3%.
At 9-year follow-up, mortality was twice as high in diabetic patients (35.9% vs.
17.9%) and the rates of nonfatal MI, CABG, and repeat PCI were higher in diabetics than in nondiabetics (see Fig. 2). Subsequent large series reported that the
initial mortality associated with balloon angioplasty in diabetics was similar to
nondiabetics, but long-term results were inferior due to higher rates of restenosis,

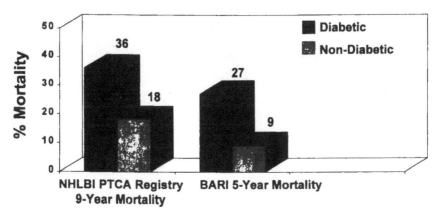

Figure 2   Mortality of patients with and without treated diabetes in the National Heart,
Lung, and Blood Institute (NHLBI) PTCA Registry (21) and in BARI (5,29).

more repeat revascularizations, and disease progression in nontarget lesions and development of new lesions in sites that were previously normal (22–26). Rozenman et al. reported restenosis occurred in 35% of nondiabetics, 36% of diabetics who were not insulin dependent, and in 61% of insulin-requiring diabetics ($p = 0.04$) (24). Barsness et al., who carefully studied paired angiograms (baseline and at 5 years) in 320 diabetic and nondiabetic patients treated percutaneously in BARI, reported more restenosis in diabetics (43% vs. 27%; $p = 0.01$) and more new lesions in diabetics (3 vs 2; $p = 0.002$), indicating an accelerated disease process in diabetics compared to nondiabetics (26). Investigators in CABRI attempted to explain poor outcomes after balloon angioplasty in diabetic patients by analyzing the amount of baseline disease and the completeness of revascularization in diabetics compared to nondiabetics; they found them to be similar, leading these investigators to believe that a greater rate of disease progression in diabetics was the reason that diabetic patients fared poorly (27). Data from EAST is also consistent with an important role of disease progression. In EAST, the survival of diabetic and nondiabetic patients treated with angioplasty was comparable for about 5 years. Subsequently, the survival curves diverged significantly, with diabetics experiencing a higher late mortality (see Fig. 3) (28). This delayed divergence of the survival curves occurred too late to be caused

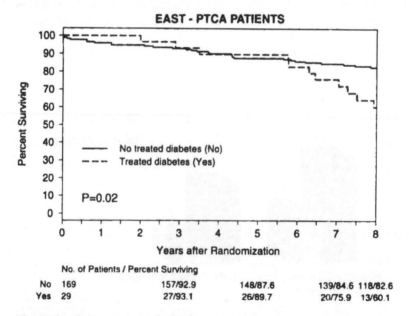

Figure 3 Eight-year survival of patients with and without treated diabetes in the Emory Angioplasty Surgery Trial (EAST) who were randomized to PTCA (28).

by postangioplasty restenosis and is best explained by more aggressive disease progression in the diabetic patients, disease progression that may not have been recognized because of a relative lack of symptoms in diabetic patients. The results reported from BARI, EAST, and CABRI are congruent and highlight the importance of postrevascularization medical, lifestyle, and surveillance strategies aimed at preventing and detecting atherosclerotic disease progression in all revascularized patients, but especially in the diabetic population.

B. Balloon Angioplasty Compared with CABG

BARI, the 1829-patient randomized comparison of balloon angioplasty and CABG in multivessel disease, showed that there was no difference in survival between the two revascularization methods after 7 years of follow-up in patients without treated diabetes (see Fig. 1) (5). However, in the 353 treated diabetics, an increased mortality was apparent at 5 years in the those treated with balloon angioplasty (35% vs. 19% with CABG; $p < 0.002$), and this observation resulted in an NHLBI alert which was published in September 1995, suggesting that caution be exercised in the use of balloon angioplasty in treated diabetics with two- and three-vessel coronary disease (29). Of interest is the analysis of practice patterns in the National Cardiovascular Network published by Peterson et al., showing that prior to the alert 47% of diabetics with two-vessel disease requiring revascularization underwent coronary angioplasty compared with only 14% with three-vessel disease, and this referral pattern was unchanged after the 1995 alert (30). The degree to which the new availability of the Palmaz-Schatz stent in 1995 encouraged persistence with percutaneous methods in diabetic patients is uncertain (see Sec. III. C). This report does suggest that percutaneous intervention is not frequently recommended in diabetics with three-vessel disease, and this is consistent with the 1981–1994 Emory experience where only 15% of insulin-dependent diabetics with three-vessel disease requiring revascularization underwent PTCA (22). Interestingly, in BARI there was no difference in ejection fraction at 5 years in PTCA- and CABG-treated patients even in subgroups of diabetes and three-vessel disease (31). In addition to the randomized trials comparing PCI and CABG, three large, single-center registries and a regional registry have been published and hazard ratios adjusted for baseline differences were reported (see Fig. 4) (22,25,32,33). In the Duke study, the survival of patients treated with PCI and CABG was not significantly different. In the MAHI study, survival was better with CABG, but these data were not adjusted. In the NNE experience, survival of multivessel-disease diabetics was better with CABG.

Although there is very little published outcome data regarding CABG versus PCI in single-vessel disease in the diabetic population, it appears that PCI is the dominant strategy utilized in this subgroup. Whether CABG or percutaneous revascularization should be pursued in two-vessel disease is controversial. Fac-

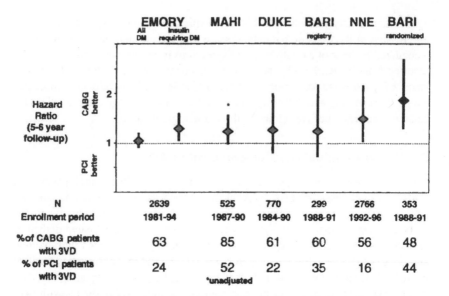

Figure 4 Hazard ratios of diabetic patients revascularized with PTCA or CABG in observational studies performed at Emory University (22), the Mid-America Heart Institute (MAHI), Duke (25), BARI Registry (34), the Northern New England (NNE) experience (33) and from the randomized BARI study (5,35). (From Ref. 33.)

tors such as LAD involvement, lesion length and complexity, number of lesions, and decreased LV function tend to lead to CABG whereas simple lesions favor the PTCA approach. In the Emory observational experience, the survival rate of insulin-treated diabetic patients with two-vessel disease was similar at 5 and 10 years for PTCA and CABG (22). In BARI, however, 7-year survival of diabetics with two-vessel disease treated with CABG was significantly better than with PTCA (5). In the BARI Registry, where revascularization therapy of diabetics was chosen by the physician for patients with two- and three-vessel disease (34), there was no difference in cardiac mortality (7.5% for PTCA and 6.0% for CABG; $p = 0.73$). Even when the predicted mortality was adjusted for baseline differences, there was no statistically significant difference between PTCA and CABG cardiac survival. In the NNE experience, survival was enhanced by CABG in diabetics with three-vessel disease (hazard ratio = 2.02; $p = 0.038$) (see Fig. 5), but not significantly improved in two-vessel disease (33 . These observations emphasize the importance of physician judgment in selecting the best revascularization therapy for a given patient.

   An important observation in BARI was the fact that the survival benefit of CABG in diabetics was conferred only to those receiving an internal mammary

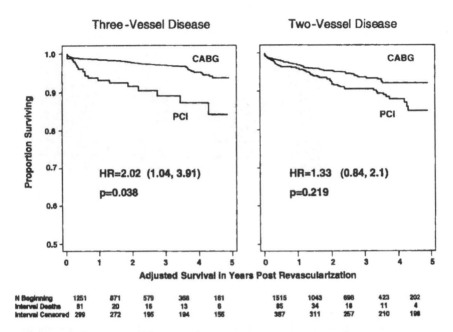

Figure 5 Survival curves for diabetic patients with three-vessel and two-vessel disease treated with PCI and CABG in the Northern New England observational study. (From Ref. 33.)

artery graft (5) (Fig. 6). Patients receiving only saphenous vein grafts had a significantly lower survival (54% vs. 83%), which was virtually identical to that of PTCA patients. Data at 5 years from the BARI randomized trial indicated that insulin-treated diabetics had significantly worse outcomes with PTCA compared with those in diabetic patients receiving oral agents, and the benefit of CABG was more apparent (34). When BARI randomized and registry patients were analyzed together, mortality rates over 5 years of follow-up were similar with CABG and PTCA among diabetics taking oral hypoglycemic drugs (35), but insulin-treated diabetics had a higher mortality and cardiac mortality with PTCA compared to CABG (relative risks 1.78 and 2.63, respectively; $p < 0.001$). Not surprisingly, diabetics with ≥ 4 significant lesions had worse outcomes with PTCA; 5-year mortality with PTCA was 43.4% compared to 24.6% following PTCA in patients with <4 significant lesions (34). The respective mortality rates following CABG were 21.6% and 17.1% for patients with ≥ 4 lesions and <4 lesions. The lack of a significant mortality benefit of CABG in diabetics with <4 lesions provides a rationale for selection of percutaneous revascularization, especially when anatomy is favorable, and there is good recognition of ischemic symptoms, the relief

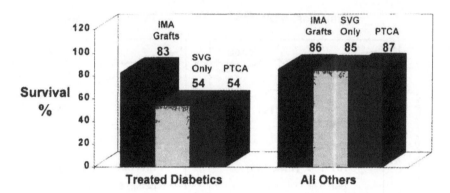

Figure 6 Survival at 7 years following randomization in BARI for patients receiving internal mammary artery (IMA) grafts, saphenous vein grafts (SVG) without IMA, and patients randomized to PTCA (5).

of which would be beneficial and whose return would signal the need for reevaluation (see Sec. III. D).

Long-term follow-up of diabetic patients in BARI provided insight into clinical factors that alter outcome. In addition to insulin dependence, patients with ST elevation, congestive heart failure, older age, and black race had higher mortality (35) and renal function was found to have a major impact. Seven-year mortality was 14% in nondiabetics with creatinine ≤1.5 mg/dL, 30% in diabetics with creatinine ≤1.5 mg/dL, and a striking 70% in diabetics with creatinine >1.5 mg/dL (see Fig. 7) (36). Mehran et al. reported that diabetes and renal insufficiency conferred additive and disastrous postprocedure prognosis following coronary angioplasty (1-year death or MI in 26%) (37). Marso et al. identified proteinuria as a marker for diabetic nephropathy and a key determinant of outcome following coronary angioplasty in diabetics (38). Two-year mortality was 7.3% for nondiabetics, 9.1% for diabetics without proteinuria, but 16.2% for diabetics with 1+ or 2+ proteinuria, and 43% for diabetics with ≥3+ proteinuria ($p <$ 0.001). Less than 25% of patients in the Marso et al. report received ACE inhibitors that have been shown to delay progression of renal insufficiency and reduce long-term morbidity and mortality in this difficult patient subset (39,40).

C. Stents

As a result of convincing randomized trials and ease of clinical use, stents are currently used in over 70% of percutaneous coronary interventions, reducing the need for emergency CABG and subsequent revascularization. Savage et al. used the randomized Stress I and II trials to compare outcomes of stenting with balloon

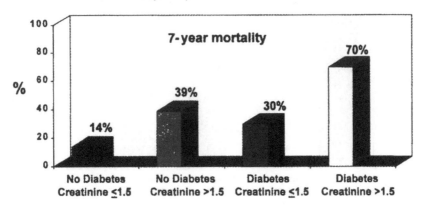

Figure 7 Seven-year mortality of patients in randomized BARI based on diabetes and renal function (creatinine ≤1.5 vs. >1.5) (36).

angioplasty in diabetics, finding that stents significantly improved procedural success (100% vs. 82%; $p < 0.01$) and acute lumen gain (1.61 mm vs. 1.06 mm; $p < 0.0001$) and reduced restenosis (24% vs. 60%; $p < 0.01$) and target vessel revascularization (13% vs. 31%; $p = 0.03$) (41). Similarly, Van Belle et al. in an observational study reported restenosis in 25% of stented diabetics compared to 63% in balloon-treated patients (42). In over 700 stented patients at Emory, Blankenbaker et al. noted that diabetics had more heart failure, hypertension, and multivessel disease and that diabetics during follow-up had more adverse events (hazard ratio 2.97; $p = 0.038$) and reduced 2-year survival (82% vs. 93%; $p = 0.005$) (43). In a large contemporary experience, Dangas et al. analyzed immediate and 1-year outcomes of stenting in 89 insulin-requiring diabetics and 373 non-insulin-treated diabetics compared to 584 nondiabetics, finding no difference in angiographic success or in-hospital complications, but 1-year MACE was significantly more common in diabetics (49%, 38%, and 25% in insulin-requiring, non-insulin-requiring diabetics and nondiabetics, respectively; $p < 0.001$) as was target vessel revascularization (26%, 18%, and 11%, respectively; $p = 0.01$) (see Fig. 8) (44). Deutsch et al. showed, however, that the benefit of stenting in diabetics did not extend to vessels <3 mm in diameter where the follow-up MLD of diabetics was significantly less than nondiabetics (1.24 mm vs. 1.55 mm; $p < 0.05$) (45). However, stenting was beneficial in the GUSTO IIB, where 6-month MACE and death were significantly reduced in diabetics undergoing PCI with stents compared with balloon angioplasty (46). It appears that stents do confer significant benefit in diabetics primarily by reducing late events compared to

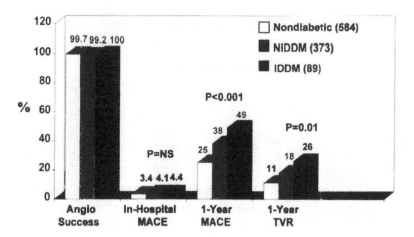

Figure 8   In-hospital and 1-year outcomes in a consecutive series of patients treated with multivessel stent implantation sorted by the absence of diabetes (nondiabetic), presence of diabetes without dependence on insulin therapy (NIDDM), and diabetes with insulin therapy (IDDM) (44).

balloon angioplasty but that the results are inferior to those in nondiabetics presumably due to the exaggerated intimal hyperplasia documented to occur in diabetics (47). The issue of post-PCI restenosis in diabetics was extensively reviewed recently (48). A very recent report from the NHLBI Dynamic Registry analyzed patients treated with PCI from July 1997 and June 1999 when 73% of patients received stents and 27% IIb/IIIa platelet receptor inhibitors. In 1056 treated diabetics, in-hospital risk was similar to nondiabetics. However, at 1 year, diabetics were at significantly greater risk of dying or undergoing repeat revascularization (49). Van Belle and colleagues showed that patency of the PTCA site was an important determinate of long-term survival (see Fig. 9) (50).

EPISTENT provided compelling data to indicate that abciximab was beneficial in diabetics undergoing stent implantation. In this randomized trial which compared outcomes in three treatment groups (stent + placebo, balloon + abciximab, and stent + abciximab), the occurrence rate of a composite endpoint of death, MI, or target vessel revascularization at 6 months was significantly reduced in the stent + abciximab group (13% vs. 25% in the stent + placebo group and 23% in the balloon + abciximab group; $p = 0.005$) (51). In diabetics, the target vessel revascularization rate for the stent + abciximab group, 8%, was less than one-half that observed in the two other groups (stent + placebo 17% and balloon + abciximab 18%, P = 0.02). It appeared that without abciximab, diabetics did not obtain the long-term reduction in TVR usually seen with stent implantation. When data from EPIC, EPILOG, and EPISTENT were pooled, abciximab de-

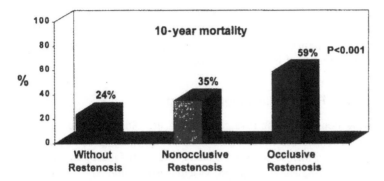

Figure 9 Ten-year mortality of 604 diabetic patients based on whether the patient was free of restenosis (without restenosis) at 6 months, had restenosis without total vessel occlusion (nonocclusive restenosis), or total occlusion (occlusive restenosis) (50).

creased the 1-year mortality from 4.5% to 2.5% (P = 0.03) (52). This is a 44% reduction in 1-year mortality. Diabetic women appear to have the most dramatic benefit with stent and abciximab (53) (see Adjunctive Therapy below).

The most potent strategy to reduce restenosis following coronary intervention, brachytherapy, appears to be equally beneficial in diabetic and non-diabetic patients. Restenosis was reduced from 37% with placebo to 18.8% (P = 0.03) in radiation-treated diabetic patients in a recently published START substudy (54).

D. Stents Versus CABG

The results in randomized trials of balloon angioplasty versus CABG (BARI, EAST, and CABRI) were congruent in showing that diabetic patients with multivessel disease treated with balloon angioplasty had more late adverse cardiac events, including death, than diabetics treated with CABG, but stents and IIb/IIIa platelet receptor inhibitors were not utilized. Two European randomized trials of stents versus CABG are currently underway, the Arterial Revascularization Therapy Study (ARTS) and Stent or Surgery (SOS). Preliminary data from ARTS in which 1205 patients were randomized to stenting or CABG were reported for 208 diabetic patients, showing that stented diabetics had higher 1-year mortality than CABG-treated diabetics (6.3% versus 3.1%) and higher 1-year MACE (38.4% versus 13.5%), but surgery patients had more strokes (6.3% versus 2.7%) (55). Analysis of cost effectiveness of CABG versus stenting in ARTS indicated that CABG was more cost effective in diabetics compared with non-diabetics (56). The trends in ARTS are similar to those seen in BARI; that is, surgery yielded lower MACE on follow-up. Detailed analysis of ARTS and SOS should provide valuable information regarding the choice of revascularization strategy, but these studies do not test the value of stenting plus abciximab, a strategy currently preferred in diabetic patients undergoing PCI.

E. Selection of Revascularization Method

Diabetics being considered for revascularization are older than nondiabetics, more likely to be female and to have more cardiac morbidity (prior MI, multilesion, multivessel, and diffuse coronary disease, and heart failure) and more comorbidity (renal insufficiency, peripheral vascular and pulmonary disease). Unfortunately, the available data are inadequate to accurately guide the clinician in the selection of optimal revascularization therapy in this patient population. What does seem clear is that balloon angioplasty alone is associated with decreased survival compared with CABG when used in patients with multivessel disease (especially when >4 lesions are treated), and very preliminary results from ARTS also recommend caution with stenting in this subgroup. As the number and complexity of lesions increase, the relative value of CABG increases. When single-lesion disease is present, CABG is rarely selected (exceptions being left main, ostial or proximal LAD unfavorable for PCI, or long or complex LAD lesions). Until more complete long-term outcome data are available from ARTS, SOS, and other trials comparing stents and CABG, physicians must make revascularization decisions in patients with multivessel disease based on incomplete study data and clinical experience. When PCI is selected, utilization of stents and abciximab provide significant advantages. CABG is indicated for many patients with multivessel disease involving the proximal LAD who are suitable for LIMA–LAD graft (see Fig. 10). With increasing lesion complexity and number, left ventricular and renal dysfunction, and insulin requirements, CABG is favored. The primary advantage of surgery is the replacement of an atherosclerotic-prone coronary arterial segment with an arterial conduit, the LIMA, which is resistant to atherosclerosis even in the diabetic patient (57). PCI is commonly used in multivessel disease with two-vessel involvement where stenting is feasible, the LAD is spared, ≤4 lesions are present, or when a culprit lesion strategy seems best due to comorbidity, advanced age, or poor distal vessels making CABG unattractive, or when use of the IMA is not feasible. The presence of anginal symptoms that would be expected to return should restenosis occur is an asset in diabetics undergoing PCI. Careful follow-up of diabetic patients undergoing multivessel PCI is indicated because they are more likely to develop restenosis at treated sites and to experience progression of disease in untreated sites. The optimal method and time intervals for routine surveillance of these patients is uncertain. Evaluation of PCI-treated patients should be focused on the time of restenosis, that is 3 to 4 months post-intervention. For long-term follow-up of

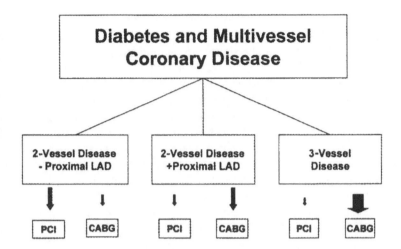

FAVOR PCI: No proximal LAD disease, single focal lesions, good LV and renal function, not insulin dependent, angina symptoms, older age, poor opportunity for IMA graft

Figure 10 Flow diagram indicating that most diabetic patients with three-vessel disease undergo CABG and that the choice of revascularization strategy is influenced by multiple factors including proximal LAD disease, lesion complexity, and other clinical features.

revascularized diabetic patients, the recommendations of the consensus panel for annual cardiac testing in diabetic patients at increased risk may be a reasonable compromise (Table 2) (9), and the documented efficacy of SPECT myocardial perfusion studies has led to the use of this method in many centers (13,14). Further studies of these issues to include an analysis of cost effectiveness of routine follow-up testing in diabetic patients are clearly needed. Aggressive medical and lifestyle measures are essential and discussed below.

F. Value of Adjunctive Therapy During and After Revascularization

1. IIb/IIIa Inhibitors and PCI

As noted above, abciximab was shown in EPISTENT to preserve the benefit of stenting in diabetic patients by reducing the target vessel revascularization by over 50% compared to placebo (51). In addition, abciximab decreased the 1-year mortality of diabetic patients when data from three placebo-controlled trials were pooled, suggesting that abciximab therapy should be strongly considered in all diabetic patients undergoing PCI with or without stent implantation (52). In this study, mortality in diabetics who underwent multivessel PCI was reduced from 7.7% to 0.9%; $p = 0.018$ with abciximab use and mortality in insulin-treated diabetics was decreased from 8.1% to 4.2%; $p = 0.073$. A recently reported subgroup analysis from EPISTENT indicated that diabetic women, who have a higher risk of death or MI after PCI, experienced a dramatic reduction in mortality, MI, or TVR at 1 year when treated with stent and abciximab compared to stent alone or balloon with abciximab (53). The mortality in the stent + abciximab arm was zero (compared to 7.7% with stent + placebo; $p < 0.06$ and 4.4% with balloon + abciximab; $p = 0.10$). The rate of death/MI/TVR with stent + abciximab was 13.3% (compared to 34.5% and 28.9%, respectively, both $p < 0.04$) and the TVR was 4.5% (compared to 21.4% and 26.7%, respectively; both $p = 0.02$). The complementary long-term benefit of stents and abciximab make a strong case for their routine use in diabetic patients during PCI, especially when the patient is female, insulin-dependent, and/or undergoing multivessel PCI.

2. Thienopyridines, PCI, and CABG

The ADP receptor antagonists clopidogrel and ticlopidine when used in conjunction with aspirin reduce complications of stenting compared to aspirin alone and aspirin plus warfarin (58,59). Ticlopidine pretreatment before coronary stenting is associated with sustained decrease in adverse cardiac events compared with ticlopidine administered post-PCI (60). Because of fewer side effects and equal or superior efficacy, clopidogrel has become standard antiplatelet therapy for prophylaxis during PCI (58–61). Its potency has been evidenced in trials comparing it with ticlopidine and also when emergency CABG is complicated by bleeding, or clopidogrel is stopped due to side effects a few days after stent implantation leading to stent thrombosis, and with the observation that prolonged therapy exceeding 6 months prevents late–late thrombosis following stent implantation and brachytherapy. The recently reported CURE trial showing benefit of clopidogrel in acute coronary syndromes has heightened interest in the more generalized use of this agent. Its relative value in the diabetic undergoing PCI has not been thoroughly tested. Given the prothrombotic milieu typical of the diabetic patient, clopidogrel must be viewed as a very important adjunctive therapy that should be initiated as early before PCI as possible and maintained until endothelialization of the coronary stent has occurred. When used in patients after CABG, clopidogrel has been shown to be more effective than aspirin, resulting in a 43% reduction in vascular death ($p = 0.03$) (63).

3. Glycemic Control After Revascularization

The randomized United Kingdom Prospective Diabetes Study (UKPDS) confirmed that glycemic control significantly reduced microvascular complications of type 2 diabetes and, to a lesser and not statistically significant extent, reduced

MI- and diabetes-related death (64). Recently reported studies indicate that tight glycemic control also decreased adverse cardiac events post-PCI (65). Yumoto et al. examined glycosylated hemoglobin (HbA1c) levels in diabetic patients following stenting reporting a lower mean value in patients without restenosis (6.8% vs. 7.5%; $p = 0.012$), suggesting an important role of glycemic control in restenosis prevention (66). The optimal choice of drug therapy to achieve glycemic control has not been determined. In the subset of patients undergoing PCI for acute MI, concern has been expressed regarding an early increased mortality in patients treated with sulfonylureas (67,68). Data from Takago and colleagues suggests that hyperinsulinemia in diabetic patients resulted in increased intimal hyperplasia within coronary stents (69) and that use of triglitozone, an agent that increases insulin sensitivity, reduced intimal hyperplasia (70). The ongoing BARI 2D trial in which patients undergoing PCI and medical therapy will be randomized to insulin-providing and insulin-sensitizing treatment strategies may provide some insight into the optimal agent for the post-PCI diabetic patient. Benefits of glycemic control in diabetics following CABG have not been carefully studied.

4. Lipid Lowering After Revascularization

Long-term follow-up data from BARI, EAST, and CABRI indicate that after PCI, progression of coronary disease in diabetics is accelerated compared to nondiabetics both at the treated site and in untreated sites (26–28). Although cholesterol lowering did not prove efficacious in reducing post-PCI restenosis in the Lovastatin restenosis trial (71), multiple beneficial effects of cholesterol-lowering therapy have been documented in this population with coronary disease including improved endothelial function and reduced cardiac events (72). More specific to the diabetic patient, in the 4S study, lowering cholesterol resulted in reduced cardiac events (11), inducing a reduction in 5-year mortality that was greater in diabetics than in nondiabetics (43% vs. 29% decrease) (73). A greater benefit in diabetics treated with HMG COA reductase inhibitors was also observed in the CARE and LIPID trials (74,75). In diabetics undergoing stent implantation, use of statins was associated with reduced clinical events and attenuation of neointimal proliferation that appeared in part independent of their cholesterol-lowering properties (76). Statins are currently regarded as first-line drugs in diabetics with elevated levels of LDL cholesterol following PCI.

Abundant data are present in the literature to confirm an important role of elevated serum lipids including LDL cholesterol, HDL cholesterol, triglycerides, apolipoprotein B, and Lp(a) in the development of saphenous vein graft atherosclerosis leading to late cardiac events after bypass surgery (77–83). The recently reported Post-Coronary Artery Bypass Graft (Post-CABG) trial showed that aggressive therapy to lower serum cholesterol led to a reduced progression of atherosclerosis in saphenous vein grafts (84) and this study has major implications for the post-CABG patient. Further analysis of prognostic factors for atherosclerosis progression in saphenous vein grafts in patients in the post-CABG trial identified current smoking, male sex, hypertension, elevated triglycerides, and low HDL as independent predictors of graft worsening (85). The importance of vein graft atherosclerosis in the diabetic population was graphically emphasized in BARI where the 7-year survival of diabetic patients treated with CABG using only saphenous vein grafts was only 54% compared to 83% for patients receiving at least one LIMA graft (see Fig. 6). It is clear, based on BARI and previously reported work (22,34), that diabetics after CABG have a reduced longevity compared to nondiabetics, especially when dependent on saphenous vein grafts. Aggressive measures are indicated in all post-CABG patients to reduce serum LDL, elevate HDL, control blood pressure, lower triglycerides, and strongly encourage smoking cessation. The effects of rigorous glycemic control on cardiac events post-CABG have not been carefully studied.

5. ACE Inhibitors After Revascularization

The HOPE study showed that the use of ramipril in 9297 patients (38% of whom were diabetic) resulted in a significant reduction in a number of adverse endpoints, including mortality, MI, stroke, cardiac arrest, and need for subsequent revascularization (86). The beneficial effects of ACE inhibitors in diabetics may relate to their effect on oxidative stress and vasodilation. ACE inhibitors increase bradykinin levels promoting vasodilation, insulin-mediated glucose uptake, and increased nitric oxide levels (87). Use of ramipril was studied in 159 patients after elective CABG or PCI who had normal blood pressure and an ejection fraction between 30% and 50%, but no congestive heart failure, finding that the ramipril-treated group had a 58% decrease in cardiac death, MI, and CHF ($p = 0.03$) and a lower all-cause mortality ($p = 0.05$) (88).

Oosterga and colleagues studied 149 patients undergoing CABG who, like the HOPE study patients, did not have the classic indications for ACE inhibitor therapy (i.e., no hypertension or LV dysfunction). Starting 2 weeks before elective CABG, patients were randomized to receive quinapril 40 mg a day or placebo for 1 year (89). At 1 year, there was a dramatic reduction in ischemic events in the quinapril-treated patients (4% vs. 18%; $p = 0.04$). These protective effects occurred independent of any effect of quinapril on blood pressure. Studies of carotid intimal thickness in 732 patients ≥ 55 years of age who had vascular disease or diabetes and at least one additional risk factor showed that, after an average follow-up of 4.5 years, ramipril significantly slowed progression of atherosclerosis (90). These and other studies indicate that ACE inhibitors are particularly beneficial in diabetic patients with established coronary artery disease and make a strong case for their routine use when the systemic blood pressure is permissive and the drug is well tolerated. Because lipid solubility enhances tissue penetration, lipophilic ACE inhibitors (ramipril, quinapril, trandolapril, and fosinopril) may be most effective in the postrevascularization patient.

6. Beta-Blockers After Revascularization

Beta-blockers have become standard therapy following myocardial infarction in those patients with adequate left ventricular function and are used in low doses following CABG for their antiarrhythmic and anti-ischemic attributes. In diabetic patients, cardioselective beta-blockers are well tolerated and should be used in virtually all postrevascularization patients without contraindications. In the Bezafibrate Infarction Prevention (BIP) study, a substantial portion of the participants had not had prior myocardial infarction and were shown to benefit from beta blockade. Overall, beta blockade resulted in a 50% reduction in mortality in this study (10). Hypertension is prevalent in diabetic patients, and beta-blockers are first-line therapy. The importance of blood pressure control is amplified in the diabetic patients in whom a 10 mmHg reduction in blood pressure translates into an approximate 20% reduction in long-term cardiac events. Because of these potential benefits, beta-blockers are routine therapy for all patients participating in the important BARI 2D trial and should be standard therapy for all diabetic patients without contraindications following revascularization.

IV. SUMMARY AND FUTURE DIRECTIONS

It is clear that coronary atherosclerosis is prevalent, underrecognized, and a major cause of morbidity and mortality in the adult diabetic population. Preventive measures coupled with aggressive screening methods are indicated to both retard the development of CAD and to identify those patients who may benefit from life-prolonging and enhancing revascularization strategies. Although it is well established that revascularization is beneficial in the diabetic patient, it is also evident that the results obtained by revascularized diabetic patients are inferior to those achieved by nondiabetic patients. Recently reported studies have focused attention on certain aspects of revascularization that enhance outcomes (use of arterial grafts, stents, IIb/IIIa platelet receptor inhibitors), and provided some guidance regarding selection of PCI versus CABG. However, even with optimal recognition of revascularization candidates and use of optimal revascularization techniques, current studies suggest that progression of disease in diabetic patients plays a large role in limiting the long-term benefit of these procedures. Further treatment of the diabetic patient must address this issue of coronary disease progression, a topic explored in preceding chapters.

REFERENCES

1. Fein F, Scheur J. Heart disease in diabetes mellitus: theory and practice. In: Rifkin H, Porte D Jr, eds. New York: Elsevier, 1990:812–823.

2. Wingard DL, Barrett-Conner E. Heart disease in diabetes. In: National Diabetes DataGroup. Diabetes in America, 2nd ed. Washington, DC: Government Printing Office, 429–448;1995. (NIH publication number 95–1468.)

3. Kannel W. Lipids, diabetes, and coronary heart disease: insights from the Framingham Study. Am Heart J 1985;110:1100–1107.

4. Yusuf S, Zucker D, Peduzzi P, et al. Effect of coronary artery bypass graft surgery on survival: overview of 10-year results from randomized trials by the Coronary Artery Bypass Graft Surgery Trialists Collaboration [published erratum appears in Lancet 1994;344:1446]. Lancet 1994;344:563–570.

5. The BARI Investigators. Seven-year outcome in the Bypass Angioplasty Revascularization Investigation (BARI) by treatment and diabetic status. J Am Coll Cardiol 2000;35:1122–1129.

6. Zarich S, Waxman S, Freeman RT. Effect of anatomic nervous system dysfunction on the circadian pattern of myocardial ischemia in diabetes mellitus. J Am Coll Cardiol 1994;24:956–962.

7. Hammund T, Tanguay JF, Bourassa MG. Management of coronary artery disease: Therapeutic options in patients with diabetes. J Am Coll Cardiol 2000;36:355–365.

8. Stamler J, Vaccaroo, Neaton JD. Diabetes, other risk factors and 12-year cardiovascular mortality for men screened for the multiple risk factor intervention trial. Diabetes Care 1993;16:434–444.

9. Consensus Development Conference on the diagnosis of coronary heart disease in people with diabetes. Diabetes Care 1998;21:1551–1559.

10. Jonas M, Reicher-Reiss H, Boyko V. Usefulness of beta blocker therapy in patients with non-insulin dependent diabetes mellitus and coronary heart disease. Am J Cardiol 1996;77:1273–1277.

11. Pyorala K, Pedersen T, Kjekshus J for the 4S group. Cholesterol lowering with Simvastatin improves progress of diabetic patients with coronary heart disease. A Subgroup analysis of the Scandinavian Simvastatin Survival Study. Diabetes Care 1997; 20:68.

12. O'Keefe JH, Wetzel M, Moe RR, et al. Should an angiotensin-converting enzyme inhibitor be standard therapy for patients with atherosclerotic disease? J Am Coll Cardiol 2001;37:1–8.

13. Kang X, Berman D, Lewin HC. Incremental prognostic value of myocardial perfusion single photon emission computed tomography in patients with diabetes mellitus. Am Heart J 1999;138:1025–1032.

14. Giri S, Shaw LJ, Miller DD. STRESS SPECT myocardial perfusion imaging for predicting cardiac events in diabetic women. J Am Coll Cardiol 2000;35:338A.

15. Cerisier A, Brulport-Cerisier V, Estour B, et al. What strategy in totally asymptomatic diabetic patients with myocardial perfusion defect at stress SPECT imaging performed as a screening test? J Am Coll Cardiol 2001;37(suppl A):327A.

16. Gibbons RJ, Chatterjee K, Daley J, et al. ACC/AHA/ACP-ASIM Guidelines for the management of patients with chronic stable angina: a report of the American College of Cardiology/American Heart Association Task Force on Practice Guidelines (Committee on the Management of Patients With Chronic Stable Angina). J Am Coll Cardiol 1999;33:2092–2197.

17. Douglas JS Jr, Hurst JW. Limitations of symptoms in the recognition of coronary

atherosclerotic heart disease. In: Heart JW, ed. Update I The Heart. New York: McGraw Hill, 1979:3–12.

18. Braunwald E, Antman EM, Beasley JW, et al. ACC/AHA guidelines for the management of patients with unstable angina and non-ST-segment elevation myocardial infarction: a report of the American College of Cardiology/American Heart Association Task Force on Practice Guidelines (Committee on the Management of Patients With Unstable Angina). J Am Coll Cardiol 2000;36:970–1062.

19. FRragmin and Fast Revascularization during InStability in Coronary artery disease (FRISC II) Investigators). Long-term low-molecular-mass heparin in unstable angina coronary-artery disease: FRISC II prospective randomized multicenter study. Lancet 1999;354:701–715.

20. Scull GS, Martin JS, Weaver WD, et al. Early angiography versus conservative treatment in patients with non-ST elevation acute myocardial infarction. J Am Coll Cardiol 2000;35:895–902.

21. Kip KE, Faxon DP, Detre KM, et al. For the Investigators of the NHLBI PTCA Registry. Coronary angioplasty in diabetic patients: the National Heart, Lung, and Blood Institute Percutaneous Transluminal Coronary Angioplasty Registry. Circulation 1996;94:1818–25.

22. Weintraub WS, Stein B, Kosinski A, et al. Outcome of coronary bypass surgery versus coronary angioplasty in diabetic patients with multivessel coronary artery disease. J Am Coll Cardiol 1998;31:10–9.

23. Stein B, Weintraub WS, Gebhart S, et al. Short and long term outcome of diabetic patients undergoing coronary angioplasty. Circulation 1995;91:979–89.

24. Rozeman Y, Sapoznikov D, Gotsman MS. Restenosis and progression of coronary disease after balloon angioplasty in patients with diabetes mellitus. Clin Cardiol 2000;23:890–894.

25. Barsness GW, Peterson ED, Ohman EM, et al. Relationship between diabetes mellitus and long-term survival after coronary bypass and angioplasty. Circulation 1997;96:2551–2556.

26. Barsness GW, Hardison RM, Detre KM, et al. Lesion progression and restenosis in PTCA-treated diabetic and non-diabetic patients with multivessel disease. Circulation 2000;102(suppl II):479.

27. Kurbaan AS, Bowker TJ, Llsley CD, et al. Is the poorer outcome post revascularization in diabetics related to completeness of revascularization? Circulation 2000; 102(suppl II):256.

28. King SB III, Kosinski AS, Guyton RA, et al. Eight-year mortality in the Emory Angioplasty Versus Surgery Trial (EAST). J Am Coll Cardiol 2000;35:1116–1121.

29. Ferguson JJ. NHLBI BARI clinical alert on diabetics treated with angioplasty. Circulation 1995;92:3371.

30. Peterson ED, Anstrom KJ, McGuire DK. The influence of the BARI diabetic treatment alert on revascularization selection pattern: The NCN results. J Am Coll Cardiol 2000;35(suppl A):544A.

31. Gibbons RJ, Miller DD, Liu P, et al. Similarity of ventricular function in patients alive 5 years after randomization to surgery or angioplasty in the BARI trial. Circulation 2001;103:1076–1082.

32. Gum PA, O'Keefe JH Jr, Borkon AM, et al. Bypass surgery versus coronary angio-

plasty for revascularization and treated diabetic patients. Circulation 1997;96(suppl II):7–10.

33. Niles NW, McGrath PD, Malenka D, et al. Survival of patients with diabetes and multivessel coronary artery disease after surgical or percutaneous coronary revascularization: results of a large regional prospective study. J Am Coll Cardiol 2001;37: 1008–1015.

34. Detre KM, Guo P, Holubkov R, et al. Coronary revascularization in diabetic patients. A comparison of the randomized and observational components of the Bypass Angioplasty Revascularization Investigation (BARI). Circulation 1999;99:633–640.

35. Brooks MM, Jones RH, Bach RG, et al. Predictors of mortality and mortality from cardiac causes in the Bypass Angioplasty Revascularization Investigation (BARI) randomized trial and registry. Circulation 2000;101:2682–2689.

36. Szczech L, Crowley EM, Holmes DR. Chronic renal insufficiency (CRI) in the Bypass Angioplasty Revascularization Investigation (BARI). Circulation 2000; 102(suppl II):555.

37. Mehran R, Dangas G, Gruberg L, et al. The detrimental impact of chronic renal insufficiency and diabetes mellitus on late prognosis after percutaneous coronary interventions. J Am Coll Cardiol 2000;35(suppl A):73A.

38. Marso SP, Ellis SG, Tuzcu M, et al. The importance of proteinuria as a determinant of mortality following percutaneous coronary revascularization in diabetics. J Am Coll Cardiol 1999;33:1269–1277.

39. Lewis EJ, Hunsicher LG, Gain RP, et al. The effect of angiotensin-converting-enzyme inhibition on diabetic nephropathy. The Collaborative Study Group (see comments) [published erratum appears in N Engl J Med 1993;330(2):152]. N Engl J Med 1993;329:1456–1462.

40. Laffel LM, McGill JB, Gans DJ. The beneficial effect of angiotensin-converting enzyme inhibition with captopril on diabetic nephropathy in normotensive IDDM patients with microalbuminuria. North American Microalbuminuria Study Group. Am J Med 1995;99:497–504.

41. Savage MP, Fischman DL, Slota P, et al. Coronary intervention in diabetic patients: improved outcome following stent implantation versus balloon angioplasty. J Am Coll Cardiol 1997;29(suppl A):188A.

42. Van Belle E, Bauters C, Hubert E, et al. Restenosis rates in diabetic patients. A comparison of coronary stenting and balloon angioplasty in native coronary vessels. Circulation 1997;96:1454–1460.

43. Blankenbaker R, Ghazzal Z, Weintraub WS, et al. Clinical outcome of diabetic patients after Palmaz-Schatz stent implantation. J Am Coll Cardiol 1998;31(suppl A): 415A.

44. Dangas G, Kobayashi Y, D'Agate DJ, et al. Long-term results after multivessel stenting in diabetic patients. Circulation 2000;102(suppl II):731.

45. Deutsch E, Martin JL, Fischman DL, et al. The late benefit of coronary stenting in small vessels is reduced in diabetic patients. J Am Coll Cardiol 1998;31(suppl A): 275A.

46. Marso SP, Ellis SG, Bhatt DL. The stenting in diabetes debate: insight from the large GUSTO II experience with extended follow-up. Circulation 1998;98(suppl I): 78.

47. Kornowski R, Mintz GS, Kent KM, et al. Increased restenosis in diabetes mellitus after coronary interventions is due to exaggerated intimal hyperplasia. A serial intravascular study. Circulation 1997;95:1366–1369.
48. Sobel BE. Acceleration of restenosis by diabetes: pathogenetic implications. Circulation 2001;103:1185–1187.
49. Laskey W, Vlachos H, Jacobs A, et al. Outcomes in diabetic patients undergoing contemporary percutaneous catheter intervention: a report from the NHLBI Dynamic Registry. In Press.
50. Van Belle E, Ketelers R, Bauters C, et al. Patency of percutaneous transluminal coronary angioplasty sites at 6-month angiographic follow-up: a key determinant of survival in diabetics after coronary balloon angioplasty. Circulation 2001;103:1218–1224.
51. Lincoff AM, Califf RM, Moliterno DJ, et al For the evaluation of platelet IIb/IIIa inhibition in stenting investigators. Complementary clinical benefit of coronary artery stenting and blockade of platelet glycoprotein IIb/IIIa receptors. N Engl J Med 1999;341:319–327.
52. Bhatt DL, Marso SP, Lincoff M, et al. Abciximab reduces mortality in diabetics following percutaneous coronary intervention. J Am Coll Cardiol 2000;35:922–928.
53. Cho L, Marso SP, Bhatt DL, Topol EJ. Striking reduction of mortality and target vessel revascularization with stent-abciximab in diabetic women. J Am Coll Cardiol 2000;35(suppl A):35A.
54. Laskey WK, Heuser RR, Suntharalingam M, et al. Effects of $^{90}Sr/^{90}Y$ beta radiation on diabetic patients with in-stent restenosis. Circulation 2000;102(suppl II):668.
55. Serruys PW, Costa MA, Betriu A, et al. The influence of diabetes mellitus on clinical outcome following multivessel stenting or CABG in the ARTS Trial. Circulation 1999;100(suppl I):364.
56. Lindeboom WK, Van Hout BA, Backx B, et al. Comparison of effectiveness and cost effectiveness of CABG versus percutaneous intervention in diabetic patients with multivessel disease. Circulation 2000;102(suppl II):555.
57. Kuntz RE. Importance of considering atherosclerosis progression when choosing a coronary revascularization strategy. The diabetes-percutaneous transluminal coronary angioplasty dilemma. Circulation 1999;99:847–851.
58. Schomig A, Neumann FJ, Kastrati A, et al. A randomized comparison of antiplatelet and anticoagulant therapy after the placement of coronary artery stents. N Eng J Med 1996;334:1084–1089.
59. Leon MB, Baim DS, Popma JJ, et al. A clinical trial comparing three antithrombotic-drug regimens for coronary artery stenting: Stent Anticoagulation Restenosis Study Investigators. N Engl J Med 1998:339:1665–1671.
60. Steinhubl SR, Ellis SG, Wolski K, et al. Ticlopidine pretreatment before coronary stenting is associated with sustained decrease in adverse cardiac events. Data from the Evaluation of Platelet IIb/IIIa Inhibitor for Stenting (EPISTENT) Trial. Circulation 2001;103:1403–1409.
61. Muller C, Buttner HG, Peterson J, et al. A randomized comparison of clopidogrel and aspirin versus ticlopidine and aspirin after the placement of coronary artery stents. Circulation 2000;101:590–593.
62. Bhatt DL, Bertrand ME, Berger PB, et al. Reduction in major adverse cardiac events,

including mortality, after stenting using clopidogrel instead of ticlopidine. Circulation 2000;102(suppl II):565.

63. Bhatt DL, Chew DP, Hirsch AT, et al. Superiority of clopidogrel versus aspirin in patients with prior cardiac surgery. Circulation 2001;103:363–368.
64. UK Perspective Diabetes Study (UKPDS) Group. Intensive blood-glucose control with sulphonylureas or insulin compared with conventional treatment and risk of complications in patients with type 2 diabetes (UKPDS). Lancet 1998;352:837–853.
65. Al-Rashdan IR, Rankin JM, Elliott TG, et al. Glycemic control and major adverse cardiac events after PTCA in patients with diabetes mellitus. J Am Coll Cardiol 1999;33:97A.
66. Yumoto K, Kato K, Doi H, et al. The influence of diabetic control on restenosis after coronary stenting. Circulation 2000;102(suppl II):730.
67. Garratt KN, Brady PA, Hassinger NL, et al. Sulfonylurea drugs increase early mortality in patients with diabetes mellitus after direct angioplasty for acute myocardial infarction. J Am Coll Cardiol 1999;33:119–124.
68. Brady PA, Terzic A. The sulfonylurea controversy: more questions from the heart. J Am Coll Cardiol 1998;31:950–956.
69. Takagi T, Akasaka T, Kaji S, et al. Increased intimal hyperplasia after coronary stent implantation in patients with hyperinsulinemia: a serial intravascular ultrasound study. Circulation 1998;98(suppl 1):229.
70. Takagi T, Yoshida K, Akasaka T, et al. Triglitazone reduces intimal hyperplasia after coronary stent implantation in patients with type 2 diabetes mellitus: a serial intravascular ultrasound study. J Am Coll Cardiol 1999;33(suppl A):33A.
71. Weintraub WS, Boccuzzi SJ, Klein JL. Lack of effect of Lovastatin on Restenoses after coronary angioplasty N Engl J Med 1994;331:1331–1336.
72. Treasure CB, Klein JL, Weintraub WS. Beneficial effects of cholesterol-lowering therapy on the coronary endothelium in patients with coronary artery disease. N Engl J Med 1995;332:481–487.
73. Haffner SM. The Scandinavian Simvastatin Survival Study (4S) subgroup analysis of diabetic subjects: implications for the prevention of coronary heart disease. Diabetes Care 1997;20:469–471.
74. Goldberg RB, Mellies MJ, Sacks FM. Cardiovascular events and their reduction with pravastatin in diabetic and glucose-intolerant myocardial infarction survivors with average cholesterol levels. Circulation 1998;98:2513–2519.
75. The Long-Term Intervention With Pravastatin In Ischemic Disease (LIPID) Study Group. Prevention of cardiovascular events and death with pravastatin in patients with coronary heart disease and a broad range of initial cholesterol levels. N Engl J Med 1998;339:1349–1357.
76. Elsner M, Walter DH, Auch-Schwelk, et al. Statin therapy in diabetic patients is associated with reduced clinical event rates and attenuated neointimal proliferation after coronary stenting. Circulation 1999;100(suppl I):365.
77. Campeau L, Enjalbert M, Lesperance J, et al. The relation of risk factors to the development of atherosclerosis in saphenous vein bypass grafts and the progression of disease in the native circulation: a study 10 years after aortocoronary bypass surgery. N Engl J Med 1984;311:1329–1332.

78. Fox M, Gruchow H, Barboriak J, et al. Risk factors among patients undergoing repeat aorta-coronary bypass procedures. J Thorac Cardiovasc Surg 1987;93:56.

79. Van Brussel B, Plokker T, Ernst S, et al. Venous coronary bypass surgery: a 15-year follow-up study. Circulation 1993;88:87–92.

80. Neitzel G, Barboriak J, Pintar K, et al. Atherosclerosis in aortocoronary bypass grafts. Morphologic study and risk factor analysis 6 to 12 years after surgery. Arteriosclerosis 1986;6:594–600.

81. Hoff H, Beck G, Skibinski C, et al. Serum Lp(a) level as a predictor of vein graft stenosis after coronary artery bypass surgery in patients. Circulation 1988;77:1238–1244.

82. Solymoss B, Marcil M, Wesolowska E, et al. Risk factors of venous aortocoronary bypass graft disease noted at late symptom-directed angiographic study. Can J Cardiol 1993;9:80–83.

83. Campeau L, Enjalbert M, Lesperance J, et al. Atherosclerosis and late closure of aortocoronary saphenous vein grafts: sequential angiographic studies at 2 weeks, 1 year, 5 to 7 years, and 10 to 12 years after surgery. Circulation 1983;68(suppl II):61.

84. The Post Coronary Artery Bypass Graft Trial Investigators. The effect of aggressive lowering of low-density lipoprotein and low-dose anticoagulation on obstructive changes in saphenous-vein coronary-artery bypass grafts. N Engl J Med 1997;336:153–162.

85. Domanski MJ, Borkowf CB, Campeau L, et al. Prognostic factors for atherosclerosis progression in saphenous vein grafts: The Postcoronary Artery Bypass Graft (Post-CABG) Trial. J Am Coll Cardiol 2000;36:1877–1883.

86. The Heart Outcomes Prevention Evaluation (HOPE) Study Investigators. Effects of an angiotensin-converting enzyme inhibitor, ramipril, on cardiovascular events in high-risk patients. N Engl J Med 2000;342:145–153.

87. Hseuh WA. In Diabetes, Treat Hidden Heart Disease. Cleveland Clin J Med 2000;67:807–813.

88. Kjoler-hansen L, Steffensen R, Grande P. The Angiotensin-coverting enzyme inhibition Post Revascularization study. (APRES). J Am Coll Cardiol 2000;35:881–888.

89. Oosterga M, Voors A, Veeger N, et al. QUO VADIS (effects of QUinapril On Vascular ACE and Determinants of Ischemia). Circulation 1998;98(suppl I):636.

90. Lonn EV, Yusuf S, Dzavik V, et al. Effects of ramipril and vitamin E on atherosclerosis. The study to evaluate carotid ultrasound changes in patients treated with ramipril and vitamin E (SECURE). Circulation 2001;103:919–925.

15

Nonpharmacological Reduction of Cardiovascular Risk

Virginia Peragallo-Dittko
Winthrop-University Hospital, Mineola, New York

Despite the exciting developments in the treatment of diabetes and the change in focus toward aggressive management of blood glucose and lipids, one aspect of management has not changed: the patient still provides 95% of the treatment. Therefore, he or she needs to learn the appropriate skills. The patient decides whether to take the prescribed medications, what foods to eat, and whether to exercise. The care of the diabetic patient requires the expertise of many disciplines and a multidisciplinary team approach remains central to the care of the diabetic patient. The team of health professionals is broad and includes the primary care physician, diabetes nurse specialist, dietitian, and other medical professionals including specialists in endocrinology, cardiology, ophthalmology, nephrology, and neurology.

Diabetes education in the United States has benefited from many significant developments and has served as a model for other areas of patient education. One significant event was the development of the National Standards for Diabetes Patient Education Programs in 1983. The National Standards were developed by experts in diabetes care and education in response to concerns that the quantity and quality of diabetes education varied considerably throughout the U.S. The application of uniformed standards has increased the quality, availability, effectiveness, accessibility, and reimbursement of diabetes education. In 1986, the American Diabetes Association implemented a process to accredit programs that meet the National Standards. With the increase in knowledge about diabetes care and education, the National Standards have been continually revised. The National Standards for Diabetes Self-Management Education provide the structure for the process of diabetes patient education.

In the practice of diabetes education, complex subjects are broken down into simple concepts that can be tailored to the individual and made culturally relevant. The advances in the understanding of diabetes and the proliferation of pharmacological treatment options have challenged diabetes educators to create teaching tools that simplify the content, focus the teaching session on what the patient needs to know, and build a framework for linking their desired change in behavior with the pathophysiology of the disease. The health professional provides the information and support; the patient makes the choices.

The insulin resistance syndrome is the central tenet of the curriculum for patients with type 2 diabetes. The insulin resistance syndrome comprises the clinical manifestations of hyperglycemia, glucose intolerance, central obesity, hypertension, and polycystic ovary syndrome and the biochemical abnormalities of hyperinsulinemia, dyslipidemia clustered as elevated triglycerides, low high-density-lipoprotein cholesterol (HDL-C), small, dense low-density-lipoprotein (LDL) particles, and altered fibrinolysis characterized by increased plasminogen activator inhibitor-1 (PAI-1). In patient terms, high blood glucose levels of diabetes are just the tip of the iceberg; elevated lipid levels and high blood pressure need to be treated as well. In other words, treatment of diabetes involves more than just blood glucose control. Together with a discussion of a patient's lab values, the iceberg could be used to explain why three different types of diabetes medications, two high blood pressure medications, and a lipid-lowering agent are needed to treat insulin resistance syndrome. Similarly, when an obese patient with elevated lipids and hemoglobin A1c proudly tells you that he ''hasn't eaten anything sweet in years,'' the need for consultation with a dietitian becomes apparent. A dietitian would take into account blood glucose, lipids, and obesity when working with this patient to create a meal plan filled with choices. Although the patient's effort to avoid sweets was important, especially in light of his elevated triglyceride level and obesity, there is more to know about treating diabetes through meal planning than just avoiding sweets.

I. NUTRITIONAL REDUCTION OF CARDIOVASCULAR RISK

In 1994, the Nutrition Recommendations for the treatment of diabetes were revised to reflect the research on glycemic indexing of foods and the impact of carbohydrate on blood glucose. Many existing beliefs were refuted and revised. For example, the long-held idea that people with diabetes should not eat sweets was refuted by research findings (1,2). Instead of focusing on the type of carbohydrate (CHO) ingested (i.e., simple or complex carbohydrates) the patient is taught to consider the portion size or amount of carbohydrate eaten at a meal. This translates into a meal plan that is more versatile and adaptable to an individual's usual habits. Under the former recommendations, a patient may have been prescribed the following carbohydrate servings for a dinner meal: 1 cup pasta (2 starch/bread servings, 30 g CHO), 1 small apple (1 fruit serving, 15 g CHO), and 8 oz. skim milk (1 milk serving, 12 g CHO). According to the revised recommendations, the patient could choose the foods listed above or choose 2 cups of pasta (60 g CHO). If the patient's weight and blood lipids were within range, the patient could choose 1½ cups of pasta and ½ cup of sweetened ice cream! By focusing on the total carbohydrates at a meal, the patient has more options and the meal plan can be adapted to his needs.

There are three key messages that are often lost in the translation of the revised recommendations. The first is that the portions of carbohydrate are critical. This is not an all-you-can-eat meal plan. Patients need to learn the portion of food equal to a carbohydrate choice. The portion of ice cream is one-half cup not one-half gallon. The second is that small portions of sweetened foods can be substituted for a carbohydrate choice only if the patient's blood lipids and weight are at or near goal. The third is that to truly evaluate a recommended meal plan, the patient needs to monitor pre- and postprandial blood glucose. Pasta with 4 oz. ice cream for dessert may meet the textbook guidelines but dramatically raise the patient's postprandial blood glucose.

If the term ADA diet has been retired, then a preprinted, 1800 calorie, diabetic diet is a dinosaur. Medical nutrition therapy for diabetes has evolved from the structure and formulas of the exchange system for meal planning with a specified macronutrient composition (i.e., 50% carbohydrate, 20% protein, 30% fat) to individualized meal plans based on the patient's lab values, usual eating habits, cultural preferences, and realistic weight goals. To meet the patient's nutritional needs, consultation with a dietitian is essential. For example, a hyperglycemic, insulin-requiring patient of reasonable body weight with lipid levels within range may follow a traditional Chinese diet that includes at least 2 cups of rice (90 g CHO) at every meal. In the past, the patient's cultural habits would have been ignored and the patient would have been counseled to limit the rice to 1 cup (45 g CHO) or substitute another source of carbohydrate. The patient, however, would have continued to eat the larger portions. Since the revision of the nutrition recommendations, the dietitian would counsel the patient to measure the portions of rice to assure consistency and would suggest an increase in the insulin dose to reduce the postprandial rise in blood glucose. This meal plan is limited, yet reasonable and culturally relevant.

The goals of medical nutrition therapy for diabetes are straightforward:

1. To restore and maintain as near-normal blood glucose levels as feasible by balancing food with insulin and activity levels.

Table 1 Category of Risk Based on Lipoprotein Levels in Adults with Diabetes

Risk	LDL cholesterol	HDL cholesterol*	Triglyceride
High	≥130	<35	≥400
Borderline	100–129	35–45	200–399
Low	<100	>45	<200

Data are given in milligrams per deciliter. *For women, the HDL cholesterol values should be increased by 10 mg/dL.
Source: Ref. 18.

2. To provide assistance in attaining optimal lipid levels (recommended values are shown in Table 1).
3. To provide appropriate calories for maintaining or attaining reasonable weights for adults, normal growth and development rates for children and adolescents, and adequate calories and nutrients during catabolic stress, pregnancy, and lactation.
4. To prevent and treat the acute and chronic complications of diabetes.
5. To improve overall health through optimal nutrition.

The nutrition-related strategies for achieving blood glucose goals and reducing cardiovascular risk are more complex and are based on the patient's needs. As research continues to clarify why weight loss is difficult for many persons (3,4), the emphasis for those with type 2 diabetes has shifted from weight loss to achieving and maintaining blood glucose and lipid goals. Moderate caloric restriction (250 to 500 calories per day less than the average daily intake as calculated from the diet history) and a nutritionally adequate meal plan accompanied by an increase in physical activity will produce a gradual and sustained weight loss. It is important to consider that a hypocaloric diet (independent of weight loss) is associated with increased sensitivity to insulin and that significant improvements in blood glucose levels generally occur before much weight is actually lost (5,6). Thus the patient who eats 3500 calories per day may be prescribed a 2500-calorie meal plan that includes reasonable portions of food instead of a 1500-calorie meal plan that is promptly abandoned.

Moderate weight loss of 10 to 20 lb. (5 to 10 kg), regardless of starting weight, has been shown to reduce hyperglycemia, dyslipidemia, and hypertension (3,7). However, if a patient has not been able to lose weight within 6 months and blood glucose levels have not improved, oral diabetes agents and/or insulin should be prescribed (8). In the past, patients would remain with elevated blood glucose levels for years until they achieved weight loss. In the current age of "treat to target," if a patient cannot achieve weight loss within 6 months, then pharmacological therapy is indicated. Even though weight loss is the preferred treatment strategy, medications can be discontinued but microvascular and macrovascular disease cannot be reversed.

The recommended fat content of the diabetes meal plan is also based on an individual patients's lipid levels, blood glucose levels, and weight goal. In general, it is recommended that saturated fat intake comprise less than 10% of daily calories, and dietary cholesterol intake be less than 300 mg or less daily (9). Patients who are at a reasonable body weight and have normal lipid levels are encouraged to follow the recommendations of the National Cholesterol Education Program (NCEP) in order to reduce their risk for cardiovascular disease. In individuals over age 2, limiting fat intake to less than 30% of daily calories, with saturated fat restricted to less than 10% of total calories, polyunsaturated fat less than 10% of daily calories, and monounsaturated fat in the range of 10% to 15% of daily calories is recommended. For patients with type 2 diabetes and elevated LDL cholesterol, further restriction of saturated fat to 7% of total calories and dietary cholesterol to less than 200 mg per day is recommended.

The amount of fat that a patient chooses to consume is often linked not only to ethnic foods but regional American foods as well. In some parts of the country, a typical breakfast includes sausage, eggs, biscuits, and gravy. Although the dietitian can offer breakfast choices lower in fat, some patients are not willing to change. For them, the goal may be to limit the high-fat breakfast to three times per week instead of every day. Patients with diabetes who have not had the benefit of counseling by a dietitian commonly limit their carbohydrate intake in a fruitless effort to lower their blood glucose levels and are left with a diet high in fat from animal protein, dairy-fat-containing foods, and oils.

People with diabetes voice the common frustration that there is nothing left to eat since carbohydrate, fat, sodium, and alcohol are restricted. A moderate sodium intake (no more than 3000 mg/day) is recommended. For those with hypertension, sodium intake is limited to less than 2400 mg/day. The decision to include moderate amounts of alcohol in the meal plan is based on the patient's triglyceride levels, weight goals, usual habits, culture, and other medications. Based on an assessment of a patient's laboratory values, usual eating habits, cultural preferences, and weight goals, a meal plan can be created that includes a variety of foods in reasonable portions.

There is much more that a patient with diabetes needs to know about what to eat. Table 2 lists both the skills that a patient needs to make management decisions and to solve problems. Because not every patient has the ability or the interest to learn new skills, some patients may be better served with focused educational sessions or lists of acceptable foods.

Table 2 Management and Problem-Solving Skills

Management skills (information required to make decisions to achieve management
  goals)
• Food sources of carbohydrate, protein, fat
• How to use nutrition facts on food labels
• Meal planning and insulin adjustments for
    illness
    delay or change in meal times
    drinking alcoholic beverages
    eating sugar-containing foods
    exercise
    travel
    competitive athletics
    holidays
• Treatment and prevention of hypoglycemia
• Nutritional management during short-term illness
• How to use blood glucose monitoring for problem solving
• Behavior change strategies
• Working rotating shifts, if needed

Improvement of lifestyle (problem-solving skills)
• Eating away from home
• Brown bag lunches
• Special occasions (birthdays, holidays, etc.)
• Grocery shopping
• Recipe modifications, menu ideas, cookbooks
• Vegetarian food choices
• Ethnic foods
• Use of convenience food
• Canning and freezing
• How to fit foods with fat replacers and sugar substitutes into the meal plan

Source: Ref. 19. (Reprinted with permission from the American Association of Diabetes Educators.)

II. BLOOD GLUCOSE MONITORING: AN UNDERUTILIZED MANAGEMENT TOOL

Self-monitoring of blood glucose (SMBG) has demonstrable clinical and educational utility for all patients with diabetes. The clinical usefulness of SMBG data
has made SMBG a standard of care. Dose titration is dependent on the data the
patient provides. Without such data, dose increases are made blindly, leaving
the patient prone to hypoglycemia. Documentation of blood glucose trends often
reveals asymptomatic hypoglycemia, and the data generated by SMBG have been

found to be clinically useful in the management of intercurrent illness in a population at risk for acute metabolic decompensation.

Many patients are trained in the mechanics of using a meter but not in how to use the data. With education, the critical uses of SMBG data by patients include enabling them to identify and treat hypoglycemia; make decisions concerning food choices or medication adjustments when exercising; determine the glycemic effect of foods and portion sizes; and manage intercurrent illness.

Diabetes educators use SMBG as the tool linking the principles of self-management with daily decision making. Learning about food products or portions is facilitated by tying the food to the postprandial blood glucose result. For example, a patient with a fasting blood glucose of 127 mg/dL chooses a bagel (60 g CHO) and 8 oz. orange juice (30 g CHO) for breakfast. But 2 h later his blood glucose is 398 mg/dL. However, a postprandial blood glucose of 159 mg/dL is measured after a breakfast consisting of an English muffin (30 g CHO) and 8 oz. Tropicana Twister Light® grapefruit juice (10 g CHO). Counseling about the need to lower the carbohydrate content of breakfast will be more effective when the patient sees the effect of his food choices on his blood glucose.

Asymptomatic patients with type 2 diabetes often see no need to change their eating habits until they measure and record elevated blood glucose readings. For patients who counter, "but I feel fine," SMBG can open the door to their education. SMBG data are used by educators to identify and influence psychosocial adaptations. It can influence self-efficacy as patients report increased confidence in their problem-solving abilities (10).

With the proliferation of blood glucose monitoring products and lancing devices, the diabetes educator often serves as a product expert linking the best product to the patient's needs. Meters and strips are designed to use nanoliters of blood and the newest products use the forearm as a site for sampling blood. The complaint of sore fingers can be minimized by helping the patient choose a realistic monitoring schedule that provides essential data and minimizes the number of skin punctures.

Most people with diabetes would benefit from more frequent blood glucose monitoring. Surprisingly, the discomfort of skin punctures is only one of the barriers to more frequent monitoring. The most common barriers involve the psychosocial issues associated with the results, such as the frustration associated with elevated readings, the need to make a decision when faced with a number, and the technological reminder of the reality of diabetes. Although many patients eagerly await FDA approval of a noninvasive glucose monitoring device that will provide ongoing, easily obtainable and accessible information about glucose levels, one can only speculate about the impact of noninvasive monitoring on blood glucose control. For health professionals, it will be challenging to match treatment modalities with automatic, nonepisodic blood glucose readings.

The Gluco Watch Biographer is a transdermal, noninvasive glucose monitoring prescription device approved by the FDA for adults aged 18 years and older. It is not meant to replace a blood glucose meter but is used in conjunction with it to provide more information about glucose levels. The Gluco Watch Biographer employs reverse iontophoresis and uses an extremely low electric current to pull glucose through the skin. The glucose is then collected and converted into an electric signal that is converted into a glucose reading. Worn like a watch, it measures and displays glucose levels as often as every 20 min for up to 12 h. An alarm sounds if readings are too high, too low, or declining rapidly. This feature is especially beneficial for those patients with hypoglycemic unawareness.

The data provided by self-monitoring of blood glucose are combined with the hemoglobin Alc and fructosamine results. Meters are available for self-monitoring of fructosamine levels and serum beta-hydroxybuterate levels. These products may be prescribed for those patients who are involved in rapid dose titration or who are ketosis prone. Both the necessary tools and self-management education are available for aggressive management of diabetes. Dose titration for the symptomatic, hyperglycemic patient is achieved long before the 3-month follow-up visit.

The hemoglobin Alc (HbAlc) remains the standard for monitoring blood glucose control. The American Diabetes Association Standards of Medical Care promote a goal of 7% or less (normal range 4.0 to 6.0%) for the hemoglobin Alc based on the results of randomized, controlled, clinical trials—most notably the Diabetes Control and Complications Trial (DCCT). Results in this trial demonstrated conclusively that the risk of development or progression of retinopathy, nephropathy, and neuropathy is reduced 50 to 75% by intensive treatment regimens when compared with conventional treatment regimens in patients with type 1 diabetes. These benefits were observed with an average HbAlc of 7.2% in intensively treated groups of patients. The reduction in risk of these complications correlated continuously with the reduction in HbAlc produced by intensive treatment. This relationship implies that near-normalization of glycemic levels may prevent complications. The largest and longest study of patients with type 2 diabetes, the United Kingdom Prospective Diabetes Study (UKPDS), conclusively demonstrated that improved blood glucose control in these patients reduces the risk of developing retinopathy and nephropathy. Epidemiological analysis of the UKPDS data showed a continuous relationship between the risk of microvascular complications and glycemia and also showed that aggressive control of blood pressure significantly reduced strokes, diabetes-related deaths, heart failure, and visual loss. For every percentage point decrease in HbAlc (e.g., 9% to 8%) there was a 35% reduction in the risk of microvascular complications.

The nondiabetic reference range for the HbAlc in the DCCT was 4.0 to 6.0%. Because different assays can give varying glycated hemoglobin values, one cannot always compare results from different laboratories. It is especially frustrating when the laboratory reports the reference range as less than 7% based on the American Diabetes Association management goals but their actual reference range of 5.0 to 8.0% is not listed on the printout. A result of 7.8% from one laboratory would be considered elevated, and the same result from another laboratory would be considered within range. It is helpful to be aware of the potential differences among laboratories as medications have been changed and doses adjusted based on results compared from two laboratories using different assays.

When discrepancies arise between the patient's reported blood glucose readings and the HbAlc, a fructosamine level may be ordered since it reflects the most recent 3 weeks of blood glucose control. Sometimes the patient's reported readings and the HbAlc do not match because the patient's blood glucose monitoring technique was inaccurate or the test strips were stored improperly. The most common reason why the results do not match is because the patient is not monitoring postprandial blood glucose. Most patients check their fasting blood glucose only. Because they are not monitoring after meals, they will not record their highest readings and will not be able to see the effects of their food choices on their blood glucose levels. The dosages of many medications should be titrated based on postprandial readings, as there is evidence that any variety of treatment modalites targeting postprandial blood glucose will lower HbAlc (11).

IV. LIFESTYLE MODIFICATIONS: SMOKING CESSATION AND EXERCISE

Much of the work documenting the impact of smoking on health does not discuss results on subsets of subjects with diabetes, suggesting that the identified risks are at least equivalent to those found in the general population. Other studies of individuals with diabetes consistently report a heightened risk of morbidity and premature death associated with the development of macrovascular complications among smokers. Although smokers have repeatedly heard of the pulmonary effects of smoking, the cardiovascular burden of diabetes, especially in combination with smoking, has not been communicated effectively to either people with diabetes or health care providers.

Despite demonstrated efficacy of smoking cessation counseling, only about 50% of patients with diabetes are advised to quit smoking by their health care providers (12). Treatment characteristics that have been identified as critical to achieving cessation include counseling by multiple health care providers, use of individual or group counseling strategies, use of interventions including problem-solving skills or skills training with social support, and use of pharmacotherapy such as nicotine replacement therapy. Recommendations regarding smoking and diabetes are listed in Table 3.

Exercise is generally regarded as one of the pivotal diabetes management tools. Results in several long-term studies (13–15) demonstrate sustained im-

Table 3 Recommendations Regarding Diabetes and Smoking

Assessment of smoking status and history

Systematic documentation of a history of tobacco use must be obtained from all adolescent and adult individuals with diabetes.

Counseling on smoking prevention and cessation

All health care providers should advise individuals with diabetes not to initiate smoking. This advice should be consistently repeated to prevent smoking and other tobacco use among children and adolescents with diabetes under age 21.

Among smokers, cessation counseling must be completed as a routine component of diabetes care.

Every smoker should be urged to quit in a clear, strong, and personalized manner that describes the added risks of smoking for people with diabetes.

Every diabetic smoker should be asked if he or she is willing to quit at this time.

If no, initiate brief and motivational discussion regarding the need to stop using tobacco, the risks of continued use, and encouragement to quit as well as support when ready.

If yes, assess preference for and initiate either minimal, brief, or intensive cessation counseling and offer pharmacological supplements as appropriate.

Effective systems for delivery of smoking cessation

Training of all diabetes health care providers in the Agency for Health Care Policy and Research Guidelines regarding smoking should be implemented.

Follow-up procedures designed to assess and promote quitting status must be arranged for all diabetic smokers.

Source: Ref. 12.

provement in glucose control while a regular exercise program is maintained. Because of the increased incidence of cardiovascular disease in patients with diabetes, the role of exercise in reducing modifiable risks has primary importance. The potential benefits of exercise for people with diabetes include:

1. Improved strength and physical work capacity.
2. Increase in high-density lipoproteins (HDL), particularly in the presence of weight loss.
3. Reduction in plasma cholesterol, triglycerides, and low-density lipoproteins (LDL).
4. Increased insulin sensitivity.
5. Reduced hyperinsulinemia.
6. Enhanced fibrinolysis.
7. Favorable changes in body composition (i.e., reduction of body fat and weight and increase in muscle mass).
8. Improved control of hypertension with pharmacological agents.

9. Improved quality of life and self-esteem, and reduced psychological stress.

The primary side effect of acute exercise is hypoglycemia. Patients require specific guidelines either to increase carbohydrate consumption or to decrease medication based on the intensity of exercise and relationship of the planned exercise to the timing of the next meal. For those attempting to lose weight, medication adjustment is chosen over adding extra calories. For some, exercise after a meal without medication adjustment is preferred. Postexercise, late-onset hypoglycemia (PEL) occurs several hours following an exercise session and is a significant concern for those treated with insulin or insulin secretagogues. Postexercise late-onset hypoglycemia can be the result of acutely increased insulin mobilization and sensitivity, increased glucose utilization, replenishment of glycogen stores, and defective counterregulatory mechanisms. Patients need to learn how to prevent PEL by remembering to supplement carbohydrates during the postexercise phase, to reduce the dose of insulin that peaks during the postexercise phase, and to monitor blood glucose frequently.

The American Diabetes Association recommends a graded exercise test for patients at high risk for underlying cardiovascular disease based on the following criteria (16): age >35 years; type 2 diabetes of >10 years duration; type 1 diabetes of >15 years duration; presence of any additional risk factor for coronary artery disease; presence of microvascular disease (including microalbuminuria); peripheral vascular disease; and autonomic neuropathy.

Rhythmic exercises with the use of the lower extremities, such as walking or cycling, are safely recommended. Patients with established cardiovascular disease usually require supervision in a monitored cardiac rehabilitation program. Unfortunately, little is known about how to increase or maintain participation in exercise programs. Relapse is common and all health care providers play a role in supporting patients in their efforts at exercise.

V. QUALITY OF LIFE AND OBSTACLES TO CARE

The delivery of diabetes care and education has undergone a paradigm shift from giving advice and blaming the patient for failure to providing patients with the choice of aggressive, individualized treatment and an education plan tailored to their needs. This shift has melded health care providers and patients as partners in managing a devastating disease. The demands for daily self-management of diabetes are so formidable that each component of the diabetes education curriculum includes discussion of the psychosocial needs of the patient. The embarrassment of hypoglycemia and resultant fear, the social aspects of eating and dealing with well-meaning family members who comment on food choices, the sense of failure associated with elevated blood glucose readings despite a sincere effort, and the frustrations of needing medication when self-image associates pill taking with the sick role are a few examples of the psychosocial complexities. Effective diabetes education begins with listening to the patient and his perception of life with diabetes.

Health care professionals can identify with patients who cannot manage to follow every single diabetes management recommendation because we cannot follow them either. Regardless of type of management, such as fee-for-service or managed care, chart reviews suggest that only about 50% of patients are asked to have their HbA1c measured even once a year, despite a recommendation for screening every 6 months. An even smaller proportion of patients are being screened on an annual basis for such complications as hyperlipidemia, retinopathy, proteinuria, or foot pathology. The compelling evidence that tight control of blood glucose, blood pressure, and lipids provides measurable improvement in outcomes warrants new initiatives. For both patients and health professionals, the opportunities and challenges are abundant.

REFERENCES

1. Bantle JP, Swanson JE, Thomas W, Laine DC. Metabolic effects of dietary sucrose in type II diabetic subjects. Diabetes Care 1993;16:1301–1305.
2. Peterson DB, Lambert J, Gerring S, Darling P, Carter RD, Jelfs R, Mann JI. Sucrose in the diet of diabetic patients—just another carbohydrate? Diabetologia 1986;29:216–220.
3. Brownell KD, Wadden TA. Etiology and treatment of obesity: understanding a serious, prevalent, and refractory disorder. J Consult Clin Psychol 1992;60:505–517.
4. Foreyt JP. Issues in the assessment and treatment of obesity. J Consult Clin Psychol 1987;55:677–684.
5. Wing RR, Blair EH, Bononi P, Marcus MD, Watanabe R, Bergman RN. Caloric restriction per se is a significant factor in improvements in glycemic control and insulin sensitivity during weight loss in obese NIDDM patients. Diabetes Care 1994;17:30–36.
6. Kelley DE, Wing R, Buonocore C. Sturis J, Polonsky K, Fitzsimmons M. Relative effects of calorie restriction and weight loss in non-insulin-dependent diabetes mellitus. J Clin Endocrinol Metab 1993;77:1287–1293.
7. Wing RR, Koeske R, Epstein LH, Nowak MP, Gooding W, Becker D. Long-term effects of modest weight loss in type II diabetic patients. Arch Intern Med 1987;147:1749–1753.
8. Watts NB, Spanheimer RG, DiGirolamo M, Gebhart SS, Musey VC, Siddiq YK, Phillips LS. Prediction of glucose response to weight loss in patients with non-insulin-dependent diabetes mellitus. Arch Intern Med 1990;150:803–806.
9. Franz MJ, Horton ES Sr, Bantle JP, Beebe CA, Brunzell JD, Coulston AM, Henry

RR, Hoogwerf BJ, Stacpook PW. Nutrition principles for the management of diabetes and related complications: a technical review. Diabetes Care 1994;17:490–518.

10. Rubin RR, Peyrot M, Saudek, CD. The effect of a diabetes education program incorporating coping skills training on emotional well-being and diabetes self-efficacy. Diabetes Educ 1993;19:210–214.

11. Bastyr III EJ, Stuart CA, Brodows RG, Schwartz S, Graf CJ, Zagar A, Robertson KE. Therapy focused on lowering postprandial glucose, not fasting glucose, may be superior for lowering HbA1c. Diabetes Care 2000;23:1236–1241.

12. Haire-Joshu D, Glasgow RE, Tibbs, TL. Smoking and diabetes. Diabetes Care 1999; 22:1887–1898.

13. Eriksson KF, Lindgarde F. Prevention of type II diabetes mellitus by diet and physical exercise. The 6 year Malmo Feasibility Study. Diabetologia 1991;34:891–898.

14. Schneider SH, Khachadurian AK, Amorosa LF, Clemow L, Ruderman NB. Ten-year experience with an exercise-based outpatient lifestyle modification program in the treatment of diabetes mellitus. Diabetes Care 1992;15(suppl 4):1800–1810.

15. Vanninen E, Uusitupa M, Siitonen O, Laitinen J, Lansimies E. Habitual physical activity, aerobic capacity, and metabolic control in patients with newly diagnosed type II diabetes mellitus: effect of a 1-year diet and exercise intervention. Diabetologia 1992;35:340–346.

16. American Diabetes Association. Diabetes mellitus and exercise. Diabetes Care 2000; 23:S50–S54.

17. Expert Panel on Detection, Evaluation, and Treatment of High Blood Cholesterol in Adults. Executive summary of the third report of the National Cholesterol Education Program (NCEP) expert panel on detection, evaluation, and treatment of high blood cholesterol in adults (Adult Treatment Panel III). JAMA 2001; 285:2486–2497.

18. American Diabetes Association. Management of dyslipidemia in adults with diabetes. Diabetes Care 2001;24:S58–S61.

19. Franz MJ, Kulkarni K, Daly AS, Gillespie SJ. In: Funnell MM, Hunt C, Kulkarni K, Rubin RR, Yarborough PC, eds. A Core Curriculum for Diabetes Education, 3rd ed. Chicago: American Association of Diabetes Educators, 1998:211.

16

Future Directions: Elucidation of Mechanisms as Targets for Therapy

David J. Schneider and Burton E. Sobel
University of Vermont, Burlington, Vermont

Optimal treatment of patients with diabetes requires an understanding of the mechanisms underlying the disease. Treatment must be designed not only to control hyperglycemia but also to prevent or retard complications that result from diverse processes underlying the development of diabetes. This chapter will focus on the therapeutic promise of elucidation of such processes and their cardiovascular consequences.

All diabetic subjects exhibit hyperglycemia. Yet hyperglycemia is only the tip of an iceberg of abnormalities in carbohydrate, lipid, and protein metabolism. Although insulin deficiency is the hallmark of type 1 diabetes, 90% of diabetic subjects suffer from type 2 diabetes, a disorder of dysinsulinemia. For decades before its onset, insulin resistance and compensatory increases in the concentration of insulin and its precursors in blood are present, particularly postprandially. Impaired glucose tolerance occurs eventually as compensatory mechanisms fail. Early treatment may delay the onset of frank diabetes and prevent or retard the development of cardiovascular complications.

Diabetes per se, independent of coexistent cardiovascular risk factors, accelerates the progression of cardiovascular disease. In addition, diabetes acts synergistically with other determinants of cardiac risk such as hypertension and hyperlipidemia. The specific pathways involved must be identified to optimize prevention of the resultant cardiovascular sequelae.

I. TREATMENT OF THE HORMONAL AND METABOLIC ABNORMALITIES OF DIABETES

Control of hyperglycemia retards progression of microvascular disease in both type 1 and type 2 diabetes. Accordingly, stringent glycemic control is imperative. Yet glycemic control exerts only a modest impact in retarding progression of macrovascular disease. Clearly other steps are needed.

The recently initiated BARI 2D trial has been designed to provide information useful in this regard. Patients are being assigned randomly to stringent and comparable glycemic control with regimens that are either insulin-sensitizing (focusing on glitazones and metformin) or inulin-providing (focusing on insulin and sulfonylureas) regimens. Thus, the potential value of reduction of insulin resistance is being assessed. The effects of the two approaches on activation of coagulation, platelets, and fibrinolysis will be clarified as well.

Because patients with type 2 diabetes are insulin-resistant, provision of exogenous insulin may be the most successful means for providing an adequate supply of substrate for energy in injured cells. By contrast, provision of additional insulin may have potentially deleterious effects such as promoting thrombosis. The provision of insulin may increase the potential for thrombin generation, increased reactivity of platelets, and decrease the fibrinolytic response. In combination, these effects may exacerbate thrombosis, predispose to reocclusion of infarct-related vessels, and delay resolution of thrombotic occlusion. Accordingly, treatment with insulin in the setting of acute myocardial infarction may entail risk. In addition, induction of hypoglycemic episodes may be particularly deleterious in association with myocardial ischemia. Thus, further study is needed to determine the nature of optimal metabolic control and the method by which it can best be achieved.

Nevertheless, results in the DIGAMI study demonstrated that stringent glycemic control at the time of occurrence of acute myocardial infarction reduces the incidence of subsequent cardiac events. The improved outcome is consistent with previously demonstrated beneficial effects of infusion of glucose, insulin, and potassium in nondiabetic subjects who sustain an acute myocardial infarction.

II. ATHEROGENESIS IN DIABETES

The traditional concept that atherogenesis is an orderly process of progressive luminal encroachment leading ultimately to occlusion has been refined. Both plaque evolution and occlusion of vessels often reflect precipitous and often repeated rupture of vulnerable atherosclerotic plaques. Thus, rupture of vulnerable plaques is the most common proximate cause of acute coronary syndromes. Such plaques are characterized by a high lipid content, a thin, relatively acellular cap, a paucity of vascular smooth muscle cells, and inflammatory cells, particularly macrophages, in the shoulder regions. The substrate for plaque rupture is a lipid-laden, often necrotic core with an overlying acellular fibrous cap. Initiators of rupture can be intrinsic to the plaque, such as activation of matrix metalloproteinases by macrophages in the shoulder region, or extrinsic, such as high shear forces exerted by nonlaminar flow of blood. Diabetes accelerates evolution of vulnerable plaques. How it does so is being explored vigorously so that novel and effective prophylactic and therapeutic targets can be identified.

Diabetic subjects (regardless of symptoms) should be treated to lower LDL cholesterol below 100 mg/dL to reduce the evolution of vulnerable plaques. Because diabetes is associated with increased small dense LDL and oxidized LDL, each atherogenic treatment should be designed to reduce their concentrations.

Paradoxically, migration of smooth muscle cells into the neointima may protect against plaque vulnerability. Thus, increased cellularity of the cap region appears to reduce the risk of plaque rupture. Cell surface proteolysis mediated by plasminogen activators (urokinase type and tissue type) is critical in migration. Accordingly, the balance between plasminogen activators and their primary inhibitor, plasminogen activator inhibitor type-1 (PAI-1), is likely to be one determinant of neointimal cellularity. Patients with diabetes have increased concentrations of PAI-1 in blood and in vessel walls. Modulation of expression of these proteins is likely to become a target for treatment.

Inflammation, reflected by markers in blood such as C-reactive protein, is increased in subjects predisposed to plaque rupture. Diabetes appears to intensify inflammation and the deleterious effects of inflammation. Elucidation of interactions between diabetes and inflammation should lead to novel treatment strategies to prevent or retard coronary atherogenesis sequelae such as acute coronary syndromes precipitated by plaque rupture.

The prevalence of hypertension in diabetic subjects is high. This condition increases external mechanical forces on vulnerable plaques and promotes plaque rupture or erosion. Altered flow attributable to atherosclerotic plaque contributes. The association between hypertension and plaque rupture underlies the need for aggressive control of blood pressure (to a target of less than 130/85). Even more aggressive control may be beneficial in reducing the incidence of cardiac events. Therapy with ACE inhibitors and/or angiotensin-1 receptor blockers may be particularly useful because of its nephroprotective effects. In addition, it may normalize deranged fibrinolysis attributable to angiotensin-dependent synthesis of PAI-1.

III. ATHEROGENESIS IN THE PREDIABETIC STATE

The 15% incidence of cardiac death in the first 10 years after the diagnosis of diabetes emphasizes the profound acceleration of progression of atherosclerosis that occurs long before diabetes becomes overt. The prediabetic state provides particularly fertile ground for germination of vulnerable plaques. Thus, a focus on treatment in the prediabetic state is likely to be important in preventing cardiovascular events later in ultimately diabetic subjects. One example is women with the polycystic ovary syndrome. These subjects are insulin-resistant and often have postprandial hyperglycemia. They are also often hypertensive. They are at increased risk for coronary artery disease. Accordingly, therapy designed to ameliorate insulin resistance is under intense investigation.

IV. THROMBOSIS COMPLICATING PLAQUE RUPTURE

Diabetes increases the risk of thrombosis complicating plaque rupture. Accordingly, diabetic compared with nondiabetic subjects are more likely to be the victims of acute coronary syndromes including myocardial infarction and unstable angina and of sudden cardiac death secondary to thrombosis in response to plaque rupture. Exaggerated thrombosis can predispose to recurrent events and to accelerated progression of atherosclerosis. Accordingly, mechanisms of prothrombosis must be delineated and their therapeutic implications exploited.

Diabetes exerts complex and diverse effects leading to activation of coagulation. Thrombin generation and activity are increased, platelets are primed, and the fibrinolytic response is impaired because of increased expression of PAI-1. The causes are attributable to both hormonal and metabolic abnormalities characteristic of diabetes. Accordingly, optimal treatment of diabetes that achieves metabolic control and normalizes the hormonal abnormalities should attenuate the prothrombotic state.

In the BARI 1 study, percutaneous coronary intervention in patients with diabetes was found to be followed by increased cardiac mortality over 5 years. One mechanism contributing to the negative outcome may have been the exaggerated thrombotic response to vessel injury. Results in subsequent studies have shown that treatment with powerful antiplatelet agents (glycoprotein IIb-IIIa inhibitors) reduces the incidence of complications after coronary intervention and in patients with acute coronary syndromes. Beneficial effects are particularly pronounced in diabetic subjects. A reduction in mortality 6 months after coronary intervention is evident in diabetic subjects treated with abciximab during the procedure. Treatment with tiroliban of patients with acute coronary syndromes reduces markedly their risk of complications over the next 30 days.

V. CARDIOMYOPATHY AND DIABETES

Induction of cardiomyopathic changes in hearts of animals rendered insulin deficient is a well-recognized phenomenon. Accordingly, the term "diabetic cardiomyopathy'' has been extant for decades. Implicated derangements include impaired function of the sarcoplasmic reticulum, an organelle responsible for the uptake and release of intracellular calcium and, therefore, pivotal in modulating cardiac contractility. However, cardiomyopathy changes may not be related exclusively to metabolic derangements typical of insulin deficiency. They occur also in hearts of patients with type 2 diabetes whose hyperglycemia is well controlled.

Abnormalities in myocardial ultrasonic backscatter are seen in diabetic subjects even when ventricular systolic and diastolic function are normal. Such changes have been attributed to intramyocardial edema, alterations in the nature and deposition of collagen, and accumulation of advanced glycation products.

Patients with diabetes who sustain acute myocardial infarction exhibit greater impairment in ventricular function and more severe congestive heart failure normalized for infarct size than do nondiabetic subjects. Factors implicated in causing such derangements include limitation of energy supply attributable to insulin resistance in the myocardium and diminished availability of intracellular glucose and its metabolites for oxidative phosphorylation, impaired calcium cycling associated with abnormalities in the sarcoplasmic reticulum calcium-sensitive ATPase, and contributions of advanced glycation end products to cross-linking structural proteins and augmenting myocardial stiffness.

Elucidation of specific mechanisms responsible for cardiomyopathic changes associated with diabetes should enhance prevention and treatment of ventricular functional impairment under basal conditions and in response to myocardial insults.

VI. SUMMARY

A worldwide epidemic of diabetes is in progress. In the United States alone, over 16 million subjects have the disease. Many more are insulin-resistant. The progression of cardiovascular disease is accelerated by diabetes itself and by its interactions with other determinants of cardiac risk. Further elucidation of mechanisms responsible will undoubtedly lead to improved treatment designed to diminish the progression of cardiovascular disease that is all too prominent in diabetes.

SUGGESTED READING

1. Bucala R, Makita Z, Zoschinsky T, Cerami A, Vlassara H. Lipid advanced glycosylation: pathway for lipid oxidation in vivo. Proc Natl Acad Sci USA 1993; 90: 6434–6438.

2. Carmeliet P, Moons L, Lijnen R, et al. Inhibitory role of plasminogen activator inhibitor-1 in arterial wound healing and neointimal formation. A gene targeting and gene transfer study in mice. Circulation 1997; 96:3180–3191.
3. Davies MJ, Woolf N, Katz DR. The role of endothelial denudation injury, plaque fissuring and thrombosis in the progression of human atherosclerosis. Atheroscler Rev 1991; 23:105–113.
4. Davies MJ, Richardson PD, Woolf N, Kratz DR, Mann J. Risk of thrombosis in human atherosclerotic plaques: Role of extracellular lipid, macrophage, and smooth muscle content. Br Heart J 1993; 69:377–381.
5. Ehrmann DA, Schneider DJ, Sobel BE, Cavaghan MK, Imperial J, Rosenfield RL, Polonsky KS. Troglitazone improves defects in insulin action, insulin secretion, ovarian steroidogenesis, and fibrinolysis in women with polycystic ovary syndrome. J Clin Endocrinol Metab 1997; 82:2108–2116.
6. Fontbonne A, Tchobroutsky G, Eschwege E, Richard JL, Claude JR, Rosselin GE. Coronary heart disease mortality risk: Plasma insulin level is a more sensitive marker than hypertension or abnormal glucose tolerance in overweight males. The Paris prospective study. Int J Obes 1988; 12:557–565.
7. Haffner SM, Lehto S, Ronnemaa T, et al.: Mortality from coronary heart disease in subjects with type 2 diabetes and in non-diabetic subjects with and without prior myocardial infarction. N Engl J Med 1998; 339:229–234.
8. Jaffe AS, Spadaro JJ, Schechtman K, Roberts R, Geltman EM, Sobel E. Increased congestive heart failure after myocardial infarction of modest extent in patients with diabetes mellitus. Am Heart J 1984; 108:31–37.
9. Kabbani SS, Watkins MW, Ashikaga T, Terrien EF, Holoch PA., Sobel BE, Schneider DJ. Platelet reactivity characterized prospectively: A determinant of outcome 90 days after percutaneous coronary intervention. Circulation 2001; 104:181–186.
10. Kruszynska Y, Yu JG, Sobel BE, Olefsky JM. Effects of troglitazone on blood concentrations of plasminogen activator inhibitor 1 in patients with type 2 diabetes mellitus and in lean and obese normal subjects. Diabetes 2000; 49:633–639.
11. LeWinter MM. Diabetic cardiomyopathy: An overview. Coron Artery Dis 1996; 7: 95–98.
12. Malmberg K, Norhammar A, Wedel II, Ryden L. Glucometabolic state at admission: Important risk market of mortality in conventionally treated patients with diabetes mellitus and acute myocardial infarction. Long-term results from the Diabetes and Insulin-Glucose Infusion in Acute Myocardial Infarction Study. Circulation 1999; 99:2626–2632.
13. Perez JE, McGill JB, Santiago JV, Schechtman KB, Waggoner AD, Miller JG, Sobel BE. Abnormal myocardial acoustic properties in diabetic patients and their correlation with the severity of disease. J Am Coll Cardiol 1992; 19:1154–1162.
14. Schneider DJ, Sobel BE. Synergistic augmentation of expression of plasminogen activator inhibitor type-1 induced by insulin, very-low-density lipoproteins, and fatty acids. Coron Artery Dis 1996; 7:813–817.
15. Sobel BE. The potential influence of insulin and plasminogen activator inhibitor type-1 on formulation of vulnerable atherosclerotic plaques associated with type 2 diabetes. Proc Assoc Am Physicians 1999; 111:313–318.
16. Sobel BE. Acceleration of restenosis by diabetes: Pathogenetic implications. Circulation 2001; 103:1165–1187.

17. Sobel BE, Woodcock-Mitchell J, Schneider DJ, Holt RE, Marutsuka K, Gold H. Increased plasminogen activator inhibitor type-1 in coronary artery atherectomy specimens from type 2 diabetic compared with nondiabetic patients: A potential factor predisposing to thrombosis and its persistence. Circulation 1998; 97:2213–2221.

18. The Diabetes Control and Complications Trial Research Group. The effect of intensive treatment of diabetes on the development and progression of long-term complications in insulin-dependent diabetes mellitus. N Engl J Med 1993; 329:977–986.

19. The BARI Investigators. Influence of diabetes on 5-year mortality and morbidity in a randomized trial comparing CABG and PTCA in patients with multivessel disease. The Bypass Angioplasty Revascularization Investigation (BARI). Circulation 1997; 96:1761–1769.

20. UK Prospective Diabetes Study (UKPDS) Group. Effect of intensive blood-glucose control with metformin on complications in over-weight patients with type 2 diabetes (UKPDS 34). Lancet 1998; 352:854–865.

21. UK Prospective Diabetes Study (UKPDS) Group. Intensive blood glucose control with sulphonylureas or insulin compared with conventional treatment and risk of complications in patients with type 2 diabetes (UKPDS 33). Lancet 1998; 352:837–853.

22. Warram JH, Martin BC, Krolewski AS, Soeldner JS, Kahn CR. Slow glucose removal rate and hyperinsulinemia precede the development of type II diabetes in the offspring of diabetic parents. Ann Intern Med 1990; 113:909–915.

Index

About the Editors

BURTON E. SOBEL is Amidon Professor and Chair of the Department of Medicine and Professor of Biochemistry at the University of Vermont College of Medicine and Physician-in-Chief, Fletcher Allen Health Care, Burlington, Vermont. The editor of *Medical Management of Heart Disease* (Marcel Dekker, Inc.) and the author or coauthor of over 820 publications, he has lectured at universities and conferences throughout the world. He is a member of the Royal Society of Medicine, the American Heart Association, and the American College of Cardiology. He received the A.B. degree (1958) from Cornell University, Ithaca, New York, and the M.D. degree (1962) magna cum laude from Harvard Medical School, Boston, Massachusetts.

DAVID J. SCHNEIDER is Associate Professor of Medicine and Director of the Vascular Biology Unit at the University of Vermont College of Medicine, Burlington, Vermont. He is the author or coauthor of more than 50 publications and a Fellow of the American Heart Association and the American College of Cardiology. Dr. Schneider obtained the B.A. degree (1982) magna cum laude from the University of Notre Dame, Indiana, and the M.D. degree (1986) from the University of Cincinnati College of Medicine, Ohio.